STRESS AND SURVIVAL
The emotional realities of life-threatening illness

STRESS AND SURVIVAL

The emotional realities of life-threatening illness

Edited by

CHARLES A. GARFIELD

Founder and Director, Shanti Project:
Volunteer Counseling for Patients and
Families Facing Life-Threatening Illness;
Assistant Clinical Professor of Medical Psychology,
Cancer Research Institute, Schools of Medicine
and Nursing, University of California,
San Francisco, California

THE C. V. MOSBY COMPANY

ST. LOUIS · TORONTO · LONDON   1979

Printed in the United States of America

The C. V. Mosby Company
11830 Westline Industrial Drive, St. Louis, Missouri 63141

Library of Congress Cataloging in Publication Data
Main entry under title:

Stress and survival.

  Bibliography: p.
  Includes index.
  1. Medicine and psychology—Addresses, essays,
lectures. 2. Critically ill—Psychology—Addresses,
essays, lectures. 3. Stress (Psychology)—Addresses,
essays, lectures. I. Garfield, Charles A.
[DNLM: 1. Stress, Psychological. 2. Adaption,
Psychological. 3. Terminal care. 4. Disease/Psychology.
5. Patient care team. 6. Attitude of health personnel.
BF789.S8 S914]
R726.5.S79   616′.001′9   78-31341
ISBN 0-8016-1743-X

CB/CB/B 9 8 7 6 5 4 3 2 1   03/A/317

Contributors

JAMES A. ABBOTT, M.D.

Psychiatrist, The Mental Health Clinic,
Veterans Administration Hospital,
Allen Park, California

HARRY S. ABRAM, M.D.

Department of Psychiatry, University of
Virginia School of Medicine,
Charlottesville, Virginia

N. J. C. ANDREASEN, M.D., Ph.D.

Assistant Professor, Department of Psychiatry,
University of Iowa College of Medicine,
Iowa City, Iowa

LEA BAIDER, Ph.D.

The Hebrew University, Jerusalem, Israel

GOTTHARD BOOTH

Psychoanalyst in private practice,
New York, New York

GENE A. BRODLAND, M.A., A.C.S.W.

Assistant Professor, Department of Psychiatry,
Southern Illinois University School of
Medicine, Springfield, Illinois

LARRY A. BUGEN, Ph.D.

Assistant Professor, Department of Health,
Physical Education, and Recreation,
University of Texas College of Education,
Austin, Texas

JOHN CASSEL, M.D.

Department of Epidemiology, University of
North Carolina, Chapel Hill, North Carolina

NED H. CASSEM, M.D.

Director of Residency Training,
Massachusetts General Hospital, Boston,
Massachusetts; Assistant Professor,
Department of Psychiatry, Harvard
Medical School, Boston, Massachusetts

NORMAN COUSINS

Editor, *The Saturday Review*

JUDITH GREGORIE D'AFFLITTI, M.S.N.

Consultant, Nursing Service, Veterans
Administration Hospital, West Haven,
Connecticut; Clinical Instructor, Department
of Psychiatry, Yale University School of
Medicine, New Haven, Connecticut

RICHARD C. ERICKSON, Ph.D.

Seattle Veterans Administration Hospital;
Department of Psychiatry
and Behavioral Sciences, University of
Washington Medical School,
Seattle, Washington

JOSEPH EYER

Lecturer in Biology, University of Pennsylvania,
Philadelphia, Pennsylvania

JEROME D. FRANK

The Johns Hopkins University School of
Medicine, Baltimore, Maryland

CHARLES A. GARFIELD

Founder and Director, Shanti Project: Volunteer
Counseling for Patients and Families Facing
Life-Threatening Illness; Assistant Clinical
Professor of Medical Psychology, Cancer
Research Institute, Schools of Medicine and
Nursing, University of California,
San Francisco, California

JON GARFIELD, M.A., Ph.D.

Student in Medical Sociology, University of
California, Santa Barbara, California; Health
Science teacher, University of California
Extension

MORRIS GELFMAN, M.D.

Director, Psychiatric Training and Education,
Milwaukee County Mental Health Center;
Associate Professor, Department of
Psychiatry, Medical College of Wisconsin,
Milwaukee, Wisconsin

ELLEN GOODMAN

Volunteer coordinator and counselor,
Shanti Project, Berkeley, California

NETTA GRANDSTAFF, Ph.D.

Stanford Medical Center, Palo Alto, California

THOMAS P. HACKETT, M.D.

Department of Psychiatry, Massachusetts
General Hospital, Boston, Massachusetts

DONALD HAY, M.D.

Medical and Clinical Director, Eastern Montana
Regional Mental Health Center,
Miles City, Montana

MILTON D. HEIFETZ, M.D.

Diplomat, American Board of Neurological
Surgery; Associate Clinical Professor of
Neurological Surgery, University of
Southern California, Los Angeles,
California

MICHAEL W. HURST, Ed.D.

Departments of Psychosomatic Medicine and
Behavioral Epidemiology, Boston University
Medical School, Boston, Massachusetts

BOBBIE J. HYERSTAY, M.S., Ph.D.

University of Oregon

IVAN ILLICH

Author and lecturer

C. DAVID JENKINS, Ph.D.

Departments of Psychosomatic Medicine and
Behavioral Epidemiology, Boston University
Medical School, Boston, Massachusetts

RICHARD BURNHAM JONES, M.S.

Volunteer and trainer, Shanti Project;
licensed marriage and family counselor,
Oakland, California; Faculty member, Holistic
Life University, San Francisco, California

DAVID M. KAPLAN, Ph.D.

Director, Division of Clinical Social Work,
Department of Family, Community, and
Preventive Medicine, Stanford University
Medical Center, Stanford, California

SAMUEL C. KLAGSBRUN, M.D.

Assistant Clinical Professor, Columbia
University College of Physicians and
Surgeons; Attending Psychiatrist, St. Luke's
Hospital, New York, New York

ROY KLETTI, M.A.

Clinical Psychologist, University of Iowa
College of Medicine, Iowa City, Iowa

HOWARD KOGAN, A.C.S.W.

Psychoanalytically Oriented Therapist in Private
Practice; Supervisor, Youth and Family
Counseling Agency; Teacher, New School
for Social Research, New York, New York

DONALD S. KORNFELD, M.D.

Chief, Psychiatric Consultation Service,
Columbia-Presbyterian Medical Center;
Associate Professor of Clinical Psychiatry,
Columbia University College of Physicians
and Surgeons, New York, New York

DOLORES KRIEGER, R.N., Ph.D.

Professor of Nursing, New York University,
New York, New York

†CHAUNCEY D. LEAKE, Ph.D.

Senior Lecturer, Department of Pharmacology,
University of California School of Medicine,
San Francisco, California

LAWRENCE LeSHAN, Ph.D.

Research Psychologist, McDonnell Foundation,
New York, New York

†Deceased.

CHRISTINA MASLACH, Ph.D.

Assistant Professor of Psychology, University of California, Berkeley, California

AKE MATTSSON, M.D.

Professor of Psychiatry and Pediatrics, University of Virginia Medical Center, Charlottesville, Virginia

MARTIN G. NETSKY, M.D.

Professor of Pathology, Vanderbilt University School of Medicine, Nashville, Tennessee

RUSSELL NOYES, Jr., M.D.

Associate Professor of Psychiatry, University of Iowa College of Medicine, Iowa City, Iowa

DONALD OKEN, M.D.

Professor and Chairman, Department of Psychiatry, Upstate Medical Center, State University of New York, Syracuse, New York

LINUS PAULING, Ph.D.

Educator, two-time Nobel Prize winner, Linus Pauling Institute of Science and Medicine, Menlo Park, California

KENNETH R. PELLETIER, Ph.D.

Department of Psychiatry, University of California School of Medicine, San Francisco, California

FLORENCE BRIGHT ROBERTS, B.S.N.

Assistant Professor of Nursing, University of Tennessee College of Nursing, Memphis, Tennessee

ROBERT M. ROSE, M.D.

Departments of Psychosomatic Medicine and Behavioral Epidemiology, Boston University Medical School, Boston, Massachusetts

YASUKO SAMESHIMA, R.N., Ed.D.

Research Assistant, Teachers College, Columbia University, New York, New York

HANS SELYE, C.C., M.D., Ph.D., D.Sc.

President, International Institute of Stress, Université de Montreal, Institut de Médecine et de Chirurgie Expérimentales Case, Montreal, Canada

LEONARD SHLAIN, M.D.

Clinical Instructor in Surgery, University of California School of Medicine, San Francisco, California; Cancer patient

HERBERT G. STEGER, Ph.D.

Clinical Psychologist and Assistant Professor, Department of Physical Medicine and Rehabilitation, California College of Medicine, University of California, Irvine, California

G. WAYNE WEITZ, M.S.W.

Brooklyn State Hospital, Division V Outpatient Services, Brooklyn, New York

EMILEE J. WILSON, M.D.

Staff Psychiatrist, Stress Unit, California State Prison, Vacaville, California

ROBERT WOODSON, Ph.D.

Director, Santa Barbara Pain Control Clinic, Santa Barbara, California

BERNIE ZILBERGELD, Ph.D.

Clinical Psychologist and Head, Men's Program, Human Sexuality Program, University of California School of Medicine, San Francisco, California

TO LINDA

After the thousands of dedications men have written to their wives—and vice versa—could there possibly be anything new to say?

Ten years; many laughs and tears later
A decade's friends, through some close encounters of the worst kind
We're still here—and I love you
A slow evolution we have, with uneasy change
How better to thank you than to say
I will love you deeply all the days of my life.

Preface

The subjects of this book are stress and survival. The anthology has been compiled for those who confront the emotional realities of life-threatening illness—for the nurse, physician, mental health professional, volunteer, clergy member or family member whose supportive presence, often in the most difficult of situations, is testimony to the importance of Terrence Des Pres's observation that "survival is a collective act."* A basic premise of the book is that one or more such supportive presences can markedly influence the patient's level of stress, will to live, and possibility of survival.

In selecting material for this anthology, it was necessary to examine our society's beliefs and attitudes toward psychologic and social support. I believe that whether we speak of physical survival or the emotional survival of an individual functioning with integrity, we find some styles of human relationship nourishing and others toxic. If, as members of the health team, we are to deliver the best patient care possible, it is vital that we identify those beliefs and attitudes that are most likely to affect the quality of that care, either directly or indirectly.

The archaic notion that emotional expression and support are inappropriate or unprofessional derives from a model of professional comportment devised by those who have learned to view emotion as a weakness and intellect as a weapon. It is based on an inaccurate conception of the way human beings function under stress.*

To those who seek with religious fervor the cool-headed detachment of professional performance, I suggest that "regardless of how cool one's head is, without the normal feelings shared by all those capable of reacting to stress, tragedy, involvement, etc. one's head is not only cool but cold and barren."†

In preparing this volume, it also became necessary to focus not only on the patient, the family, and their health care providers, but also on the nature of modern life. With wonderment—and a tinge of sadness—I was forced to conclude that for the first time in history what goes in our bodies may be worse nutritionally than what comes out! More subtle and equally vital is Arnold Toynbee's observation:

At the earliest moment at which we catch our first glimpse of man on earth, we find him not only on the move but already moving at an accelerating pace. This crescendo of acceleration is continuing today. In our generation it is perhaps the most difficult and dangerous of all the current problems of the race.

The primary purposes of this book, then, are:

1. "To understand the capacity of men and women to live beneath the pressure of protracted crisis, to sustain terrible damage in mind and body, and

---

*Des Pres, T.: The survivor, New York, 1976, Oxford University Press.

*Garfield, C.: Psychosocial care of the dying patient, New York, 1978, McGraw-Hill Book Co.
†Babbini, L.: Letters, Heart and Lung 5(2):328, 1976.

yet be there, sane, alive, still human.''*

2. To offer insights into the ways that emotional support may be instrumental in promoting quality of life, longevity, and, at times, survival.

3. To examine closely the optimal ways of providing emotional support to patients and families facing life-threatening illness.

My own clinical experience comes from being founder and director of the Shanti Project—a volunteer counseling service for patients and families facing life-threatening illness—and research psychologist at the Cancer Research Institute, University of California Medical Center in San Francisco. Emotional stress, the hope for survival, and the testing of each helper's psychological resources are familiar themes to anyone working in this field. A few insights have emerged with increasing intensity in the course of my work. First is the rejection of any philosophy maintaining that life or death is insignificant. Macbeth had a much different set of experiences than I when he said:

> Out, out brief candle!
> Life's but a walking shadow . . .
> . . . it is a tale.
> Told by an idiot, full of sounds and fury,
> Signifying nothing.

More familiar are the words of C. S. Lewis:

It is hard to have patience with people who say, ''There is no death,'' or ''Death doesn't matter.'' There is death. And whatever is, matters. And whatever happens has consequences, and it and they are irrevocable and irreversible. You might as well say that birth doesn't matter. I look up at the night sky. Is anything more certain that that in all those vast times and spaces, if I were allowed to search them, I should nowhere find her face, her voice, her touch? She died. She is dead. Is the word so difficult to learn?†

Second is the realization that some events that befall us are outrageously painful and unfair. However, it may be precisely these events that trigger quantum leaps in insight to higher levels of understanding. Clearly such events are unwelcome, but the difficult task of coping with them may lead us to greater emotional strength and compassion for others.

Here, in the bedroom, dead quiet reigned. Everything, down to the last trifle, spoke eloquently of the tempest undergone, of weariness, and everything rested. . . . On the bed, by the window, the boy lay open-eyed, with a look of wonder on his face. He did not move, but it seemed that his open eyes became darker and darker every second and sank into his skull. Having laid her hands on his body and hid her face in the folds of the bed-clothes, the mother now was on her knees before the bed. Like the boy she did not move, but how much living movement was felt in the coil of her body and in her hands! . . . The doctor stopped by his wife, thrust his hands into his trouser pockets and bending his head to one side looked fixedly at his son. His face showed indifference; only the drops which glistened on his beard revealed that he had been lately weeping. The repulsive terror of which we think when we speak of death was absent from the bedroom. In the pervading dumbness, in the mother's pose, in the indifference of the doctor's face was something attractive that touched the heart, the subtle and elusive beauty of human grief, which it will take men long to understand and describe, and only music, it seems, is able to express. Beauty too was felt in the stern stillness. Kirlov and his wife were silent and did not weep, as if they confessed all the poetry of their condition. As once the season of their youth passed away, so now in this boy their right to bear children has passed away, alas! forever to eternity. The doctor is forty-four years old, already grey and looks like an old man; his faded sick wife is thirty-five. Andrey was not merely the only son, but the last.*

Last is a belief in the exquisite beauty and resilience of the human spirit.

The longer I live, the more do human beings appear to be fascinating and full of interest . . .

---

*Des Pres, op. cit.
†Lewis, C. S.: A grief observed, New York, 1961, The Seabury Press, Inc.

*Chekhov, A.: Enemies.

foolish and clever, mean and almost saintly, diversely unhappy—they're all dear to my heart; it seems to me that I do not properly understand them and my soul is filled with an inextinguishable interest in them. Many of them whom I knew are dead, I'm afraid that except me there is no one who will tell their story as I would like to do and dare not; it will seem as though such men had never existed on earth at all.*

I am grateful to those individuals whose friendship and support helped me to complete this volume during a period of personal stress and survival:

Linda Beech, Ellen Goodman, and John Golenski for their excellent work with Shanti Project clients and volunteers and for their dedication to the project far beyond the call of duty.

Michael and Justine Toms, Emmett Jones and Judy Metzger, Dale Larson, Dick Kalish, Polly Doyle, Shelly and Sylvia Korchin, and Paul and Ruth von Blum for lovingly demonstrating that intelligence and decency can co-vary during times of extreme stress.

John and Andree Moran, Bruce and Gloria Lawrence, Frank and Sarah Geer, Enrico Jones, Howard Kreitsek, and Lee Lundell whose presence at key moments made all the difference in the world.

Mrs. Carl W. Stern, Martin Paley and the San Francisco Foundation, Dr. Robert Glaser and the Kaiser Family Foundation, Jane Lehman and the Arca Foundation, Wally Haas, Jr., and the Evelyn and Walter Haas, Jr., Fund, Julie Bloomfield and the William Babcock Memorial Endowment, Larry Kramer and the Louis R. Lurie Foundation, and Ed Nathan and the Zellerbach Family Fund for their awareness of the needs of patients and families facing life-threatening illness, support of the Shanti Project, and personal encouragement.

All Shanti volunteers, past and present, whose dedicated work constitutes an inspiring demonstration of human kindness.

Dr. Robert Butler and his colleagues at the National Institute on Aging for supporting my postdoctoral research training in the area of psychosocial care of the dying patient.

Drs. Samuel Silverstein and Ralph Simon and their colleagues at the National Institute of Mental Health for supporting our training film entitled "Counseling the Terminally Ill."

My parents, Sylvia and Edward Garfield, whose unconditional love and friendship make adherence to the biblical mandate, "Honor thy father and thy mother" the sincerest of pleasures.

My brother, Jon Garfield, for caring so much about his contribution to this volume and for reminding me of the dangers of naive choices of friends and work.

My special friend, Jeremiah Garfield, whose unflagging allegiance and wise midnight counsel intensified my desire to understand interspecies communication.

Ann Esposito, friend and administrative assistant, who attended expertly to the many details involved in preparing this manuscript.

Ruth Veres for her consistently excellent editorial assistance.

Those caring people working diligently in hospitals, hospices, clinics, nursing homes, and the community who understand that survival—both physical and emotional—is a collective act. In their honor, I would like to support Professor Agnew's proposal that we establish major awards, comparable to the Nobel Prize, for humanism in the health care field.* Conversely, I would also like to support his idea that we award booby prizes, attended by widespread publicity, to those institutions or individuals whose humanism is demonstrably absent or grossly suspect!

Charles A. Garfield

---

*Gorki, M.: Two stories, The Dial, 1927.

*Agnew, L.: Humanism in medicine, The Lancet, p. 596, 1977.

Contents

PART I

Introduction

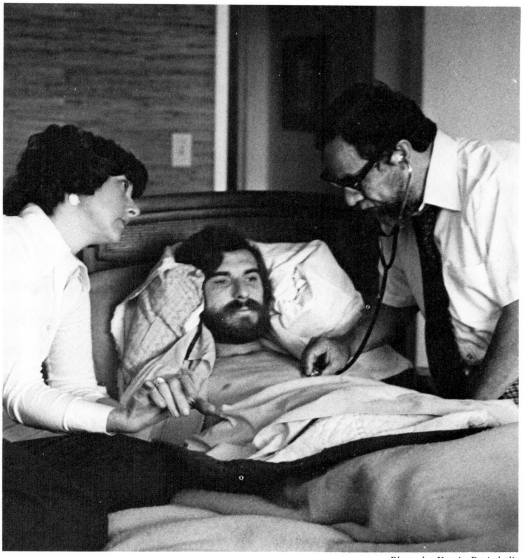

Photo by Katrin P. Achelis

1

On life in extremity: psychosocial elements of survival

CHARLES A. GARFIELD

How do human relationships reduce stress and affect the course and recovery from illness? What factors in a supportive relationship help induce health? Can the quality of a person's relationships significantly improve his or her chances of overcoming life-threatening illness? Although research on these issues is scarce, many people believe that caring, supportive relationships can appreciably increase the will to live and positively alter a patient's chances of survival.

Any understanding of the psychosocial aspects of survival requires an appreciation of the nature of life in extremity. What is the experience of the seriously ill patient attempting to cope with a life-threatening illness? What energies or coping styles does the patient employ to fight the ever-present possibility of death? What ways of relating to life in extremity make survival most probable? What can we as helpers do to mobilize best the psychosocial resources for survival?

To learn about life in extremity, I turned first to literature of the Holocaust—first-hand accounts and secondary analyses of life in the concentration camps—and then to a remarkable book by Terrence Des Pres called *The Survivor*. The following is a distillation of some of the more important observations made by Des Pres about the survivors of the camps. Many of these observations are applicable to patients and families facing life-threatening illness. Obviously the two situations differ in some fundamental ways. However, important analogies exist concerning the nature of life in extremity and the psychosocial elements of survival.

1. The extreme situation is not an event, not a period of crisis with a beginning, middle, and end, but rather, a state of existence. People spend themselves in that endless empty time, day upon day, without the encouragement of visible progress, without hope of positive end in sight, and always with the knowledge that death may win.

2. The survivor is not merely a victim; he refuses to see his victimization as total. He fights as best he can and does not consent to death in any form. He does not accept the logic of the situation imposed upon him.

3. The survivor must be prepared to run risks that keep him alive by bringing him closer to death.

4. The survivor is aware of the drift toward fatal indifference and the moment when a simple expression of care pulls him together! *Nobody survived without help.* Some minimal fabric of care, some margin of giving and receiving, is essential to life in extremity. In a literal sense therefore the survivor owes his life to his comrades. *Survival is a collective act.*

5. We cannot understand the survivor's

3

behavior apart from its context. We cannot ignore the simple fact that the survivor's situation is itself abnormal.

6. Permanently exhausted, the survivors were often sick; a night's sleep was 4 or 5 hours at most. Under such stress, we might expect a retreat into unconsciousness, into coma, as when a person faints from shock or excess pain. Where did the strength to get up come from? At any moment of relaxed striving, sleep could become part of the slide toward death, a surrender of the will to shove on. Every morning a survivor's will had to be renewed; it was not through some secret fortitude of the heart, but through the physical act of getting up.

7. Survivors acquire a capacity for realism, impersonal and without the least illusion. "The more we gained in experience, our insights sharpened, our vigilance developed and our reactions quickened. We acquired a greater capacity for adapting ourselves to conditions."

8. In extremity the function of intelligence is not to judge one's chances, which are nearly zero, but to make the most of each day's opportunity for getting through that day.

9. Life in extremity reveals in its movements a definite rhythm of decline and renewal. Survivors not only wake, but reawake, fall low and begin to die, and turn back to life.

10. When the body lies shrunken to a childish form, when arms and legs have become like thin twigs, when the mouth is parched and puckered, when every bit of food causes a return of dysentery, when the very smell of the camp soup brings on nausea, when there is no help, no care, no medicine—whence comes this magic will to live? Where is it born? In which recess of the human body does it bud and blossom so strongly that it can conquer death in its many shapes? Whence comes that imperishable willpower to find the means of defense?

11. The survivor's experience is evidence that the need to help is as basic as the need for help. This fact points to the radically social nature of life in extremity and explains an unexpected but very widespread activity among survivors: A major form of behavior is gift giving. The survivors were continually giving and sharing little items with each other—there was just the delight of being able to give something; it did not matter what as long as it was rare and distinctly a gift. Perhaps the most striking thing about this kind of giving, apart from the extreme gratitude it could generate, is the fact that pity played no part.

12. When men and women know they are dying, the smallest favors can shake the frail world of their being with seismic force. The power of such moments is enormous, and the bonds thus created go far deeper than guilt or pride or ordinary obligations.

13. Compassion means to "suffer with." It is an act of imaginative entrance into the world of another's pain and is proper on the part of those who do not themselves bear the same kind or degree of suffering. Through compassion we close the distance between one condition and another. As long as the division between unearned luck and unearned disaster remains a structure of our common world, compassion has about it the nature of a moral imperative, but only for those whom fate has not tried.

14. As Kostoglotov in Solzhenitsyn's *Cancer Ward* says, "I have often wondered before, and now particularly I wonder: What, after all, is the highest price one should pay for life? How much should one pay, how much is too much?" The question is always there, and each turn of events requires a new answer. So it is when Kostoglotov enters the cancer ward. His chance for a bit more life depends on a hormone treatment that will deprive him of his virility, and this is the decision he must face: "To become a walking husk of a man—isn't that an exorbitant price? It would be a mockery. Should I pay it?"

What is basic to Des Pres's observations is that a relationship exists between the emotional state of the individual and his physical status; that is, to an often remarkable degree, specific psychologic and social facts in a patient's world can powerfully and positively influence survival. Dr. Eugene P. Pendergrass,[4] an oncologist and past president of the American Cancer Society, in his presidential address in 1959 stated:

Anyone who has had an extensive experience in the treatment of cancer is aware that there are great differences among patients. . . . I personally have observed cancer patients who have undergone successful treatment and were living and well for years. Then, an emotional stress such as the death of a son in World War II, the infidelity of a daughter-in-law, or the burden of long unemployment seem to have been precipitating factors in the reactivation of their disease which resulted in death. . . . There is solid evidence that the course of disease in general is effected by emotional distress. . . . Thus, we, as doctors, may begin to emphasize treatment of the patient as a *whole* as well as the disease from which the patient is suffering. We may learn how to influence general body systems and through them modify the neoplasm which resides within the body.

As we go forward . . . searching for new means of controlling growth both within the cell and through systemic influences, it is my sincere hope that we can widen the quest to include the distinct possibility that within one's mind is a power capable of exerting forces which can either enhance or inhibit the progress of this disease.

Dr. Bruno Klopfer[2] in his presidential address in 1957 to the Society for Projective Techniques offered the following dramatic case example:

Mr. Wright had a generalized far advanced malignancy involving the lymph nodes, lymphosarcoma. Eventually the day came when he developed resistance to all known palliative treatments. Also, his increasing anemia precluded any intensive efforts with X-rays or nitrogen mustard, which might otherwise have been attempted. Huge tumor masses, the size of oranges, were in the neck, axillas, groin, chest and abdomen. The spleen and liver were enormous. The thoracic duct was obstructed, and between 1 and 2 liters of milky fluid had to be drawn from his chest every other day. He was taking oxygen by mask frequently, and our impression was that he was in a terminal state, untreatable, other than to give sedatives to ease him on his way.

In spite of all this, Mr. Wright was not without hope, even though his doctors most certainly were. The reason for this was, that the new drug that he had expected to come along and save the day had already been reported in the newspapers! Its name was "Krebiozen" (subsequently shown to be a useless, inert preparation).

Then he heard in some way, that our clinic was to be one of a hundred places chosen by the Medical Association for evaluation of this treatment. We were allotted supplies of the drug sufficient for treating twelve selected cases. Mr. Wright was not considered eligible, since one stipulation was that the patient must not only be beyond the point where standard therapies could benefit, but *also* must have a life expectancy of at least 3, and preferably 6 months. He certainly didn't qualify on the latter point, and to give him a prognosis of more than 2 weeks seemed to be stretching things.

However, a few days later, the drug arrived, and we began setting up our testing program which, of course, did *not* include Mr. Wright. When he heard we were going to begin treatment with Krebiozen, his enthusiasm knew no bounds, and as much as I tried to dissuade him, he begged so hard for this "golden opportunity," that against my better judgment, and against the rules of the Krebiozen committee, I decided I would have to include him.

Injections were to be given three times weekly, and I remember he received his first one on a Friday. I didn't see him again until Monday and thought as I came to the hospital he might be moribund or dead by that time, and his supply of the drug could then be transferred to another case.

What a surprise was in store for me! I had left him febrile, gasping for air, completely bedridden. Now, here he was, walking around the ward, chatting happily with the nurses, and spreading his message of good cheer to any who would listen. Immediately I hastened to see the others who had received their first injection at the same time. No change, or change for the worse was noted. Only in Mr. Wright was there brilliant improvement. The tumor masses had melted like snowballs on a hot stove, and in only these few days, they were half their original size! This is, of course, far more rapid regression than most radiosensitive tumors could display under heavy X-ray given every day. And we already knew his tumor was no longer sensitive to irradiation. Also, he had had no other treatment outside of the single useless "shot."

This phenomenon demanded an explanation, but not only that, it almost insisted that we open our minds to learn, rather than try to explain. So, the injections were given 3 times weekly as planned, much to the joy of the patient, but much to our bewilderment. Within 10 days he was able to be discharged from his "deathbed," practically all signs of his disease having vanished in this short time. Incredible as it sounds, this "terminal" patient, gasping his last breath through an oxygen mask, was now not only breathing normally, and fully active, he took off in his plane and flew at 12,000 feet, with no discomfort!

This unbelievable situation occurred at the beginning of the "Krebiozen" evaluation, but within two months, conflicting reports began to appear in the news, all of the testing clinics reporting no results. At the same time, the originators of the treatment were still blindly contradicting the discouraging facts that were beginning to emerge.

This disturbed our Mr. Wright considerably as the weeks wore on. Although he had no special training, he was, at times, reasonably logical and scientific in his thinking. He began to lose faith in his last hope which so far had been life-saving and left nothing to be desired. As the reported results became increasingly dismal, his faith waned, and after two months of practically perfect health, he relapsed to his original state, and became very gloomy and miserable.

But here I saw the opportunity to *double-check* the drug and maybe too, find out how the quacks can accomplish the results that they claim (and many of their claims are well substantiated). Knowing something of my patient's innate optimism by this time, I deliberately took advantage of him. This was for purely scientific reasons, in order to perform the perfect control experiment which could answer all the perplexing questions he had brought up. Furthermore, this scheme could not harm him in any way, I felt sure, and there was nothing I knew anyway that could help him.

When Mr. Wright had all but given up in despair with the recrudescence of his disease, in spite of the "wonder drug" which had worked so well at first, I decided to take the chance and play the quack. So deliberately lying, I told him not to

believe what he read in the papers, the drug was really most promising after all. "What then," he asked, "was the reason for this relapse?" "Just because the substance deteriorates on standing," I replied. "A new super-refined, double-strength product is due to arrive tomorrow which can more than reproduce the great benefits derived from the original injections."

This news came as a great revelation to him, and Mr. Wright, ill as he was, became his optimistic self again, eager to start over. By delaying a couple of days before the "shipment" arrived, his anticipation of salvation had reached a tremendous pitch. When I announced that the new series of injections were about to begin, he was almost ecstatic and his faith was very strong.

With much fanfare, and putting on quite an act (which I deemed permissible under the circumstances), I administered the first injection of the doubly potent, *fresh* preparation—consisting of *fresh water* and nothing more. The results of this experiment were quite unbelievable to us at the time, although we must have had some suspicion of the remotely possible outcome to have even attempted it at all.

Recovery from his second near-terminal state was even more dramatic than the first. Tumor masses melted, chest fluid vanished, he became ambulatory, and even went back to flying again. At this time he was certainly the picture of health. The water injections were continued, since they worked such wonders. He then remained symptom-free for over two months. At this time the final AMA announcement appeared in the press—"Nationwide tests show Krebiozen to be a worthless drug in treatment of cancer."

Within a few days of this report Mr. Wright was readmitted to the hospital *in extremis*. His faith was now gone, his last hope vanished, and he succumbed in less than two days.

In time we will learn more about the psychosomatic conditions that enhance survival. We will understand better the psychophysiologic variables that promote health and even the kinds of human relationships that emotionally and physically enhance life the most. For now, in the words of C. S. Lewis, "Whatever is, matters. And whatever happens has consequences." In the final analysis, what may matter most is the love that we have given and received and the quality of care that we have offered our patients and each other.

When we honestly ask ourselves which persons in our lives mean the most to us, we often find it is those who, instead of giving much advice, solutions, or cures, have chosen rather to share our pain and touch our wounds with a gentle and tender hand. The friend who can be silent with us in a moment of despair or confusion, who can stay with us in an hour of grief and bereavement, who can tolerate not knowing, not curing, not healing, and face with us the reality of our powerlessness, that is the friend who cares.[3]

Thus the most important insight gained from my work with those who have survived, as well as those who have not, is best expressed by a difference of opinion between Goethe and the Spanish writer Unamuno. Goethe, as he lay dying, was heard to say, "Light, light, the world needs more light." It was not until much later that Unamuno replied, "Goethe was wrong. What he should have said was, 'Warmth, warmth, the world needs more warmth.' We shall not die from the darkness but from the cold."

REFERENCES

1. Des Pres, T.: The survivor, New York, 1976, Oxford University Press, Inc.
2. Klopfer, B.: Psychological variables in human cancer, Journal of Projective Techniques **21:**331-340, 1957.
3. Nouwen, H.: Out of solitude, Notre Dame, Indiana, 1959, Ave Maria Press.
4. Pendergrass, E.: Presidential address, American Cancer Society, 1959.

PART II

The relation of social and psychologic factors to illness

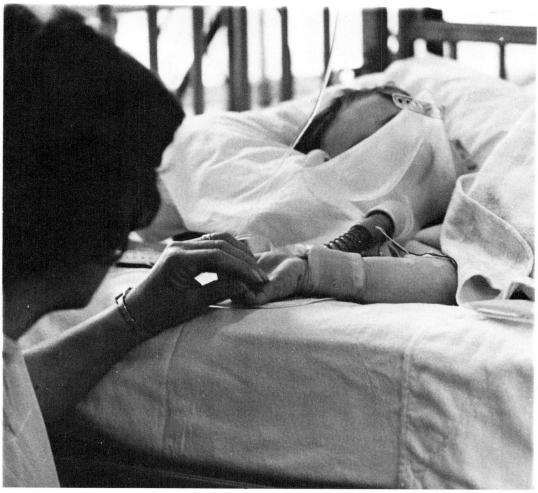

Photo by Arlene Bernstein

2

Stress without distress

HANS SELYE

When I received Dr. Garfield's invitation to participate in this conference, I felt strongly motivated to attend because I wanted to share my own experiences and struggles against disease with physicians and other health care workers dealing with terminally ill patients. I myself have survived two complete arthrectomies for osteoarthritis and the mental as well as physical anguish following surgery involving an "incurable" reticulosarcoma.

I began to develop an osteoarthritis of the hip joint when I was 50 years old. My surgeon, Dr. F. E. Stinchfield, recommended an operation that, at the time, was very dangerous. He would expose and remove all the bony irregularities and cover the joint surface with a metallic cap. Afraid of becoming nothing more than a burden to my family and myself, I agreed to the surgery.

As a result of the operation, I developed a severely bleeding stress ulcer. Nevertheless I continued to perform a daily regimen of exercises to maintain the motility of the painful artificial hip. I eventually recovered and was able to return to my routine, proud to have licked the disease.

I was really desperate when, a few years later, it became apparent that an osteoarthritis had attacked my other hip. Still determined not to become an invalid, I once again agreed to undergo surgery. This time a somewhat improved technique was used: the head of my hipbone was completely sawed off along with the socket from my pelvis. The surgeon replaced them with

plastic objects, permanently inserted in my bones like fillings in a tooth. Once again I went through the prolonged, painful exercise period, calling upon all my motivation to get me through the difficult time. Finally I was ready to get back to work, able to move about unaided.

Several years went by with few problems until, once again, I found myself needing surgery. This turned out to be a much more dangerous situation. An egg-shaped tumor had developed under the skin of my thigh, and it was diagnosed as a reticulosarcoma. I had it removed immediately by a Montreal surgeon, Dr. J. E. Tabah, and his team. After the operation they severely irradiated the surrounding area with a cobalt bomb. I insisted on knowing my chances for a lasting recovery. Dr. Tabah spoke frankly, admitting that this type of cancer spreads rapidly and almost always kills within a year except in rare cases when the surgeon succeeds in removing all the cancer cells.

It is difficult to live normally when you are treated like a man condemned to die, so I told no one outside my immediate family about my predicament. I immersed myself in my work, summoning all my strength to get on with living and avoid brooding. A year went by, then two, and it turned out that I was that fortunate exception. Now, years after the discovery of my cancer, I know the danger, though slight, still exists. My artificial hips could break down; my cancer could regain its vitality. In any case I shall eventually die of old age. But nothing could deprive me of those years during

11

which I enjoyed a life full of pleasure and satisfaction. As I have often said, "It is not what happens to you, but the way you take it."

Few people like to think about death, and the prolongation of life is one of the most ancient ambitions of man. Yet to really love life is to accept death, as the latter is the natural endpoint of the former. In the words of Montaigne, "The ceaseless labor of man's whole life is to build the house of death."

Death is inevitable, but it is quite possible not to worry about it all the time. Having faced death before, I am fully determined to go on working as long as my health permits and I constantly make plans that could not possibly be accomplished in less than 10, 20, or more years. Of course I know that I shall never finish these projects, but it gives me great satisfaction to think of myself dying suddenly in the middle of an enterprise for which I feel great enthusiasm and which had developed to the point where it can be carried further by my successors.

Between the time when I first conceived the notion of stress and the present day, 50 years have passed, and these were really years of intense effort. Still, I do not consider my work on stress to be finished—far from it! I know very well that I shall never see the end of this study, for we are constantly faced with new ways of looking at almost every biologic problem. I think I can safely say, without exaggerating the vitality of this work, that it will go on forever, as long as biology and medicine exist, just like the study of metabolism, heredity, or growth.

In 1926 when stress was still a mystery and I was a second-year medical student, I first came across the "syndrome of just being sick." I wondered why the most diverse diseases produced so many common signs and symptoms. Whether a man suffers from severe blood loss, an infection, or advanced cancer, he loses his appetite, strength, and ambition; usually he also loses weight and even his facial expression betrays his illness. I felt sure that the syndrome of just

being sick, which is essentially the same no matter what disease we have, could be analyzed and expressed scientifically.

This possibility fascinated me. With the enthusiasm of youth I wanted to start work right away, but my background as a second-year medical student did not reach far enough and I got no farther than the formulation of an idea. The more I learned about the details of medicine, the more I forgot my broad but imprecise plan to tackle the syndrome of just being sick.

Years later under auguries more auspicious for research, I encountered the problem again. I was working as a young assistant in the biochemistry department of McGill University in Montreal, trying to find a new sex hormone in extracts of cattle ovaries. I injected the extracts into rats to see if their organs would show changes that could not be attributed to a known hormone.

Much to my satisfaction, the first and most impure extracts changed the rats in three ways: (1) the adrenal cortex became enlarged, (2) the thymus, the spleen, the lymph nodes, and all other lymphatic structures shrank, and (3) deep, bleeding ulcers appeared in the stomach and in the upper gut.

Because the three types of change were closely interdependent, they formed a definite syndrome. The changes varied from slight to pronounced depending on the amount of extract I injected.

At first I ascribed all these changes to a new sex hormone in my extract. But soon I found that all toxic substances—extracts of kidney, spleen, or even a toxin not derived from living tissue—produced the same syndrome. Gradually my classroom concept of the syndrome of just being sick came back to me. I realized that the reaction I had produced with my impure extracts and toxic drugs was an experimental replica of the syndrome of just being sick. Adrenal enlargement, gastrointestinal ulcers, and thymicolymphatic shrinkage were the omnipresent signs of damage to the body when under disease attack. Thus the three changes became the objective indices of stress and the basis for the development of the entire stress concept.

In my first paper on the syndrome of stress,[2] I suggested the term "alarm reaction" for the animal's initial response because I thought that the syndrome probably represented a general call to arms of the body's defensive forces.

However, the alarm reaction evidently was not the entire response. Further experiments showed that continuous exposure to any noxious agent capable of setting off this alarm reaction is followed by a stage of adaptation or resistance. Apparently disease is not just suffering, but it is a fight to maintain the homeostatic balance of our tissues when they are damaged. No living organism can exist continuously in a state of alarm. Any agent so damaging that continuous exposure to it is incompatible with life causes death within hours or days of the alarm reaction. However, if survival is possible, the alarm reaction gives way to what we call the *stage of resistance.*

What happens in the resistance stage is in many instances the exact opposite of events in the alarm reaction. For instance, during the alarm reaction, the adrenal cortex discharges into the bloodstream secretory granules that contain hormones. Consequently the gland is depleted of its stores. In the resistance stage an abundant reserve of secretory granules accumulates in the cortex. Again, in the alarm reaction the blood volume diminishes and body weight drops; during the stage of resistance the blood is less concentrated and body weight returns to normal.

Curiously, after prolonged exposure to any noxious agent, the body loses its acquired ability to resist and enters the *stage of exhaustion.* This third stage always occurs as long as the stress is severe enough and is applied long enough because the adaptation energy or adaptability of a living being is always finite.

All these findings made it necessary to coin an additional all-embracing name for the syndrome. I called the entire response

the general adaptation syndrome (GAS: *general,* because it is produced only by agents that have a general effect upon large portions of the body; *adaptative,* because it stimulates defenses and thereby helps inure the body to hardship; *syndrome,* because its signs are coordinated and partly dependent on each other). This whole syndrome then evolves through three stages: (1) the alarm reaction, (2) the stage of resistance, and (3) the stage of exhaustion.

An important part of the defense mechanism in the resistance stage is the pituitary, which secretes the so-called adrenocorticotrophic hormone (ACTH) that in turn stimulates the adrenal cortex to produce corticoids. Most important of these adaptive hormones are the glucocorticoids, such as cortisone, which inhibit tissue inflammation, and the mineralocorticoids, which promote inflammation. These hormones allow the body to defend its tissues by inflammation or to surrender them by inhibiting inflammation.

Various derangements in the secretion of adaptive hormones in the resistance stage result in what we call diseases of adaptation. These diseases are not caused by any particular pathogen, but rather result from a faulty adaptive response to the stress induced by some pathogen. For example, the excessive production of a proinflammatory hormone in response to some mild local irritation could damage organs far from the original site of an injury. In this sense the body's faulty adaptive reactions seem to initiate or encourage various maladies. These could include emotional disturbances, headaches, insomnia, sinus attacks, high blood pressure, gastric and duodenal ulcers, certain rheumatic or allergic afflictions, and cardiovascular and kidney diseases.

For many years, we overcame two other obstacles to the concept of a single stereotyped response to stress. One obstacle was that qualitatively different types of agents of the same stressor potency do not elicit exactly the same overall syndrome. For example, cold causes shivering, heat produces sweating, epinephrine increases blood sugar, and insulin decreases it. All of these stressors have different specific effects, but their nonspecific effects are essentially the same: they all elicit the GAS, that is, adrenal cortex enlargement, shrinking of the thymus, deep bleeding ulcers.

The second obstacle was that the same stressor appeared to have different effects on different individuals, but we traced this difference to conditioning factors that can selectively enhance or inhibit a particular stress effect. This conditioning may be internal, resulting from genetic predisposition, age, or sex, or external, resulting from certain hormone treatments, drugs, or diet. Because of such conditioning, a normally tolerable degree of stress can adversely affect a predisposed region upon which a biologic agent acts, causing a disease of adaptation.

There is ample evidence that nervous and emotional stimuli (rage, fear, pain, etc.) can act as stressors, eliciting the GAS. Animals conditioned with corticoids and natrium salts undergo heart failure when we expose them to purely nervous stimuli. On the other hand, pretreatment with neurogenic stressors protects an animal's heart under nervous stimuli that would otherwise prove fatal. Neurogenic stressors can also protect against inflammatory and hypersensitivity reactions, mainly through the pituitary-adrenocortical axis. Psychosomatic medicine shows that mental attitudes can produce bodily changes. Common examples are stomach ulcers or heightened blood pressure caused by emotional upsets.

In a series of experiments, the Medical Research Group of the Swedish Army sought to determine whether psychologic stimuli can provoke biochemical and physiologic reactions that lead to internal disorders. The Swedish experimenters[1] subjected 32 senior officers (average age, 56 years) to the stress of alternating for 75 hours between staff work and 3-hour sessions at an electronic shooting range. The officers were not allowed to relax or sleep, use stimulants, smoke, or go for walks. Although the experiment provoked emotional reactions of only moderate intensity, the subjects underwent significant biochemical changes.

In a similar, considerably more trying experiment, 31 soldiers stayed at the shooting range for the entire 75 hours. Although their average age was only 29, their emotional and biochemical reactions were much more pronounced. One officer experienced temporary claustrophobia and panic. His epinephrine excretion was very high; he suffered headaches, blurred vision, and palpitations; and his pulse exceeded 100 beats per minute.

In both experiments approximately 25 percent of the subjects developed pathologic electrocardiographic patterns. Only after several days of rest did their electrocardiographs return to normal. The experiments prove that relatively brief stints of stress, below the intensity that most people ordinarily experience at some time in their lives, can provoke pathologic changes in our body. If they are repeated often or are allowed to persist for long periods, they might cause disease.

On the opposite question of whether bodily changes and actions affect mentality, we have almost no systematic research. Of course I do not refer to the potential psychologic effects of physical brain damage. But it is a fact that looking fit helps us to be fit. A pale, unwashed, unshaven tramp in dirty rags actually resists physical or mental stresses more effectively after a shave, some sun, a bath, and a change into crisp new clothes.

Man has long been aware of physical and mental strain, the relationships between bodily and mental reactions, and the importance of defensive, adaptive responses. But stress first became meaningful to me when I found that we can dissect it by modern research methods and identify the components of the stress response in chemical and physical terms. Then I was able to use the concept of stress to solve purely medical problems as well as problems of everyday life.

From what the laboratory and the clinical

study of somatic diseases has taught us concerning stress, we have tried to arrive at a code of ethics based not on traditions of our society, inspiration, or blind faith in the infallibility of a particular prophet, religious leader, or political doctrine, but on the scientifically verifiable laws that govern the body's reactions in maintaining homeostasis and living in satisfying equilibrium with its surroundings.

In a recent book, *Stress without Distress,*[3] on the behavioral implications of the stress concept and in my autobiography[4] I attempted to show in more detail how we can adjust our personal reactions to enjoy fully the eustress of success and accomplishment without suffering the distress commonly generated by frustrating friction and purposeless aggressive behavior against our surroundings.

It is a biologic law that man—like the lower animals—must fight and work for some goal that he considers worthwhile. We must use our innate capacities to enjoy the eustress of fulfillment. Only through effort, often aggressive egoistic effort, can we maintain our fitness and assure our homeostatic equilibrium with the surrounding society and the inanimate world. To achieve this state, our activities must earn lasting results; the fruits of work must be cumulative and must provide a capital gain to meet future needs. To succeed, we have to accept the scientifically established fact that man has an inescapable natural urge to work egoistically for things that can be stored to strengthen his homeostasis in the unpredictable situations with which life may confront him. These are not instincts we should be ashamed of or combat. We can do nothing about having been built to work; work is primarily for our own good. Organs that are not used (muscles, bones, even the brain) undergo inactivity and atrophy. Every living being looks out first of all for itself. There is no example in Nature of a creature guided exclusively by altruism and the desire to protect others. In fact, a code of universal altruism would be highly immoral since it would expect others to

look out for us more than for themselves.

"Love thy neighbor as thyself" is a command filled with wisdom, but as originally expressed it is incompatible with biologic laws; we do not need to develop an inferiority complex if we cannot love all our fellowmen on command. Neither should we feel guilty because we work for treasures that can be stored to ensure our future homeostasis. Hoarding is a vitally important biologic instinct that we share with animals such as ants, bees, squirrels, and beavers.

How can we develop a code of ethics that accepts egoism and working to hoard personal capital as morally correct? That is what I attempted to explain in *Stress without Distress,*[3] and here I shall summarize the main conclusions in the form of three basic guidelines.

1. *Find your own natural predilections and stress level.* People differ with regard to the amount and kind of work they consider worth doing to meet the exigencies of daily life and to assure their future security and happiness. In this respect, all of us are influenced by hereditary predispositions and the expectations of our society. Only through planned self-analysis can we establish what we really want; too many people suffer all their lives because they are too conservative to risk a radical change and break with traditions.

2. *Learn altruistic egoism.* The selfish hoarding of the goodwill, respect, esteem, support, and love of our neighbor is the most efficient way to give vent to our pent-up energy and create enjoyable, beautiful, or useful things.

3. *Earn your neighbor's love.* This motto, unlike love on command, is compatible with man's structure, and, although it is based on altruistic egoism, it could hardly be attacked as unethical. Who would blame him who wants to assure his own homeostasis and happiness by accumulating the treasure of other people's benevolence towards him? Yet this makes him virtually unassailable, for nobody wants to attack and destroy those upon whom he depends.

These are the three main principles derived from observations on the basic mechanisms that maintain homeostasis in cells, people, and entire societies and that help them face the stressors encountered in their constant fight for survival, security, and well-being. Once understood and clearly formulated we can use them best by conscious control.

Man, with his highly developed central nervous system, is especially vulnerable to psychic insults, and there are various little tricks to minimize these. Here are a few that I have found useful.

Whatever situation you meet in life, consider first whether it is really worth fighting for. Do not forget what Nature has taught us about the importance of carefully adjusting syntoxic and catatoxic attitudes to any problems of a cell, a man, or even a society.[3]

Try to keep your mind constantly on the pleasant aspects of life and on actions that can improve your situation. Try to forget everything that is irrevocably ugly or painful. This is perhaps the most efficient way of minimizing stress by what I have called voluntary mental diversion. As a wise German proverb says, "Imitate the sundial's way: Count only the pleasant days."

When faced with a task that is very painful yet indispensable to achieve your aim, don't procrastinate; cut right into an abscess to eliminate the pain, instead of prolonging it by gently rubbing the surface. Nothing paralyzes your efficiency more than frustration; nothing helps it more than success. Even after the greatest defeats the depressing thought of being a failure is best combatted by taking stock of all your past achievements, which no one can deny you. Such conscious stocktaking is most effective in reestablishing the self-confidence necessary for future success. There is something even in the most modest career that we are proud to recall—you would be surprised to see how much this can help when everything seems hopeless.

Admit that there is no perfection, but in each category of achievement something is tops; be satisfied to strive for that.

Do not underestimate the delight of real simplicity in your life style. Avoidance of all affections and unnecessary complications earns as much goodwill and love as pompous artificiality earns dislike.

Realize that men are not created equal, though they should of course have a birthright to equal opportunities. After birth, in a free society, their performance should determine their progress. There will always be leaders and followers, but the leaders are worth keeping only as long as they can serve the followers by acquiring their love, respect, and gratitude.

Finally do not forget that there is no ready-made success formula that would suit everybody. We are all different and so are our problems. The only thing we have in common is our subordination to those fundamental biologic laws that govern all living beings including man. As Sir Francis Bacon said, "In order to dominate Nature, we must obey her." I should like to add "and in order to obey her we must understand her laws." Hence I think a natural code of behavior based on the strictly scientific clarification of nonspecific adaptive mechanisms comes closest to what can be offered as a general guideline for conduct.

REFERENCES

1. Levi, L.: Emotional stress and biochemical reactions as modified by psychotropic drugs with particular reference to cardiovascular pathology (Pamphlet of Department of Medicine and Psychiatry, Stockholm), International Symposium on Psychotropic Drugs in Internal Medicine, Baie Domizia, Italy, International Congress Series No. 182, pp. 206-220, Amsterdam, 1968, Excerpta Medica.
2. Selye, H.: A syndrome produced by diverse nocuous agents, Nature **138:**32, 1936.
3. Selye, H.: Stress without distress, Philadelphia, 1974, J. B. Lippincott Co.
4. Selye, H.: The stress of my life, Toronto, 1977, McClelland & Stewart, Ltd.

3

The relation of psychological stress to onset of medical illness

MICHAEL W. HURST, C. DAVID JENKINS, and ROBERT M. ROSE

INTRODUCTION

Physicians and related health-care providers have become increasingly aware of the importance of psychological factors in the course and outcome of medical illness. However, there is much less agreement about the influence of psychological factors on the onset and development of medical illness. This chapter focuses on the relationship between psychological stress and the onset of medical illness.

There are a multitude of psychological factors such as personality, psychodynamics, psychopathology, previous family history, psychological stress, physiological stress, and the like that might be considered. This chapter specifically focuses on psychological stress. We must be careful to delineate what we mean by stress inasmuch as this concept is defined differently by leading experts (1-3).

One model of psychological stress postulates an event or situation that precipitates an emotional response such as anxiety or depression (4). The events must be appraised as harmful, threatening, challenging, and relevant to the individual in order to elicit the emotional response (5). This model is also concerned with the potential role of coping and adaptation in determining the intensity and type of emotional response (6). In sum, this model defines psychological stress in terms of emotional responses.

The second model holds that certain stimulus situations impose a psychological stress on an individual because they elicit attempts at adjustment (7). In other words, this model defines psychological stress in terms of the occurrence of certain stimulus situations rather than in terms of emotional response. If individuals are similar in how they rank various life events in terms of adjustment, then we may postulate that such events impose equivalent psychological stress for different individuals.

Recent work has shown that individuals of the United States, Norway, Finland, Japan, Denmark, and Sweden tend to rate a list of 40-50 stimulus life events in almost exactly the same way (8-10). For example, the death of a spouse is uniformly seen as an event that would cause a tremendous amount of adjustment, whereas a vacation would not. This second model therefore would imply that the amount of adjustment required defines the stressfulness of the event.

The relationship of psychological stress to mental illness has been extensively studied and many current reviews are available (7, 11). The relationship of psychological stress to certain physical illnesses is less well known and documented. Two physical disease clusters—heart disease and cancer—are leading causes of death in the United

States. Psychological stress has been implicated in their onset over the years. Recent literature has been particularly intriguing.

This chapter focuses specifically on the relationship of psychological stress to the onset of cardiovascular and neoplastic diseases. Each of the disease categories is then considered from the two approaches to definition of psychological stress: emotional responses and life event stimulus situations. Finally, conclusions and suggestions for research and practice are offered, based on the preceding review.

HEART DISEASE

This section concentrates on those psychosocial variables that qualify under the rubric of "stress" as defined above. These include disturbing life changes on the stimulus side of the equation and unpleasant effects on the response side. We have specifically excluded consideration of predisposing personal traits such as the "coronary-prone behavior pattern," which has been well established as a risk factor to coronary heart disease.

Anxiety and depression studies

Classical symptoms of anxiety include tenseness, sleep problems, irritability, numbness, restlessness, pains, and vague fears (12). Symptoms of depression include sadness, sleep problems, loss of appetite, irritability, restlessness, fatigue, and lack of interest (12). Since the symptoms overlap a great deal, we will view anxiety and depression together as emotional responses indicative of psychological stress.

Theil et al (13) studied 50 patients with myocardial infarctions (MI) and 50 age-matched, healthy, nonpatient controls. The patients with MI scored significantly higher on anxiety and depression scales than the controls. Specifically, they reported significantly more feelings of nervousness, sleep disturbances, and shortness of breath. Theil and his co-workers probed further in interviews with the patients and controls. They found that many of the MI patients reported

being particularly anxious and depressed prior to their MI. Unfortunately, the significance of these findings may be overestimated, since the controls were healthy subjects rather than patients with other diseases. In addition the experience of MI may have biased the recall of anxiety and depression symptoms.

Two prospective studies have confirmed the importance of sleep disturbances prior to MI. Friedman et al (14) studied thousands of Health Plan records in the Kaiser-Permanente medical program. The patients had responded to a 155-item questionnaire earlier in the program. Lack of energy, feeling blue, and many minor physical complaints were reported significantly more often by those who later developed MI than by persons who remained free of heart disease. Friedman also found that persons who reported trouble falling asleep or staying asleep were more likely to be in the group that later developed MI than in a control group remaining free of coronary heart disease (CHD). However, when all the subjects who had symptoms at initial exam suggestive of possible myocardial ischemia were removed from the analysis, the differences between those who did and did not later develop MI were diminished.

Thomas & Greenstreet (15) administered several biographical and psychological questionnaires to first- and second-year medical students. They contacted these individuals, or their families in cases of death, 11 to 27 years after graduation to determine their health status. The investigators found that medical students who had reported being fatigued upon awakening incurred MI proportionately more often in later years than those students who did not have this sleep complaint.

Kavanagh & Shepard (16) also noted that increased tiredness and a deterioration in general health was reported in the week prior to MI by 102 survivors of the event. This study, however, had no control group.

Greene et al (17) reported that sudden coronary death was frequently preceded by a period of depression followed by an abrupt change to a state of arousal. The arousal was marked by increased work, anxiety, or anger. The MI followed shortly upon the reactive arousal period. These clinical results were limited by the lack of specific measures of depression, anxiety, and anger, as well as by the fact that no control group was included.

A prospective Israeli study (18) reported that a three-item anxiety index was prospectively associated with the incidence of angina pectoris (AP). High-anxiety subjects developed twice the incidence of AP as did low-anxiety subjects. This was a statistically significant difference. However, in this study the anxiety assessment was not predictive of MI.

A controlled study by Eastwood & Trevelyan (19) screened 2200 English citizens who were on medical practitioners' lists. Psychological screening inventories and interviews were administered to identify persons with psychiatric problems. Chronic mild anxiety and depression were the main symptoms of the group so identified. They were matched with control subjects from the same medical lists who did not manifest these symptoms. Both groups were given thorough cardiological examinations. Significantly more diagnoses of "possible and probable CHD" were found in the anxiety-depression group than in the control group. This difference held true for both males and females.

In sum, recent clinical and prospective studies suggest that either newly-evidenced anxiety and depression or exacerbated chronic anxiety and depression may heighten the probability of onset of CHD and particularly of AP. However, the evidence fails to distinguish whether these manifestations of psychological stress are long-term precursors or short-term precipitants of CHD. Also, it has not been established that either of these manifestations interact with recognized risk factors such as high serum cholesterol, high blood pressure, cigarette smoking, obesity, or the coronary-prone behavior pattern (Type A).

Life event studies

In the following studies, and those reported later in the section on cancer, the Schedule of Recent Experiences (20) or a similar scale has been used. Subjects indicate the occurrence of life events (such as loss of job, buying a house, death in the family, and so forth) for given periods of time such as the past 6 months, 7-12 months ago, 13-18 months ago, and 19-24 months ago. Each event is assigned Life Change Units (LCUs) according to previous studies and the LCUs are summed for each time period. A typical listing of events and LCU is given in Holmes & Masuda (21). The sum of occurrences and/or the sum of LCU can be considered an estimate of psychological stress.

Rahe & Lind (22) obtained a list of 67 persons who had died a sudden cardiac death in Stockholm, Sweden, during a three-month period in 1968. A total of 39 next-of-kin participated in this study. They completed the Schedule of Recent Experiences (SRE) on behalf of the deceased. The investigators found a statistically significant increase in the total LCU for the sudden-death patients in the year prior to death, compared to the two years before that year. The final six months before death showed the highest levels of LCU. These findings held true for patients who did and did not have prior CHD histories. This seemingly impressive finding is greatly marred by the lack of a control group, since the increase in LCU as time approached the present could merely be a result of better memory in the next-of-kin for recent as compared to past periods.

Three very similar studies have presented comparable findings. Theorell & Rahe (23) studied 54 post-MI patients. Again there was a significant rise in the total LCU in the six months preceding the MI. This was true only for those patients with no previous history of MI. Those with a prior history of MI had higher life change scores both in the prior six months as well as before that time. In contrast, another uncontrolled study of 30 male post-MI patients (24) found no significant difference in the mean level of life change in the final six months. Rahe et al (25) studied 279 survivors of MI. They, too, completed the SRE. Subjects were divided into two groups: one MI group was characterized by a good health history for the two years prior to MI, the other by a poor health history for the same period of time. The group with illness prior to the MI had twice the total amount of life change over each six-month period in the two years as did the group without an illness history. Some of the difference between these groups may have resulted from the fact that several SRE events are health changes. Hence the group with prior illness would be expected to have a higher life change total than the healthier group. Both groups, however, did show a significant rise in LCU during the final six months prior to the MI.

The above studies are suggestive but not conclusive. They are severely handicapped by their retrospective designs. The results are highly dependent on recall, which may be influenced by the occurrence of MI. In addition, the studies all lack comparison groups that would control for type and occurrence of illness as well as for decreases in recall as a function of elapsed time.

Theorell, Lind & Floderus (26) attempted to overcome these limitations using a prospective design with 6579 male construction workers in Sweden. Follow-up reviews of medical records were completed for all workers 12-15 months after the completion of the SRE. Subjects with first MI events ($N=32$) were compared to all other subjects after excluding those with cardiovascular disease known at intake. There was no significant difference between the mean levels of life change between the MI group and all others.

Although these life change studies might suggest some causal role of stressful life situations in the onset of heart disease, other explanations for the reported results can be offered. Selective or diminished recall of life events over extended periods of time would account for the significant difference

in life change totals of the final six months prior to MI compared to results from a year earlier.

A person-specific or environmentally specific adjustment for a given life event may be more important than the generalized adjustment value assigned from studies of large populations of persons, most of whom have not recently experienced the events they are rating. This possible alternative is given credence by Lundberg, Theorell & Lind (27). They found that the sum of an individual's own retrospective assessments of distress associated with each life event was, in fact, more strongly discriminating between the MI and the comparison group than the use of individual ratings of adjustment demanded by the life events or average assessments by the total group of either distress or adjustment. Thus, the occurrence of events commonly believed to demand adjustment may be less important in the onset of heart disease than the occurrence of events that the individual finds personally upsetting.

In other words, systemic emotional arousal (2) engendered by events relevant to the individual (5), or in which the individual is engaged/involved (28), may constitute the most important aspect of psychological stress in the onset of heart disease. This suggestion finds some support in a recent study of patients with congestive heart failure.

Perlman et al (29) noted four studies examining the relationship between emotional factors and the onset of congestive heart failure. Two studies seemed to indicate a strong emotional precipitating factor and two did not. One of the reasons suggested for this discrepancy in results was "different definitions of emotional stress." Another was the "depth of patient and family interviews." Perlman et al interviewed each of 105 congestive heart failure patients for 1½-2 hr. An age- and sex-matched group of 50 consecutive patients with no history of congestive heart failure was also interviewed. The interviewer was unaware of the patient diagnoses. Relatives were interviewed and asked the same questions as the patients.

The definition of emotional/psychological stress for this study was unique. To quote the authors,

> For this study an emotional or psychological factor was defined as any event or circumstances that represented trauma or produced a strong emotional reaction in the patient. Only events and reactions that occurred not more than 3 days before the onset of symptoms and hospitalization were considered. Chronic anxiety states of mind . . . were not included. Changes in the patients' affect during the relating of the event and the effects it had on his behavior before hospitalization were more crucial than the nature of the event itself.

This definition encompassed each aspect of Mason's (1,2) Lazarus's (5), and Singer's (28) components of psychological stress. Although the Perlman study was retrospective, the definition and results are instructive. Fifty-one of the 105 congestive heart patients (49%), but only 12 of 50 (24%) control patients, experienced a clearly identifiable emotional event in the three days preceding hospitalization. This difference was significant at the 0.01 level. In this case the period of recall was so short that memory should not have been a confounding factor in the results. However, there may have been a differential propensity to report such events between the two groups rather than an actual difference in occurrences.

No matter how one examines the data, it seems that both perspectives of psychological stress suggest an important role for psychological distress in the onset of heart disease. Until more evidence of a substantial and controlled nature is available, we cannot say how important psychological stress is, compared to physiological risk factors or to other psychosocial factors such as the coronary-prone behavior pattern. It may well turn out to be the case that psychological stress is a catalyst for other risk factors rather than a true participant in the disease process. On the other hand, chronic and repeated exposure to stress may have direct physiological consequences that play a role in the etiology of heart disease (30).

Cancer: anxiety and depression studies

Early in this chapter we noted that one perspective on psychological stress suggested that anxiety and depression would indicate the presence or operation of psychological stress on a person. Review of the recent heart disease literature suggested that persons suffering from anxiety and depression were more likely to experience the onset of CHD than persons who were not anxious and depressed. This kind of more carefully controlled comparison study has not been done for cancer. The lower incidence of cancer and the tremendous difficulty inherent in trying to ascertain the patient's psychological state prior to the development of cancer has discouraged prospective studies along these lines. However, it is worthwhile to examine some of the conclusions made by researchers.

LeShan (31) reviewed literature published from 1902-1957. The great majority of studies were clinical in nature and based on the personal experiences of the reporting physicians. One of the main themes of all these studies was that depression, hopelessness, and undischarged grief seemed to be significant precursors of the discovery of cancer. LeShan also pointed out that many studies suggested that depression and hopelessness were reactions to the unreplaced loss of an emotionally close relationship. Studies conducted by LeShan & Worthington (32-34) seemed to indicate that this loss of a particularly intense personal relationship could be placed prior to the probable onset of the disease. The development of the depressive symptoms seemed to occur just prior to the appearance of the cancer. However, all of the studies reviewed by LeShan were retrospective and the vast majority were uncontrolled. Hence these conclusions are more provocative than conclusive.

Greene (35) reported on a series of three studies with leukemia and lymphoma patients that he and his co-workers had conducted over several years. Over one hundred patients had been studied by the time of Greene's summary report. He and his workers felt that depressive and anxious reactions to losses and separations were symptoms particularly associated with the onset of leukemia or lymphoma.

In their initial comments to a paper devoted to ego defenses in the etiology of cancer, Bahnson & Bahnson (36) noted that loss and depression seemed to be significant antecedents to the onset of cancer. However, they further cautioned that these conditions and emotional states may be necessary but not sufficient conditions for the onset of malignant neoplasms.

Hagnell (37) reported on a prospective study of the personality of 2550 Swedish citizens who were followed for ten years. He found a significant difference in the premorbid personalities of those who did and those who did not develop cancer. Unfortunately, the assessment procedure was based on an unusual personality theory that is not comparable to any other system. However, the ''substable'' personality, characteristic of those who developed cancer, had a major component related to depression. The ''substable'' person tended to lose energy and withdraw emotional expression when depressed. A liberal interpretation suggests that this type of person suffered from a more severe form of clinical depression than those persons characterized as ''superstable'' (cool, analytical, and aloof).

At least one, if not the only, prospective study of the role of anxiety and depression in the onset of cancer has been reported recently. Thomas & Greenstreet (15) followed up on 1076 graduates of the Johns Hopkins Medical School. Initial testing was completed in the first two years of medical school. The follow-up data was collected 11-27 years after initial testing. They found that those nine who later developed cancer had consistently lower depression, anxiety, and anger at initial testing than those students who died of suicide, or developed mental illness, hypertension, or coronary

occlusions. These students also were significantly lower in anxiety and depression than the normal controls (disease-free at follow-up).

This prospective finding clearly echoed the findings of Kissen (38); Kissen, Brown & Kissen (39); and Abse et al. (40). These investigators had consistently found that cancer patients (and lung cancer patients in particular) had significantly lower neuroticism scores than other patient groups as well as normal controls. These studies tested patients admitted for diagnostic work-ups. Testing was done prior to diagnosis. Control patients were those whose work-ups resulted in nonmalignant diagnoses. The neuroticism measure used by these investigators is equivalent to an assessment of physical complaints and anxiety.

Thus, the results of the prospective and carefully controlled studies contradict the clinical and retrospective uncontrolled studies. Both theoretical (36) and descriptive (38) explanations have been offered that might resolve the contradiction. However, the explanations have not been replicated in other settings, let alone put to the test of a prospective study.

From the point of view of psychological stress in the onset of cancer, it seems to us that the literature points very strongly to the need for prospective studies that include at least three elements for prediction, namely, assessments of psychological factors, physiological risk factors, and longitudinal stimulus event histories. Only then may it be possible to unravel the role of psychological stress in the onset of cancer.

Life event studies

In his review of 7 studies, LeShan (31) concluded: ''The most consistently reported, relevant psychological factor has been the loss of a major emotional relationship prior to the first-noted symptoms of the neoplasm.'' A closer examination of the studies he reviewed in coming to this conclusion indicated that these losses might have occurred anywhere between six months and eight years before the probable onset of symptoms. Kavetsky, Turkevich & Balitsky (41) reported similar findings and conclusions by many Russian clinicians. They also reported that the Russians tended to explain these findings in terms of endocrine or metabolic changes that occurred under conditions of psychological stress.

In the section on anxiety and depression, we noted two studies by LeShan & Worthington (32, 34) that indicated that a significantly greater proportion of cancer patients than controls (both disease-free and noncancer patients) revealed a history of a loss of a particularly intense emotional relationshp prior to the diagnosis of cancer. This deduction was made on the basis of a projective test that was administered to all the research subjects.

These suggestive results led to an epidemiological study of mortality rates for groups of people that could be expected to differ in terms of the loss of an important emotional relationship (42). Widowed persons were predicted to have the highest cancer mortality rate; divorced persons the next highest; then married persons; and finally single persons. LeShan then reviewed several reports of female cancer mortality rates and regrouped the data to reflect age-adjusted mortality rates for the widowed, divorced, married, and single groups. In the five studies he reviewed, LeShan "found no statistical studies whose results were inconsistent with the hypotheses." These results seem quite suggestive. However, it is important to note that the results were only for women and were based on data from 1900-1932. We do not know if this finding would continue to hold true in more recent times or if it applies to men. This might be a fruitful area of investigation.

Greene's (35) summary report of three studies involving 100 leukemia and lymphoma patients suggested an etiological role for anxiety and depression. The most common precipitants for these reactions were death and threat of death or separation from parents, spouse, children, or other signifi-

cant persons. The retrospective interview examination covered the four-year prodromal period before the apparent onset of the cancer. The loss experience most often occurred around 12 months prior to onset.

Bahnson & Bahnson (36) also reported on a series of studies they had conducted. Ninety-nine cancer patients suffering from various cancers were studied by means of an unstructured interview. Thirty-eight normal males served as control subjects. The interviewers were aware of patient diagnoses. The implications of the results of this study seemed to be that the cancer patients experienced an unresolved loss of a dependency relationship one to two years prior to the onset of the neoplasm.

Thus, LeShan (42), Green (35), and Bahnson & Bahnson (36) all reported similar findings. Their data suggested that the loss of a particularly intense dependency relationship occurred shortly before the onset of cancer.

A more direct life event approach was applied by Schmale & Iker (43). They reported on a series of three investigations with a total of 51 women. The women had been referred for a cone biopsy due to positive Pap tests. They had no gross evidence of cervical disease. An open-ended interview and psychological tests were administered before the biopsy results were known to the subject, her physician, the pathologist, or the investigators. The biopsy results indicated that 19 women had cervical cancer.

The interview protocols were rated for the presence of feelings of hopelessness in response to a life event in the six months prior to the first positive Pap smear. According to this criteria, 18 subjects were predicted to have cancer. Thirty-three were predicted to not have cancer because they had not developed the hopelessness reaction. Eleven of the 18 predicted to have cancer did, in fact, have it. Of the 33 predicted not to have it, 25 did not. An error in interpretation led the researchers to conclude that these results were nonsignificant. However, our own calculations show that the predictions were significantly accurate at a high level of confidence (chi-square-6.76, $df=1$, p less than 0.01). In addition, those who actually had cancer had significantly higher depression scores on a personality test.

On the other hand, Muslin, Gyarfas & Pieper (44) studied 165 women admitted for breast biopsies. A questionnaire was completed and an interview was conducted before the results of the biopsy were known to subjects or investigators. The interview was rated for the presence or absence of "a permanent loss of a first degree relative or other person whom the subject specifically stated was emotionally important to her." Subjects were grouped into pairs of benign and malignant lesions with each pair being matched for age, race, marital status, and socioeconomic status. It was possible to produce 37 matched pairs by this method.

The interviews revealed an excess of 17% more separation losses among the cancer subjects while the questionnaire revealed only an 8% excess in comparison to the matched controls. The differences between loss rates of the cancer patients and controls was nonsignificant.

Grissom, Weiner & Weiner (45) studied 30 lung cancer patients, 30 emphysema patients, and 30 disease-free veterans. Group smoking histories were matched by subject selection procedures. The SRE and the Tennessee Self Concept questionnaires were administered to all of the subjects. The LCU totals for the year prior to admission to the Veterans Administration hospital for diagnostic purposes were not statistically different among any of the groups.

Thus, for lung and breast cancers there has been a lack of definitive evidence that increased life event stress plays a role in the onset of the neoplasm, while there has been some consistent suggestion that life event stress may be related to the onset of cervical cancer, leukemia, and lymphoma. Since all of the studies were retrospective, Grinker's (46) caution seems pertinent: "There is always danger of attributing characteristics to a particular event if a dis-ease process such as carcinoma develops somewhere in the adjacent time span. . . ." On the other hand, we do not fully concur with Crisp's (47) or Brown's (48) suggestions that clinicians and researchers should be more concerned with course and outcome than with etiology. Their position has fewer inherent difficulties from a research and rehabilitation standpoint, but it tends to rule out control and prevention.

IMPLICATIONS AND CONCLUSIONS

Research and clinical evidence suggests that psychological stress may be important in the onset of heart and neoplastic diseases. Yet most of the evidence is based on retrospective and/or uncontrolled studies. The few prospective studies that have been undertaken seem to contradict or diminish the significance of the retrospective findings, particularly for cancer studies. Overall, the results of studies on the relationship of psychological stress to the onset of medical illness have suggested a complex interaction of factors rather than a simple causal link.

This complicated state of affairs does not seem to hold with respect to the course and outcome of cancer or cardiac patients. Depression, hopelessness, and anxiety have been shown to adversely affect the course and outcome of cancers in several recent studies (48-53). Similar findings have been reported for cardiac patients (54) and for patients with congestive heart failure (29). These course and outcome studies are implemented more easily and at less expense than studies on etiology and onset. They suggest a strong role for psychiatric consultation and liaison in the rehabilitation of cardiovascular and neoplastic patients. But we are left with the question of what to do to prevent the disease in the first place.

At this stage of research in the area, the most appropriate conclusion is that more research is needed. Long-term prospective studies with carefully defined and selected controls are needed. Consistent and replicable assessments and definitions of psychological stress would help alleviate difficulties in interpretation of results. Simultaneous testing of psychological, physical, and historical factors in a repeated prospective design would augment the explication of the interaction between stress and disease onset. Caution, reliability, and scientific rigor have been neglected too long in this important area.

REFERENCES

1. Mason, J. W. 1975. A historical view of the stress field, Part I. *J. Hum. Stress* 1:6-12.
2. Mason, J. W. 1975. A historical view of the stress field, Part II. *J. Hum. Stress* 1:22-36.
3. Selye, H. 1975. Confusion and controversy in the stress field. *J. Hum. Stress* 1:37-44.
4. Rosenwald, G. C. 1961. The assessment of anxiety in psychological experimentation: a theoretical reformulation and test. *J. Abnorm. Soc. Psychol.* 62:666-73.
5. Lazarus, R. S. 1971. The concepts of stress and disease. *Society, Stress and Disease,* ed. L. Levi, 1:53-58. London: Oxford Univ. Press.
6. Coelho, G. V., Hamburg, D. A., Adams, J. E., eds. 1974. *Coping and Adaptation.* New York: Basic.
7. Dohrenwend, B. S., Dohrenwend, B. P., eds. 1974. *Stressful Life Events: Their Nature and Effects,* New York: Wiley.
8. Rahe, R. H. 1969. Life crisis and health change. *Psychotropic Drug Response: Advances in Prediction,* ed. P. R. May, R. Whittenborn, 92-125. Springfield, Ill: Thomas.
9. Rahe, R. H., Bennett, L., Romo, M., Siltanen, P., Arthur, R. J. 1973. Subject's recent life changes and coronary heart disease in Finland. *Am. J. Psychiatry* 130:1222-26.
10. Rahe, R. H., Lundberg, U., Theorell, T., Bennett, L. K. 1971. The social readjustment rating scale: A comparative study of Swedes and Americans. *J. Psychosom. Res.* 15:241-49.
11. Levi, L., ed. 1971. *Society, Stress and Disease, Vol. I: The Psychosocial Environment and Psychosomatic Diseases.* London: Oxford Univ. Press.
12. Freedman, A. M., Kaplan, H. I., Saddock, B. J. 1972. *Modern Synopsis of the Comprehensive Textbook of Psychiatry.* Baltimore: Williams & Wilkins.
13. Thiel, H. G., Parker, D., Bruce, T. A. 1973. Stress factors and the risk of myocardial infarction. *J. Psychosom. Res.* 17:43-57.
14. Friedman, G. D., Ury, H. K., Klatsky, A. L., Siegelaub, M. S. 1974. A psychological questionnaire predictive of myocardial infarction. *Psychosom. Med.* 36:327-43.
15. Thomas, C. B., Greenstreet, R. L. 1973. Psycho-

biological characteristics in youth as predictors of five disease states: suicide, mental illness, hypertension, coronary heart disease, and tumor. *Johns Hopkins Med. J.* 132:16-43.
16. Kavanaugh, T., Shepard, R. J. 1973. The immediate antecedents of myocardial infarction in active men. *Can. Med. Assoc. J.* 109:19-22.
17. Greene, W. A., Goldstein, S., Moss, A. J. 1972. Psychosocial aspects of sudden death. *Arch. Intern. Med.* 129:725-31.
18. Medalie, J. H., Snyder, M., Groen, J. J. et al. 1973. Angina pectoris among 10,000 men: five-year incidence and univariate analysis. *Am. J. Med.* 55:583-94.
19. Eastwood, M. R., Trevelyan, H. 1971. Stress and coronary heart disease. *J. Psychosom. Res.* 15:289-92.
20. Holmes, T. H., Rahe, R. H. 1967. The social readjustment rating scale. *J. Psychsom. Res.* 11:213-18.
21. Holmes, T. H., Masuda, M. 1974. Life change and illness susceptibility. *Stressful Life Events: Their Nature and Effects,* ed. B. S. Dohrenwend, B. P. Dohrenwend, 45-72. New York: Wiley.
22. Rahe, R. H., Lind. E. 1971. Psychosocial factors and sudden cardiac death: a pilot study. *J. Psychosom. Res.* 15:19-24.
23. Theorell, T., Rahe, R. H. 1971. Psychosocial factors and myocardial infarction. I. An inpatient study in Sweden. *J. Psychosom. Res.* 15:25-31.
24. Rahe, R. H., Paasikivi, J. 1971. Psychosocial factors and myocardial infarction. II. An outpatient study in Sweden. *J. Psychosom. Res.* 15:33-39.
25. Rahe, R. H., Romo, M., Bennett, L., Siltanen, P. 1973. *Subjects' recent life changes and myocardial infarction in Helsinki.* San Diego: US Navy Med. Neuropsychiatr. Res. Unit. Mimeographed.
26. Theorell, T., Lind, E., Floderus, B. 1975. *Life events and prospective near-future serious illness with special reference to myocardial infarction studies on middle-aged building construction workers.* Stockholm: Lab. Clin. Res., Karolinska Inst. Mimeographed.
27. Lundberg, U., Theorell, T., Lind, E. 1975. Life changes and myocardial infarction: individual differences in life change scaling. *J. Psychosom. Res.* 19:27-32.
28. Singer, M. T. 1973. Engagement-involvement: a central phenomenon in psychophysiological research. Presented at Meet. Am. Psychosom. Soc., Denver, Colo.
29. Perlman, L. V., Ferguson, S., Bergum, K., Isenberg, E. L., Hammarsten, J. F. 1975. Precipitation of congestive heart failure: social and emotional factors. *Ann. Intern. Med.* 75:1-7.
30. Levi, L. 1973. Stress, distress, and psychosocial stimuli. *Occup. Mental Health* 3:2-10.
31. LeShan, L. 1959. Psychological states as factors in the development of malignant disease: a critical review. *J. Natl. Cancer Inst.* 22:1-18.

32. LeShan, L., Worthington, R. E. 1955. Some psychologic correlates of neoplastic disease. *J. Clin. Exp. Psychopathy* 16:281-88.

33. LeShan, L., Worthington, R. E. 1956. Some recent life history patterns observed in patients with malignant disease. *J. Nerv. Ment. Dis.* 124:460-65.

34. LeShan, L., Worthington, R. E. 1956. Loss of cathexes as a common psychodynamic characteristic of cancer patients. *Psychol. Rep.* 2:183-93.

35. Greene, W. A. 1966. The psychosocial setting of the development of leukemia and lymphoma. *Ann. NY Acad. Sci.* 125:794-801.

36. Bahnson, C. B., Bahnson, M. B. 1966. Role of the ego defenses: denial and repression in the etiology of malignant neoplasm. *Ann. NY Acad. Sci.* 125:827-45.

37. Hagnell, O. 1966. The premorbid personality of persons who develop cancer in a total population investigated in 1947 and 1957. *Ann. NY Acad. Sci.* 125:846-55.

38. Kissen, D. M. 1966. The significance of personality in lung cancer in men. *Ann. NY Acad. Sci.* 125:820-26.

39. Kissen, D. M., Brown, R. I., Kissen, M. 1969. A further report on personality and psychosocial factors in lung cancer. *Ann. NY Acad. Sci.* 164:535-45.

40. Abse, D. W., et al 1974. Personality and behavioral characteristics of lung cancer patients. *J. Psychosom. Res.* 18:101-13.

41. Kavetsky, R. E., Turkevich, N. M., Balitsky, K. P. 1966. On the psychophysiological mechanism of the organism's resistance to tumor growth. *Ann. NY Acad. Sci.* 125:933-45.

42. LeShan, L. 1966. An emotional life-history pattern associated with neoplastic disease. *Ann. NY Acad. Sci.* 125:780-93.

43. Schmale, A., Iker, H. 1966. The psychological setting of uterine cervical cancer. *Ann. NY Acad. Sci.* 125:807-13.

44. Muslin, H. L., Gyarfas, K., Pieper, W. J. 1966. Separation experience and cancer of the breast. *Ann. NY Acad. Sci.* 125:802-6.

45. Grissom, J. J., Weiner, B. J., Weiner, E. A. 1975. Psychological correlates of cancer. *J. Consult. Clin. Psych.* 43:113-14.

46. Grinker, R. R. 1966. Psychosomatic aspects of the cancer problem. *Ann. NY Acad. Sci.* 125:876-82.

47. Crisp, A. H. 1970. Some psychosomatic aspects of neoplasia. *Br. J. Med. Psychol.* 43:313-31.

48. Brown, F. 1966. The relationship between cancer and personality. *Ann. NY Acad. Sci.* 125:865-73.

49. Stavraky, K. M., Buck, C. N., Lott, J. S., Wanklin, J. M. 1968. Psychological factors in the outcome of human cancer. *J. Psychosom. Res.* 12:251-59.

50. Achte, K., Vauhkonen, M.-L. 1970. Psychic factors in cancer: psychiatric approach, Part I. In *Cancer and Psyche,* Monogr. Psychiatr. Clin. Helsinki, pp. 7-44. Helsinki: Kunnallispaino.

51. Viitamaki, R. O. 1970. Pychological determinants of cancer: Psychometric approach, Part II. See Ref. 50, pp. 45-142.

52. Davies, R. K., Quinlan, D. M., McKegney, F. P., Kimball, C. P. 1973. Organic factors and psychological adjustment in advanced cancer patients. *Psychosom. Med.* 35:464-71.

53. Schonfield, J. 1972. Psychological factors related to delayed return to an earlier life style in successfully treated cancer patients. *J. Psychosom. Res.* 16:41-46.

54. Kimball, C. P., Quinlan, D., Osborne, F., Woodward, B. 1973. The experience of cardiac surgery: V. Psychological patterns and prediction of outcome. *Psychother. Psychosom.* 22:310-19.

4

Medical nemesis

IVAN ILLICH

Within the last decade medical professional practice has become a major threat to health. Depression, infection, disability, dysfunction, and other specific iatrogenic diseases now cause more suffering than all accidents from traffic or industry. Beyond this, medical practice sponsors sickness by the reinforcement of a morbid society which not only industrially preserves its defectives but breeds the therapist's client in cybernetic way. Finally, the so-called health-professions have an indirect sickening power—a structurally health-denying effect. I want to focus on this last syndrome, which I designate as medical Nemesis. By transforming pain, illness, and death from a personal challenge into a technical problem, medical practice expropriates the potential of people to deal with their human condition in an autonomous way and becomes the source of a new kind of un-health.

Much suffering has always been man-made: history is the record of enslavement and exploitation. It tells of war, and of the pillage, famine, and pestilence which come in its wake. War between commonwealths and classes has so far been the main planned agency of man-made misery. Thus, man is the only animal whose evolution has been conditioned by adaptation on two fronts. If he did not succumb to the ele-

ments, he had to cope with use and abuse by others of his kind. He replaced instincts by character and culture, to be capable of this struggle on two frontiers. A third frontier of possible doom has been recognized since Homer; but common mortals were considered immune to its threat. Nemesis, the Greek name for the awe which loomed from this third direction, was the fate of a few heroes who had fallen prey to the envy of the gods. The common man grew up and perished in a struggle with Nature and neighbour. Only the élite would challenge the thresholds set by Nature for man.

Prometheus was not Everyman, but a deviant. Driven by Pleonexia, or radical greed, he trespassed the boundaries of the human condition. In hubris or measureless presumption, he brought fire from heaven, and thereby brought Nemesis on himself. He was put into irons on a Caucasian rock. A vulture preys at his innards, and heartlessly healing gods keep him alive by regrafting his liver each night. The encounter with Nemesis made the classical hero an immortal reminder of inescapable cosmic retaliation. He becomes a subject for epic tragedy, but certainly not a model for everyday aspiration. Now Nemesis has become endemic; it is the backlash of progress. Paradoxically, it has spread as far and as wide as the franchise, schooling, mechanical acceleration, and medical care. Everyman has fallen prey to the envy of the gods. If the species is to survive it can do so only by learning to cope in this third group.

Reprinted from Lancet **1**:918-921, 1974. Abridged from a lecture given in Edinburgh on April 26 and in Nottingham on May 1, 1974. The lecture is based on the book *Medical Nemesis*.

INDUSTRIAL NEMESIS

Most man-made misery is now the by-product of enterprises which were originally designed to protect the common man in his struggle with the inclemency of the environment and against wanton injustices inflicted by the élite. The main source of pain, disability, and death is now an engineered—albeit non-intentional—harassment. The prevailing ailments, helplessness and injustice, are now the side-effects of strategies for progress. Nemesis is now so prevalent that it is readily mistaken for part of the human condition. The desperate disability of contemporary man to envisage an alternative to the industrial aggression on the human condition is an integral part of the curse from which he suffers. Progress has come with a vengeance which cannot be called a price. The down payment was on the label and can be stated in measurable terms. The installments accrue under forms of suffering which exceed the notion of "pain."

At some point in the expansion of our major institutions their clients begin to pay a higher price every day for their continued consumption, in spite of the evidence that they will inevitably suffer more. At this point in development the prevalent behaviour of society corresponds to that traditionally recognised in addicts. Declining returns pale in comparison with marginally increasing disutilities. *Homo economicus* turns into *Homo religiosus*. His expectations become heroic. The vengeance of economic development not only outweighs the price at which this vengeance was purchased; it also outweighs the compound tort done by Nature and neighbours. Classical Nemesis was punishment for the rash abuse of a privilege. Industrialised Nemesis is retribution for dutiful participation in society.

War and hunger, pestilence and sudden death, torture and madness remain man's companions, but they are now shaped into a new *Gestalt* by the Nemesis overarching them. The greater the economic progress of any community, the greater the part played by industrial Nemesis in the pain, discrimination, and death suffered by its members.

Therefore, it seems that the disciplined study of the distinctive character of Nemesis ought to be the key theme for research amongst those who are concerned with health care, healing, and consoling.

TANTALUS

Medical Nemesis is but one aspect of the more general "counter-intuitive misadventures" characteristic of industrial society. It is the monstrous outcome of a very specific dream of reason—namely, "tantalizing" hubris. Tantalus was a famous king whom the gods invited to Olympus to share one of their meals. He purloined Ambrosia, the divine potion which gave the gods unending life. For punishment, he was made immortal in Hades and condemned to suffer unending thirst and hunger. When he bows towards the river in which he stands, the water recedes, and when he reaches for the fruit above his head the branches move out of his reach. Ethologists might say that Hygienic Nemesis has programmed him for compulsory counter-intuitive behaviour. Craving for Ambrosia has now spread to the common mortal. Scientific and political optimism have combined to propagate the addiction. To sustain it, the priesthood of Tantalus has organised itself, offering unlimited medical improvement of human health. The members of this guild pass themselves off as disciples of healing Asklepios, while in fact they peddle Ambrosia. People demand of them that life be improved, prolonged, rendered compatible with machines, and capable of surviving all modes of acceleration, distortion, and stress. As a result, health has become scarce to the degree to which the common man makes health depend upon the consumption of Ambrosia.

CULTURE AND HEALTH

Mankind evolved only because each of its individuals came into existence protected by various visible and invisible cocoons. Each one knew the womb from which he had come, and oriented himself by the stars under which he was born. To be human and to become human, the individual of our species has to find his destiny in his unique struggle with Nature and neighbour. He is on his own in the struggle, but the weapons and the rules and the style are given to him by the culture in which he grew up. Each culture is the sum of rules with which the individual could come to terms with pain, sickness, and death—could interpret them and practise compassion amongst others faced by the same threats. Each culture set the myth, the rituals, the taboos, and the ethical standards needed to deal with the fragility of life—to explain the reason for pain, the dignity of the sick, and the role of dying or death.

Cosmopolitan medical civilisation denies the need for man's acceptance of these evils. Medical civilisation is planned and organised to kill pain, to eliminate sickness, and to struggle against death. These are new goals, which have never before been guidelines for social life and which are antithetic to every one of the cultures with which medical civilisation meets when it is dumped on the so-called poor as part and parcel of their economic progress.

The health-denying effect of medical civilisation is thus equally powerful in rich and in poor countries, even though the latter are often spared some of its more sinister sides.

THE KILLING OF PAIN

For an experience to be pain in the full sense, it must fit into a culture. Precisely because each culture provides a mode for suffering, culture is a particular form of health. The act of suffering is shaped by culture into a question which can be stated and shared.

Medical civilisation replaces the culturally determined competence in suffering with a growing demand by each individual for the institutional management of his pain. A myriad of different feelings, each expressing some kind of fortitude, are homogenised into the political pressure of anaesthesia consumers. Pain becomes an item on a list of complaints. As a result, a new kind of horror emerges. Conceptually it is still pain, but the impact on our emotions of this valueless, opaque, and impersonal hurt is something quite new.

In this way, pain has come to pose only a technical question for industrial man—what do I need to get in order to have my pain managed or killed? If the pain continues, the fault is not with the universe, God, my sins, or the devil, but with the medical system. Suffering is an expression of consumer demand for increased medical outputs. By becoming unnecessary, pain has become unbearable. With this attitude, it now seems rational to flee pain rather than to face it, even at the cost of addiction. It also seems reasonable to eliminate pain, even at the cost of health. It seems enlightened to deny legitimacy to all non-technical issues which pain raises, even at the cost of disarming the victims of residual pain. For a while it can be argued that the total pain anaesthetised in a society is greater than the totality of pain newly generated. But at some point, rising marginal disutilities set in. The new suffering is not only unmanageable, but it has lost its referential character. It has become meaningless, questionless torture. Only the recovery of the will and ability to suffer can restore health into pain.

THE ELIMINATION OF SICKNESS

Medical interventions have not affected total mortality-rates: at best they have shifted survival from one segment of the population to another. Dramatic changes in the nature of disease afflicting Western societies during the last 100 years are well documented. First industrialisation exacerbated infections, which then subsided. Tuberculosis peaked over a 50–75-year period and declined before either the tubercle bacillus had been discovered or antituberculous programmes had been initiated. It was replaced in Britain and the U.S. by major malnutrition syndromes—rickets and pellagra—which peaked and declined, to be replaced by disease of early childhood, which in turn gave way to duodenal ulcers in young men. When that declined the modern epidemics took their toll—coronary heart-disease, hypertension, cancer, arthritis, diabetes, and mental disorders. At least in the U.S., death-rates from hypertensive heart-disease seem to be declining. Despite intensive research no connection between these changes in disease patterns can be attributed to the professional practice of medicine.

Neither decline in any of the major epidemics of killing diseases, nor major changes in the age structure of the population, nor falling and rising absenteeism at the workbench have been significantly related to sick care—even to immunisation. Medical services deserve neither credit for longevity nor blame for the threatening population pressure.

Longevity owes much more to the railroad and to the synthesis of fertilisers and insecticides than it owes to new drugs and syringes. Professional practice is both ineffective and increasingly sought out. This technically unwarranted rise of medical prestige can only be explained as a magical ritual for the achievement of goals which are beyond technical and political reach. It can be countered only through legislation and political action which favours the deprofessionalisation of health care.

The overwhelming majority of modern diagnostic and therapeutic interventions which demonstrably do more good than harm have two characteristics: the material resources for them are extremely cheap, and they can be packaged and designed for self-use or application by family members. The price of technology that is significantly health-furthering or curative in Canadian medicine is so low that the resources now squandered in India on modern medicine would suffice to make it available in the entire sub-continent. On the other hand, the skills needed for the application of the most generally used diagnostic and therapeutic aids are so simple that the careful observation of instruction by people who personally care would guarantee more effective and responsible use than medical practice can provide.

The deprofessionalisation of medicine does not imply and should not be read as implying negation of specialised healers, of competence, of mutual criticism, or of public control. It does imply a bias against mystification, against transnational dominance of one orthodox view, against disbarment of healers chosen by their patients but not certified by the guild. The deprofessionalisation of medicine does not mean denial of public funds for curative purposes, it does mean a bias against the disbursement of any such funds under the prescription and control of guild-members, rather than under the control of the consumer. Deprofessionalisation does not mean the elimination of modern medicine, nor obstacles to the invention of new ones, nor necessarily the return to ancient programmes, rituals, and devices. It means that no professional shall have the power to lavish on any one of his patients a package of curative resources larger than that which any other could claim on his own. Finally, the deprofessionalisation of medicine does not mean disregard for the special needs which people manifest at special moments of their lives; when they are born, break a leg, marry, give birth, become crippled, or face death. It only means that people have a right to live in an environment which is hospitable to them at such high points of experience.

THE STRUGGLE AGAINST DEATH

The ultimate effect of medical Nemesis is the expropriation of death. In every society the image of death is the culturally conditioned anticipation of an uncertain date. This anticipation determines a series of behavioural norms during life and the structure of certain institutions.

Wherever modern medical civilisation has penetrated a traditional medical culture, a novel cultural ideal of death has been fostered. The new ideal spreads by means of technology and the professional ethos which corresponds to it.

In primitive societies death is always conceived as the intervention of an actor—an enemy, a witch, an ancestor, or a god. The Christian and the Islamic Middle Ages saw in each death the hand of God. Western death had no face until about 1420. The Western ideal of death which comes to all equally from natural causes is of quite recent origin. Only during the autumn of the Middle Ages death appears as a skeleton with power in its own right. Only during the 16th century, as an answer European peoples developed the "arte and crafte to knowe ye Will to Dye." For the next three centuries peasant and noble, priest and whore, prepared themselves throughout life to preside at their own death. Foul death, bitter death, became the end rather than the goal of living. The idea that natural death should come only in healthy old age appeared only in the 18th century as a class-specific phenomenon of the bourgeois. The demand that doctors struggle against death and keep valetudinarians healthy has nothing to do with their ability to provide such service: Ariès has shown that the costly attempts to prolong life appear at first only among bankers whose power is compounded by the years they spend at a desk.

We cannot fully understand contemporary social organisation unless we see in it a multi-faceted exorcism of all forms of evil death. Our major institutions constitute a gigantic defence programme waged on behalf of "humanity" against all those people who can be associated with what is currently conceived of as death-dealing social injustice. Not only medical agencies, but welfare, international relief, and development programmes are enlisted in this struggle. Ideological bureaucracies of all colours join the crusade. Even war has been used to justify the defeat of those who are blamed for wanton tolerance of sickeness and death. Producing "natural death" for all men is at the point of becoming an ultimate justification for social control. Under the influence of medical rituals contemporary death is again the rationale for a witch-hunt.

CONCLUSION

Rising irreparable damage accompanies industrial expansion in all sectors. In medicine these damages appear as iatrogenesis. Iatrogenesis can be direct, when pain,

sickness, and death result from medical care; or it can be indirect, when health policies reinforce an industrial organisation which generates ill-health: it can be structural when medically sponsored behaviour and delusion restrict the vital autonomy of people by undermining their competence in growing up, caring, ageing: or when it nullifies the personal challenge arising from their pain, disability, and anguish.

Most of the remedies proposed to reduce iatrogenesis are engineering interventions. They are therapeutically designed in their approach to the individual, the group, the institution, or the environment. These so-called remedies generate second-order iatrogenic ills by creating a new prejudice against the autonomy of the citizen.

The most profound iatrogenic effects of the medical technostructure result from its non-technical social functions. The sickening technical and non-technical consequences of the institutionalisation of medicine coalesce to generate a new kind of suffering—anaesthetised and solitary survival in a world-wide hospital ward.

Medical Nemesis cannot be operationally verified. Much less can it be measured. The intensity with which it is experienced depends on the independence, vitality, and relatedness of each individual. As a theoretical concept it is one component in a broad theory to explain the anomalies plaguing health-care systems in our day. It is a district aspect of an even more general phenomenon which I have called industrial Nemesis, the backlash of institutionally structured industrial hubris. This hubris consists of a disregard for the boundaries within which the human phenomenon remains viable. Current research is overwhelmingly oriented towards unattainable "breakthroughs." What I have called counterfoil research is the disciplined analysis of the levels at which such reverberations must inevitably damage man.

The perception of enveloping Nemesis leads to a social choice. Either the natural boundaries of human endeavour are estimated, recognised, and translated into politically determined limits, or the alternative to extinction is compulsory survival in a planned and engineered Hell.

In several nations the public is ready for a review of its health-care system. The frustrations which have become manifest from private-enterprise systems and from socialised care have come to resemble each other frighteningly. The differences between the annoyances of the Russian, French, Americans, and English have become trivial. There is a serious danger that these evaluations will be performed within the coordinates set by post-cartesian illusions. In rich and poor countries the demand for reform of national health care is dominated by demands for equitable access to the wares of the guild, professional expansion and sub-professionalisation, and for more truth in the advertising of progress and lay-control of the temple of Tantalus. The public discussion of the health crisis could easily be used to channel even more power, prestige, and money to biomedical engineers and designers.

There is still time in the next few years to avoid a debate which would reinforce a frustrating system. The coming debate can be reoriented by making medical Nemesis the central issue. The explanation of Nemesis requires simultaneous assessment of both the technical and the non-technical side of medicine—and must focus on it as both industry and religion. The indictment of medicine as a form of institutional hubris exposes precisely those personal illusions which make the critic dependent on the health care.

The perception and comprehension of Nemesis has therefore the power of leading us to policies which could break the magic circle of complaints which now reinforce the dependence of the plaintiff on the health engineering and planning agencies whom he sues. Recognition of Nemesis can provide the catharsis to prepare for a non-violent revolution in our attitudes toward evil and pain. The alternative to a war against these ills is the search for the peace of the strong.

Health designates a process of adapta-tion. It is not the result of instinct, but of autonomous and live reaction to an experienced reality. It designates the ability to adapt to changing environments, to growing up and to ageing, to healing when damaged, to suffering and to the peaceful expectation of death. Health embraces the future as well, and therefore includes anguish and the inner resource to live with it.

Man's consciously lived fragility, individuality, and relatedness make the experience of pain, of sickness, and of death an integral part of his life. The ability to cope with this trio in autonomy is fundamental to his health. To the degree to which he becomes dependent on the management of his intimacy he renounces his autonomy and his health *must* decline. The true miracle of modern medicine is diabolical. It consists of making not only individuals but whole populations survive on inhumanly low levels of personal health. That health should decline with increasing health-service delivery is unforeseen only by the health manager, precisely because his strategies are the result of his blindness to the inalienability of health.

The level of public health corresponds to the degree to which the means and responsibility for coping with illness are distributed amongst the total population. This ability to cope can be enhanced but never replaced by medical intervention in the lives of people or the hygienic characteristics of the environment. That society which can reduce professional intervention to the minimum will provide the best conditions for health. The greater the potential for autonomous adaptation to self and to others and to the environment, the less management of adaptation will be needed or tolerated.

The recovery of a health attitude towards sickness is neither Luddite nor Romantic nor Utopian: it is a guiding ideal which will never be fully achieved, which can be achieved with modern devices as never before in history, and which must orient politics to avoid encroaching Nemesis.

5

Social stress and medical ideology

JON GARFIELD

There is a well-known laboratory experiment in which hungry animals are manipulated with food incentives into a relentless struggle to perform an impossible task. This untenable, "double-bind" situation reliably precipitates madness, ulcers, or sudden death in its victims. Were there a health policy for these animals, it should logically include strategies addressing the problem at its roots—the social context that engenders the prolonged stress and ensuing pathology. Inappropriate indeed would be approaches locating the problem solely within the afflicted organism, approaches that ignored the environment and employed only such means as antistress medication and behavior therapy to help the stressed creatures adjust to and cope with their pathogenic situation.

In subtler but highly significant ways, modern medicine falls prey to this kind of error. Focusing diagnosis and treatment almost exclusively on the afflicted individual, medicine systematically overlooks and thereby obscures social determinants of disease and death. This bias contributes to health policies that seriously underemphasize the etiologic factors arising in people's jobs, physical environment, families, and communities, that is, the socially induced stress, environmental toxins and carcinogens, and occupational hazards afflicting the modern world. For related reasons, the medical profession also tends to overlook the social and psychologic aspects of patient care.

Medicine, however, has not always operated under these restrictions. Relationships between social life and health were major concerns of nineteenth century medical practitioners. It has only been in the twentieth century that changes in medical concepts have tended to eliminate stress and other psychosocial factors from etiologic consideration.

After describing these assumptions and their impact on patient care, I will review evidence demonstrating that the stresses and strains of work and daily life are significant determinants of morbidity and mortality. I will specifically consider research on the relationships between occupational stress and coronary disease. I will also discuss the implications of such evidence for medical conception and health care strategy, arguing that it is necessary to abandon both the mechanistic and the individualistic biases of current medical ideology to accommodate what we now know about stress-related disease. Finally I will propose specific changes in working conditions, which, according to available evidence, are likely to reduce stress and therefore protect health.

SOCIAL AND FLEXNERIAN MEDICINE

The pathogenicity of stress and other social and occupational conditions was more central to medical concern in the 1800s than it has been in the present century. The classic instance emerged during the revolutionary period of 1848. The young German physician Rudolph Virchow, investigating the Silesian typhus epidemic of 1847, observed that the diseases were particularly prevalent among the impoverished.[1] He

33

went on to study the afflictions produced by the wretched social and working conditions imposed on the industrial wage laborer: "The proletariat in ever increasing degrees became the victim of diseases and epidemics, its children either died prematurely or developed into cripples."[2] Based on such observations, Virchow and other French and German physicians of the period concluded that the origins of certain diseases and epidemics were as much social and economic as they were biologic.

Termed "social medicine" by the French in 1848, this approach investigated the contributions of poverty, working conditions, nutrition, housing, and other social factors to disease and mortality. The champions of social medicine backed their convictions with political action and issued proposals for eliminating poverty and unemployment, reducing the working day, and promoting adequate housing, health standards in the work place, and reliable research on the social causes of disease. The defeat of the revolution of 1848 removed all hope of achieving social medicine's broad agenda, and a limited program of sanitary reform replaced this movement for health-promoting social change.[3]

Shifts in medical conception have made it difficult for twentieth century medical research to emphasize the social problems that vexed the physicians of the social medicine movement. Current medical theory and practice are based mainly on mechanistic and reductionist principles that do not accommodate social and psychologic factors in etiology. Pivotal in the development of modern medical belief were the doctrine of specific etiology, introduced in the late 1800s with the germ theory of disease, and the Flexner report of 1910, in which the human body was viewed as a "machine" and in which a stringently reductionist, single-causal notion of pathogenesis was promoted.

Although the germ theory and the Flexner report are considered milestones in the development of scientific medicine, the theory of specific etiology, even when it was first introduced, ran counter to available evidence.[1] Having previously documented relationships between social conditions and infectious disease, "Virchow . . . had good epidemiological reasons to remain unimpressed while presiding at the now famous meeting of the Berlin Physiological Society in 1882 where Koch first presented his report" on the single-factor etiology of tuberculosis.[1]

There were shrewd thinkers among the physicians who were not convinced that microorganisms alone could account for the causation of disease. They did not deny that microorganisms were present in diseased tissue. They emphasized rather that disease was prevalent chiefly among individuals exposed to, and suffering from the strains and stresses of life. In their opinion, microorganisms could invade and cause disease only after the tissues had been weakened by some form of physiological misery.[1]

Despite the evidence to the contrary, the specificity theory, later generalized to accommodate specific "causes" besides microorganisms, gained hegemony.

The mythology of a value-free science belied the political significance of the specificity doctrine. If germs were the *sole* cause of infectious disease, social factors could be dismissed from etiology. As the early proponent Emil Behring declared in 1893, germ theory held out the promise that "the study of infectious disease could now be pursued unswervingly without being sidetracked by social considerations and reflections on social policy."[3]

With its emphasis on specificity theory and biologic reductionism, the Flexner report legitimized a paradigm that coincided with the interest of its corporate sponsors (Rockefeller and Carnegie) in minimizing the significance of social and industrial determinants of disease.[4,5] Analyzing the Rockefeller Foundation's influence on the shift to Flexnerian medicine, Brown[5] states that with very few exceptions:

Rockefeller money did not support medical research that involved the relationship of social factors to health and disease. . . . Excluded were the contributions of socio-economic class, housing conditions, working conditions, social stress of unemployment and economic insecurity . . . to disease and health.

Flexnerian medicine, in short, "was ideologically compatible with industrial capitalism's desire to depoliticize medicine."[5] This ideologic function contributed to the report's attraction to class-conscious industrialists, and between 1910 and 1934 the nine largest foundations in the United States spent more than $154 million to reform medical education in the Flexnerian mold.[4]

Today, Western medicine remains chiefly Flexnerian and continues to obscure the social causes of disease by focusing diagnosis and treatment almost exclusively on the biologic subsystems of the individual. Pathogenic environments—hazardous and stressful working conditions, environmental carcinogens, etc.—are systematically underemphasized.[6]

FLEXNERIAN MEDICINE IN ACTION

Medical sociology has documented the indifference of doctors and hospitals to the psychosocial aspects of patient care. This indifference reflects and perpetuates medicine's neglect of those factors in etiologic considerations. In their classic study of a university hospital, Duff and Hollingshead[7] conclude:

Patients and their families had life problems which disabled in various ways but were accepted as a part of the life the patients led. *Although patients and physicians focused upon physical disease, personal and social attributes produced disability as great as that caused by physical disease.* Of the 155 patients discharged alive, 14 per cent were not disabled, 24 per cent were disabled from physical disease, 44 per cent were disabled from psychosocial disturbances, and 18 per cent were disabled from a combination of these causes. While patients sought relief from the physical and emotional pain resulting from these psychosocial disturbances, they did not expect physicians to diagnose and treat them as such.

In the face of a poor prognosis, the personal and social realities for the patient and his family

were usually discounted or ignored. All parties concerned concentrated on the treatment of the physical disease, but in these situations the impact of the illness on the patient and his family was profound and disconcerting. Patients, family members, nurses, and physicians failed to communicate; they guessed at what was being said. Isolation, suspicion, and distrust were common.

In spite of increased emphasis on behavioral and social scientific "enrichment" of medical education, medical students are socialized to think in biologic reductionist terms and become impatient with psychologic and social concerns.[7-10] The Flexnerian concept reduces health and illness to functions and malfunctions among "parts" of a mechanistically conceived body. Medical students learn to objectify patients and to call the patient a "kidney," a "case," or "clinical material."[8]

Parsons,[11] apologetically, and Freidson,[12] critically, characterize the doctor-patient relationship as impersonal, distanced, and inequitable. (Freidson discusses "professional dominance," and Parsons characterizes the sick role incumbent as helpless.) Freidson also maintains that doctors withhold information from patients, inducing "blind faith," to bolster their dominant positions and to prevent "management problems." "Insistence on faith constitutes insistence that the client give up his role as an independent adult and, by so neutralizing him, protects the esoteric foundations of the profession's institutionalized authority."[12]

Isolated from the personal and social circumstances of their patients and socialized into a predominantly mechanistic and wholly individualistic approach to medicine, physicians are likely to turn a deaf ear to evidence of psychosocial etiologic factors. According to Dreitzel[10]:

The majority of doctors . . . fail to see the patient as a person. . . . In fact, when asked if they wanted to know more about their patients as individuals, 98 per cent of the doctors said no. Doubtless this instrumentalist attitude is reinforced by the patients themselves, who often display a tendency to compensate their own feelings of powerlessness toward their social and physical environment by an almost magical belief in the curative powers of what we have termed scientist medicine. As a result the patient becomes submissive to the point of resignation, allowing the doctor to define his disease and the appropriate treatment exclusive of all social, psychological, and economic considerations. *The doctor and his patient are all too often unconscious allies in the conviction that the causes of disease are accidents of nature rather than a reflection of social institutions*—an alliance which finds its expression in the petrified authority structure of the doctor-patient relationship, particularly in the hospital (italics added).

Similarly Waitzkin and Waterman[13] contend:

> It might be argued, as Parsons implies, that the distancing mechanisms invoked by these normative patterns are necessary in a professional relationship, where the intimacy involved in history taking and the physical examination might create conflicts. On the other hand, these same normative patterns allow physicians to act more effectively as agents of social control, relatively detached from their patients' objective living conditions and emotional concerns. . . . The normative patterns described by Parsons may inhibit doctors from allying with their patients in fighting the sociopolitical conditions which often are the source of suffering and the impetus to seek certification of illness.

MEDICAL ECOLOGY AND SELF-CARE

The mechanistic and individualistic biases of Flexnerian medicine obscure social contributions to morbidity and mortality. Although currently fashionable ecologic and "holistic" approaches challenge medicine's mechanistic character, they tend to adopt its individualistic bias. The renewed emphasis on multifactorial explanations focuses increased attention on psychosocial factors in health—psychosocial factors that are generally divorced from any larger social context. Consequently the roles of personality, behavior, and life-style in disease genesis receive much attention, whereas the broader social, political, and economic conditions that promote or per-

petuate known etiologic factors are rarely considered. A truly holistic approach would look beyond the individual to address the pathogenic aspects of the social and physical environment.

Overlooking the importance of social determinants of disease, individualistic self-care strategies hold the individual solely or primarily responsible for ill health. While it is good to educate people to the benefits of seat belts and the harm in smoking, the individual cannot eliminate environmental toxins and carcinogens or create a rational and safe transportation system. Exaggerations of the individual's control over the conditions determining his or her health become a smoke screen through which fundamental social problems appear as simple matters of personal choice and life-style. McKinlay[14] discusses the tendency to blame the victim:

> To use the upstream-downstream analogy, one could argue that people are blamed (and, in a sense, even punished) for not being able to swim after they, perhaps against their volition, have been pushed into the river by the manufacturers of illness.

In recognizing the connection between stress and pathology, self-care strategies delegate to the individual the responsibility for coping with stressful jobs and social conditions. Relaxation techniques, meditation, and biofeedback are offered to help people relax in and adjust to stressful environments that are accepted as givens. Most people who try these techniques discontinue them, however, largely because of the contradiction in trying to maintain a relaxed state in a high pressure world.[15] Strategies for changing the working and living conditions that demonstrably contribute to stress pathology are rarely proposed.

A good deal of epidemiologic study, however, illustrates that social change could be an important health strategy. Research identifying stressful working conditions that contribute to coronary heart disease is an important example.

STRESS, ALIENATED LABOR, AND CORONARY DISEASE

Central to the following analysis is the contention that certain formulations of the clinical concept of "stress" have a sociologic counterpart in the concept of "alienation." This correspondence provides a conceptual basis for relating social and psychophysiologic processes. Stress, operationalized in a variety of conceptually disparate ways, has been frequently identified as a precursor of coronary disease.[16] Below I will review evidence that some of the psychosocial precursors of coronary disease originate in alienating working conditions. I argue that objectively alienating work situations, that is, work that systematically undermines the self-defined needs of workers in a manner not subject to their control, tends to result in states of chronic stress that are known precursors of coronary disease.

The concepts of stress and alienation require clarification. References to "stress" in the medical literature are vague and ambiguous. Some writers use the term to refer to an organismic state; others use it to describe an environmental factor. To prevent this ambiguity and clarify the dialectic interrelatedness of contextual and organismic conditions, I will reserve the word "stress" for organismic states while using "alienating" and "stressful" to describe contexts capable of inducing chronic stress.

Individuals experience stress when the consequences of their actions are irrelevant or contrary to their needs, intentions, or expectations. This important aspect of stress has been identified in a variety of formulations. Reviewing epidemiologic and experimental evidence that stress functions as a nonspecific pathogenic factor, Cassel[17] concludes "that at least one of the properties of stressful social situations might be that in which the actor is not receiving adequate evidence (feedback) that his actions are leading to anticipated consequences." Similarly, but in a more psychologic vein, Katz[18] contends that it is not any reaction to a stressful situation but a reaction, which

he terms "abnormal," that is likely to impair health:

In an organism stimulated by stress and mobilizing resistant forces, the organism can overcome stress if its efforts are in the direction of reducing or accomodating the stress, internal or external. On the other hand, if the organism's actions increase or perpetuate stress, the reactions can be considered "abnormal."

Although a life without stress is neither possible nor desirable, prolonged and excessive stress is associated with chronic physiologic arousal, which apparently predisposes people to coronary disease and other stress pathologies.[15]

To understand the full effects of stress, it is necessary to relate psychophysiologic conditions to social contexts. Formulations that attribute stress primarily to the individual's response patterns evoke the question of how such behavior occurs. Why would a person act in such a manner as to increase or perpetuate the condition causing his or her distress? Social circumstances can contribute, and the concept of alienation depicts social conditions capable of inducing behaviors associated with excessive and chronic stress.

"Alienation" characterizes objective situations that divorce the consequences of human activity from the needs and control of the actors. Since Marx, the concept has found its primary application in the analysis of externally controlled working conditions that undermine workers' abilities to actualize their felt needs and intentions. Alienated labor is coerced labor, planned and managed from without. Stripped of creativity and craft, it bears no intrinsic relationship to the workers' own conception of what is to be produced or how to produce it. Without control over their working conditions, workers may be required to perform nothing but boring and meaningless tasks and pressured to labor at arbitrarily defined rates, intensities, and durations. In short, alienated labor is labor that recreates the conditions of the worker's own distress.

"Alienation" bears a striking resemblance to the preceding formulations of "stress." Both concepts depict chronic conditions in which actors are unable to determine their situations or to act in accordance with their basic needs and interests.

The assembly line is a supreme example of alienated labor, for it is the virtual subjugation of human movement to the pace and rhythm of a centrally controlled apparatus. The stress and alienation of conveyer-line work are apparent: The worker becomes an extension of the machinery, losing the ability to regulate his or her own activity in the constant struggle to keep the pace the apparatus demands. The technology controls the worker, rather than the worker controlling the productive process. Kritsikis and colleagues[19] studied 150 men with angina pectoris in a population of more than 4000 industrial workers in Berlin and found that conveyer-line work and psychic overstrain connected with pressured work were associated with the disease.

Similarly, piecework—a system applying constant monetary pressure to speed up workers' activities—and other time-pressuring work situations are known to contribute to various physiologic stress indices and coronary risk factors.[20] In one study, Levi[21] compared the physiologic effects of piecework and salaried work on young female invoice clerks working in their customary work place. On the days they were paid by the piece—days described by the women as exhausting and stressful—their mean epinephrine level increased 40 percent, whereas their norepinephrine level rose 27 percent. Mjasnikov[22] has reported that high rates of essential hypertension were suffered by telephone operators working under constant pressure to complete a large number of transactions per unit of time. Friedman and co-workers[23] studied the physiologic effects of occupational stress on 40 accountants for a 5-month period and found that deadlines in the tax calendar were associated with significant increases in serum cholesterol and blood coagulation time. After reviewing the evidence, Eyer[15,24] concluded that time-pressured, externally controlled work is causally related to hypertension, coronary disease, and other stress-related diseases.

Piecework, the assembly line, and related technologies embody a specific class interest. One way employers increase their profits is to maximize the effort and the productivity of the work force. Alienation is inherent in the conditions that these technologies were designed to promote: The external control of the worker's activity to serve the employer's economic interest, irrespective of the worker's felt needs and desires. Occupational pressure and stress therefore are likely results of alienated labor.

As the popular notion suggests, overwork and its subjective correlates are clearly related to coronary disease. Russek and Zohman[25] report that 91 of 100 coronary patients studied had experienced prolonged emotional stress associated with occupational demands prior to the onset of disease, whereas only 20 percent of the control group had had comparable experiences. Of the coronary group, 25 percent had held two jobs and 46 percent had worked 60 or more hours weekly. Occupational stress was reported to be a more important risk factor than diet, smoking, lack of exercise, or family medical history. Sales[26] provides a study associating work overload and cardiovascular disease, and Biorck and others[27] and Buell and Breslow[28] have linked overtime work with coronary disease. Reporting effects of qualitative and quantitative work overload, French and Caplan[29] indicate:

Our findings from several studies show that the various forms of workload produce at least nine different kinds of psychological and physiological strain in the individual. Four of these (job dissatisfaction, elevated cholesterol, elevated heart rate, and smoking) are risk factors in heart disease. It is reasonable to predict that reducing work overload will reduce heart disease.

The worker who is denied control over the labor process can be and often is required to perform at stressful and excessive levels. These pressures result from bureaucratic control over the work process (for example, assembly line speedups, compulsory overtime, scientific management) and from psychologic manipulation of employees via applications of motivational research. In addition, economic pressures frequently force low-income workers to hold two jobs or constantly work overtime.

Psychologic tendencies to overwork, such as the subjective aspects of Type A (coronary-prone) behavior, are also encouraged by the predominant social organization of work and contingent cultural processes. That is, compulsive striving and chronic overwork are "logical" adaptations to bureaucratic organizations that stratify workers into innumerable levels and rankings. Amidst such hierarchy, (often technically unnecessary) divisions of labor function to promote the idea that work satisfaction and the "good life" are to be attained by working hard enough, long enough, and rapidly enough to achieve the next rung on the ladder. The Type A orientation is readily internalized in a culture steeped in the mythology of social mobility. Although actual mobility is rare, schools and the media foster idealizations of individuals competing to "sell themselves" on the job market, striving to outdo others for jobs, degrees, and promotions.

SUBJECTIVE ASPECTS OF ALIENATION

In common parlance "alienation" refers to subjective feelings of frustration, meaninglessness, isolation, and powerlessness. As used in social theory and here, however, the concept applies to an objective social situation that exists independent of its recognition by those in that situation. The assembly line alienates by rendering the worker powerless over the productive process whether or not the worker subjectively feels alienated. Feelings of frustration, dissatisfaction, and powerlessness are, of course, likely to arise in alienating contexts. These are the psychologic elements of alienation.

Several studies have identified psychologic precursors and correlates of coronary disease that coincide with the subjective aspects of alienation. According to Dreyfuss and co-workers,[30] men with coronary disease are likely to experience little control over their lives, to view the relationship between their efforts and achievements as uncertain, and to report conflicts in their life contexts. Wolf[31] and Cathey and others[32] associate the "Sisyphus complex," characterized by relentless, ungratifying striving and prolonged, unresolved frustrations, with myocardial infarction and sudden death. This pattern includes dissatisfaction in work as well as in leisure activity.

Research on the well-known coronary-prone or Type A behavior pattern[33] shows that coronary-prone individuals "are engaged in a relatively chronic struggle to obtain an unlimited number of poorly defined things from their environment in the shortest period of time and, if necessary, against the opposing efforts of other things or persons in the same environment." Highly committed to their "treadmill existence," Type A individuals stringently repress their often considerable frustration, hostility, and insecurity.

Thus the subjective elements of alienation—experiences of powerlessness, estrangement, and frustration—appear to be psychologic precursors of coronary disease. Job dissatisfaction, an obvious sign of worker alienation, is a case in point. Several studies associate job dissatisfaction with coronary disease.[34-36] Moreover, a 15-year prospective study of longevity reports[37]:

When the six strongest independent variables (work satisfaction, happiness rating, physical functioning, tobacco use, performance IQ, and leisure activity) are combined in a step-wise multiple regression, *work satisfaction is the best over-all predictor of the LQ* ["Longevity Quotient"] and explains about half of the final cumulative variance explained. This work satisfaction score represents a person's reaction to his general usefulness and ability to perform a meaningful social role (italics added).

Job dissatisfaction is not merely the result of individual preferences. It arises predictably from repetitive, externally controlled, uncreative working conditions. In one study, only 24 percent of a cross-section of blue-collar workers and 43 percent of a cross-section of white-collar workers reported that they would voluntarily choose the same kind of work if given another chance. On the other hand, urban university professors, mathematicians, physicists, and certain other "professionals"—people who have more autonomy in their work, higher prestige and pay, and more outlets for their skill and creativity—reported overwhelmingly (93 percent, 91 percent, 89 percent, respectively) that they would choose similar work again.[38] In short, job dissatisfaction has an objective basis; it is largely a function of social class and the degree of alienation inherent in the work situations available to people of different social strata. The well-known inverse relationship between social class and mental and physical disease[39-42] may in part reflect the social distribution of job options.

SOCIAL CHANGE AS PREVENTIVE MEDICINE

Returning to McKinlay's[14] analogy of a river as a pathogenic environment, we can see three health strategies: (1) providing technologic assistance such as lifeboats, (2) developing health education emphasizing swimming lessons, and (3) promoting efforts to attack the problem at its roots—the conditions that force people into the river. Even a cursory reading of the literature on stress-related pathology reveals that discussions of the first two types of approaches—technologic adaptation (via antistress drugs) and education or therapy to change individual behavior—virtually exhausts the current universe of discourse. With a few notable exceptions (for example, Eyer's work[15,24]), the literature rarely gives serious consideration to the strategy of changing stressful working and living conditions.

A major reason for this neglect of "social medicine" in the Virchowian sense is Flexnerian ideology and the structures of medical care that reinforce it. Medicine in the Flexnerian mold is predominantly organized around hospital-based, curative, individual therapy. Environmental, occupational, community, and preventive medicines are relatively marginal and underdeveloped. Within this structure the bulk of medicine's human and material resources are divorced from possible applications of social epidemiologic research, applications that would need to address social problems as *social,* not only as individual and biologic.

Ideologies often reflect the material interests of the groups and classes that promote them, and Flexnerian medicine, it must be recalled, was promoted at great expense by class-conscious elements of the corporate sector. As Navarro[6] notes, "an ideology that saw the 'fault' of disease as lying with the individual and that emphasized the individual therapeutic response clearly absolved the economic and political environment from responsibility for disease."

The neglect of social medicine then has a deeper explanation: When conditions sustaining healthy corporate profits and capital accumulation come into conflict with public health needs, the welfare of capital frequently gains priority. The limitations on health policy imposed in the service of the corporate sector include strong constraints on government intervention in health.[6,43] A clear illustration is industry's history of successfully undermining attempts to legislate effective regulation of industrially produced carcinogens, pollutants, and other hazards. For example, in the first 4 years of enforcement of the Occupational Safety and Health Act, the average fine was a whopping 25 dollars per violation.[44]

Contradictions between human health and corporate interest are evident in the area of stress-related disease and require solutions not contained in the Flexnerian paradigm. Compulsory overtime, for example, is staunchly defended as a "managerial prerogative" because corporations find it cheaper than hiring and training additional workers. Compulsory overtime promotes two stressful and pathogenic situations: overwork and unemployment. Overwork, as noted previously, has frequently been identified as a precursor of coronary disease.[25-29] Unemployment produces increases in blood pressure[45] and other coronary risk factors.[46] The abolition of compulsory overtime—a policy that increases the stress and powerlessness of those who must overwork and of those who remain unemployed—should be an obvious measure if the health and welfare of the many are not to be subordinated to the material interests of the powerful few.

In addition to compulsory overtime, other stressful work conditions were also developed to maximize the efficiency and productivity of the labor force. Piecework, speedups, assembly lines, and scientific management all manipulate the rate and manner in which workers produce, providing higher corporate profits but greater stress and alienation for the work force. As evidence of the pathogenicity of externally controlled, time-pressured work increases,[15,24] it becomes appropriate to consider speedups, piecework, and other time-pressuring policies as impediments to occupational health and safety.

In the long run, a potent remedy for worker alienation and other pathogenic work conditions would be the replacement of authoritarian hierarchies with participatory worker democracy. As Edwards and colleagues[47] note:

Worker control of even large-scale and complex modern enterprises can generate opportunities for pride and fulfillment arising out of participation in a common endeavor whose social purpose is understood and valued by the whole community. Thus, we believe that truly democratic control of the workplace can go a long way to reduce alienation and all of its harmful consequences.

People with democratic control over their work situations would work more cooperatively and less competitively than those subject to hierarchy. They would not knowingly impose on themselves hazardous or inordinately stressful conditions. Worker control could therefore be the most effec-

tive means of reducing occupational health problems arising from chronic stress, noise, exposure to toxins, and physical hazards.

Moreover, the evidence suggests that when work is not alienated, efficiency does not have to be coerced. The appendix to *Work in America,*[48] for example, summarizes 34 cases in which higher productivity and worker satisfaction resulted from increased worker participation. After reviewing the literature, Blumberg[49] reported that this relationship has been demonstrated with a "consistency . . . rare in social research."

It is not really difficult to explain why participation "works"; it is almost a matter of common sense that men will take greater pride and pleasure in their work if they are allowed to participate in shaping the policies and decisions which affect their work. . . . The participating worker is an involved worker, for his job becomes an extension of himself and by his decisions he is creating his work, modifying and regulating it. As he is more involved in his work, he becomes more committed to it, and, being more committed, he naturally derives more satisfaction from it.[49]

Why then do employers resist even rudimentary forms of worker control or at most experiment with the semblance, but not the substance, of democratization? They resist because democratization threatens to undermine mechanisms of social control that are required to sustain their class privileges. Bureaucratic hierarchies of status and authority reflect and reproduce the larger society's class structure; upper strata appropriate disproportionate shares of wealth and influence, whereas the majority are disciplined, "kept in their places," through authoritarian social relations. Gintis and Bowles[50] report:

Instances of even moderate worker control are instituted only in marginal areas and in isolated firms fighting for survival. When the crisis is over, there is usually a return to "normal operating procedure." The threat of workers escalating their demand for control is simply too great, and the usurpation of the prerogative of hierarchic authority is quickly slashed. Efficiency in the broader sense is subordinated to the needs of bureaucratic control.

True worker democracy therefore remains essentially an ideal to be realized in the struggle for a more equal society. Nonetheless, its embryonic forms have demonstrated that alienation is not an inevitable result of industrialization but can be largely overcome when authoritarian hierarchies give way to democratic enterprises.

If these proposals seem extreme or farfetched approaches to health problems, consider that the benefits of minimizing alienating work conditions go far beyond likely reductions in those stress-related pathologies considered.

Either the absence of work or meaningless work is creating an increasingly intolerable situation. The human costs of this state of affairs are manifested in worker alienation, alcoholism, drug addiction, and other symptoms of poor mental health.[48]

Moreover overcoming (as opposed to merely coping with) alienation and chronic stress requires no external justification and should, as Turshen[51] suggests, be considered basic to any definition of "positive health."

Physicians, health personnel, and health educators can address chronic stress and other social determinants of disease by researching and publicizing these problems and by laying to rest the individualistic and mechanistic assumptions of the Flexnerian paradigm. Of course, this does not imply that doctors should become social engineers. The notion that, because of their etiologic import, social and psychologic problems can and should fall within the province of medical decision bears the unsettling implication that medicine would increasingly shape people's lives. Instead, as Brown and Margo[52] suggest, those in health fields can work with community groups, trade unions, and others whose situations (work speedups, noise, pollution, etc.) include hazardous conditions to be challenged:

It is not social methods that must be integrated into medical work, for that leads inevitably to the ameliorative case work approach. Rather, *medicine and the other health professions must integrate their methods into the broader struggles to alter the social and physical environment.*[52]

Chronic stress and alienation warrant such efforts. Each year one in ten adults in the United States uses Valium or Librium —a technologic adaptation to stressful circumstances.[53] It is certainly time to acknowledge that fighting the conditions that force people into the "river" is at least as important as lifeboats and swimming lessons.

ACKNOWLEDGEMENTS

I am grateful to the following people for their suggestions, comments, and technical assistance: Rich Appelbaum, Stanley Aronowitz, Rick Brown, Ann Esposito, Dick Flacks, Wendy Garfield, Carol Huffine, Kathy Johnson, Richard Lichtman, Jim Ryder, Mona Sarfaty, Ruth Veres, and Norma Wikler.

REFERENCES

1. Dubos, R. J.: The gold headed cane in the laboratory. In Annual lectures, National Institutes of Health, Washington D. C., 1953, U.S. Government Printing Office, pp. 89-102.
2. Virchow, R. Quoted in Rosen, G.: The evolution of social medicine. In Freeman, H. E., Levine, S., and Reeder, L. G., eds.: Handbook of medical sociology, Englewood Cliffs, N. J., 1972, Prentice-Hall, Inc.
3. Rosen, G.: The evolution of social medicine. In Freeman, H. E., Levine, S., and Reeders, L. G., eds.: Handbook of medical sociology, Englewood Cliffs, N. J., 1972, Prentice-Hall, Inc.
4. Berliner, H. S.: A larger perspective on the Flexner report, Int. J. Health Serv. **5(4):**573-592, 1975.
5. Brown, E. R.: Rockefeller medicine men: medicine and capitalism in America, Berkeley, 1979, University of California Press.
6. Navarro, V.: Social class, political power, and the state: their implications in medicine. In Medicine under capitalism, New York, 1976, Prodist.
7. Duff, R., and Hollingshead, A. B.: Sickness and society, New York, 1968, Harper & Row, Publishers.
8. Becker, H. S., Greer, B., Hughes, E. C., and Strauss, A. L.: Boys in white: student culture in medical school, Chicago, 1961, University of Chicago Press.
9. Kleinbach, G.: Social structure and education of health personnel, Int. J. Health Serv. **4:**297-317, 1974.
10. Dreitzel, H. P.: Introduction: the social organiza-

tion of health. In Dreitzel, H. P., ed.: The social organization of health, New York, 1971, Macmillan, Inc.

11. Parsons, T.: Social structure and dynamic process: the case of modern medical practice. In The social system, New York, 1951, The Free Press.

12. Freidson, E.: Professional dominance: the social organization of medical care, New York, 1970, Atherton Press.

13. Waitzkin, H., and Waterman, B.: Social theory and medicine, Int. J. Health Serv. 6:9-23, 1976.

14. McKinlay, J. B.: A case for refocussing upstream: the political economy of illness. Unpublished paper, Boston University, 1974. Quoted in Renaud, M.: On the structural constraints to state intervention in health, Int. J. Health Serv. 5:559-571, 1975.

15. Eyer, J., and Sterling, P.: Stress-related mortality and social organization, Review of Radical Political Economy 9(1):1-44, 1977.

16. Jenkins. C. D.: Psychological and social precursors of coronary disease, New Engl. J. Med. 284:244-255; 284:307-317, 1971.

17. Cassel, J.: Psychosocial processes and "stress": theoretical formulations, Int. J. Health Serv. 4: 471-482, 1974.

18. Katz, A. H.: The social causes of disease. In Dreitzel, H. P., ed.: The social organization of health, New York, 1971, MacMillan, Inc.

19. Kritsikis, S., Heinemann, A., and Eitner, S.: Die angina pectoris im aspekt ihrer korrelation mit biologischer disposition, psychologischen und soziologischen einflussfaktoren, Deutsch. Gesundh. 23:1878-1885, 1968. Cited in Kiritz, S., and Moos, R. H.: Physiological effects of social environments, Psychosom. Med. 36:96-114, 1974.

20. Levi, L., ed.: Stress and distress in response to psychosocial stimuli. New York, 1972, Pergamon Press, Inc.

21. Levi, L.: The stress of everyday work as reflected in productiveness, subjective feelings and urinary output of adrenaline and noradrenaline under salaried and piece-work conditions, J. Psychosom. Res. 8:199-202, 1964.

22. Mjasnikov, A.: Discussion in Proceedings of Joint WHO-Czechoslovakian Cardiovascular Society Symposium on Pathogens in Essential Hypertension, Prague, 1961. Cited in Kiritz, S., and Moos, R. H.: Physiological effects of social environments, Psychosom. Med. 36:96-114, 1974.

23. Friedman, M., Rosenman, R. H., and Carroll, V.: Changes in serum cholesterol and blood clotting time in men subjected to cyclic variation of occupational stress, Circulation 17:852-861, 1958.

24. Eyer, J.: Hypertension as a disease of modern society, Int. J. Health Serv. 5:539-558, 1975.

25. Russek, H. I., and Zohman, B. L.: Relative significance of heredity, diet, and occupational stress in coronary heart disease in young adults, American Journal of the Sciences 235:266-275, 1958.

26. Sales, S.: Organization role as a risk factor in coronary disease, Admin. Sci. Quart. 14:325-336, 1969.

27. Biorck, G., Blomqvist, G., and Sievers, J.: Studies in myocardial infarction in Malmo 1935-54: II. Infarction rate by occupational group, Acta Med. Scand. 161:21-32, 1958.

28. Buell, P., and Breslow, L.: Mortality from coronary heart disease in California men who work long hours, J. Chronic Dis. 11:615-626, 1958.

29. French, J., and Caplan, R.: Organizational stress and individual strain. In Marrow, A., ed.: The failure of success, New York, 1972, AMACOM.

30. Dreyfuss, F., Shanon, J., and Sharon, M.: Some personality characteristics of middle-aged men with coronary artery disease, Psychother. Psychosom. 14:1-16, 1966.

31. Wolf, S.: Psychosocial forces in myocardial infarction and sudden death, Circulation 40(suppl. 4):74-83, 1969.

32. Cathey, C., Jones, H. B., Naughton, J., Hammersten, H. H., and Wolf, S.: The relation of life stress to the concentration of serum lipids in patients with coronary artery disease, Am. J. Med. Sci. 244:421, 1962.

33. Friedman, M.: Pathogenesis of coronary artery disease, New York, 1960, McGraw-Hill Book Co.

34. Lilijefors, I., and Rahe, R. H.: An identical twin study of psychosocial factors in coronary heart disease in Sweden, Psychsom Med. 32:525-543, 1970.

35. Sales, S. M., and House, J.: Job dissatisfaction as a possible risk factor in coronary heart disease, J. Chronic Dis. 23:861-873, 1971.

36. Theorell, R., and Rahe, R. H.: Behavior and life satisfaction characteristics of Swedish subjects with myocardial infarction, J. Chronic Dis. 25: 139, 1972.

37. Palmore, E.: Predicting longevity: a follow-up controlling for age, Gerontologist 9:247-250, 1969.

38. Kahn, R.: The work module, 1972. Cited in Work in America, Report of a Special Task Force to the Secretary of Health, Education and Welfare, Cambridge, Mass., 1973, The M.I.T. Press.

39. Antonovsky, A.: Social class, life expectancy and overall mortality, Milbank Mem. Fund Q. 45:63, 1967.

40. Antonovsky, A.: Social class and illness: a reconsideration, Sociological Inquiry 37:311-322, 1967.

41. Hollingshead, A. B., and Redlich, F. C.: Social class and mental illness: a community study, New York, 1958, John Wiley & Sons, Inc.

42. Kosa, J., Antonovsky, A., and Zola, I. K., eds.: Poverty and health: a sociological analysis, Cambridge, Mass., 1969, Harvard University Press.

43. Renaud, M.: On the structural constraints to state intervention in health, Int. J. Health Serv. 5:559-571, 1975.

44. Berman, D. M.: Why work kills. A brief history of occupational safety and health in the United States, Int. J. Health Serv. 7:63-87, 1977.

45. Kasl, S. V., and Cobb, S.: Blood pressure changes in men undergoing job loss: a preliminary report, Psychosom. Med. **32:**19-38, 1970.

46. Kasl, S. V., Cobb, S., and Brooks, G.: Changes in serum uric acid and cholesterol levels in men undergoing job loss, J.A.M.A. **206:**1500-1507, 1968.

47. Edwards, R. C., Reich, M., and Weisskopf, T. E.: Alienation. In Edwards, R. C., Reich, M., and Weisskopf, T. E., eds.: The capitalist system, Englewood Cliffs, N. J., Prentice-Hall, Inc.

48. Work in America, Report of a special task force to the Secretary of Health, Education and Welfare, Cambridge, Mass., 1973, the M.I.T. Press.

49. Blumberg, P.: Industrial Democracy: The sociology of participation, New York, 1968, Schocken Books, Inc.

50. Gintis, H., and Bowles, S.: Capitalism and alienation. In Edwards, R. C., Reich, M., and Weisskopf, T. E., eds.: The capitalist system, Englewood Cliffs, N. J., 1972, Prentice-Hall, Inc.

51. Turshen, M.: The political ecology of disease, Review of Radical Political Economics **9**(1):45-60, 1977.

52. Brown, E. R., and Margo, G. E.: Health education: can the reformers be reformed? Int. J. Health Serv. **8:**3-26, 1978.

53. Waldron, I.: Increased prescribing of Valium, Librium, and other drugs—an example of the influence of economic and social factors on the practice of medicine, Int. J. Health Serv. **7:**37-62, 1977.

6

Psychosocial processes and "stress": theoretical formulation

JOHN CASSEL

Despite widespread belief that psychosocial processes may be important in disease etiology, attempts to document the role of such factors in epidemiologic studies have led to conflicting and often confusing results. It is the thesis of this paper that this is largely a result of inadequacies in our theoretical framework. The point of view is presented that this stems from an uncritical subscription to and often erroneous interpretation of "stress" theory, a failure to recognize that psychosocial processes are unlikely to be directly pathogenic (in the way that, for example, a microorganism is) and unlikely to be unidimensional. An alternative point of view with data from animal and human studies is presented, and the implications for research strategy and the delivery of health care are discussed.

In the pursuit of one of its central objectives, epidemiologic enquiry has consistently sought to identify those factors in man's environment that influence his health. For most of its recorded history the focus has been on physicochemical factors, supplemented, since the discovery of microorganisms, by microbiologic agents thought to be directly pathogenic to the human organism. The increasing recognition of the inability of these factors to explain the occurrence of many diseases of modern societies, or at best to afford a very partial explanation, has led to a search for new categories of environmental factors potentially capable of producing disease. Guided by the elaboration of the stress concept of disease, as originally formulated by the work of Cannon (1), Selye (2), and Wolff

(3), recent investigators have postulated that one of the hitherto overlooked features of the environment of potential importance in disease etiology is the presence of other members of the same species. In other words, the concept of the environment for epidemiologic purposes has been expanded from the physical and microbiologic to include the social.

Despite increased efforts, however, attempts to document the role of social factors in the genesis of disease have led to conflicting, contradictory, and often confusing results. There is today no unanimity of opinion that social factors are important in disease etiology, or, if they are, which social processes are deleterious, how many such processes there are, and what the intervening links between such processes and disturbed physiologic states may be. In part this unsatisfactory state of affairs is a function of the methodologic difficulties in-

Reprinted from International Journal of Health Services **4**:471-482, 1974.

45

herent in such studies, particularly the difficulties of measuring in any precise form such relatively intangible processes. To a larger extent, and underlying these methodolgic difficulties are, I believe, inadequacies in our theoretical or conceptual framework. The purpose of this paper is to make these inadequacies as explicit as possible, present an alternative point of view and some of the evidence supporting this view, and discuss the research and intervention strategies that such a view would dictate.

As indicated above, much of the research into the role of social factors in disease etiology has been based upon implicit or explicit notions derived from stress theory. While there can be no doubt that the concept of stress has made a significant contribution to our ideas about the nature of disease and its causes, the uncritical subscription to these ideas and the often erroneous interpretation of the theory as propounded by its originators have frequently led to inappropriate research strategy and contradictory findings.

First it is important to recognize the semantic difficulties surrounding the use of the word "stress." In the hands of Selye and Wolff, the originators of this term as applied in a scientific sense to medicine, stress was envisaged as a bodily state, not a component of the environment. Thus Wolff (4) states,

I have used the word stress in biology to indicate that state within a living creature which results from the interaction of the organism with noxious stimuli or circumstances, i.e. it is a dynamic state within the organism; it is not a stimulus assault, load symbol, burden, or any aspect of environment, internal, external, social or otherwise.

While both Selye and Wolff demonstrated that this stress state (evidenced by neuroendocrinal changes) can be produced by a variety of noxious stimuli, physical as well as psychologic, neither investigator attempted to define the characteristics or the properties of these nonphysical (psychologic and/or social) noxious stimuli. Despite such formulations, subsequent investigators have tended to apply the term "stress" to these postulated noxious social or psychologic stimuli, often quoting Selye or Wolff for their justification. The use of the word "stressor" to indicate the environmental noxious stimulus, and "stress state" or more frequently "stress disease" to indicate the postulated consequences of such exposure, clarifies the semantic difficulty but highlights the more important conceptual issue. Stated in its most general terms, the formulation subscribed to (often implicitly) by most epidemiologists and social scientists working in this field is that the relationship between a stressor and disease outcome will be similar to the relationship between a microorganism and the disease outcome. In other words, the psychosocial process under investigation is envisaged as a stressor capable of having a direct pathogenic effect analogous to that of a physicochemical or microbiologic environmental disease agent. The corollaries of such a formulation are that there will be etiologic specificity (each stressor leading to a specific stress disease), and there will be a dose-response relationship (the greater the stressor, the more likelihood of disease). There is serious doubt as to the utility or appropriateness of both of these notions.

The ideas that disease is produced only by exposure to the direct pathogenic action of disease agents and that if psychosocial processes can produce disease, they do so by virtue of some direct pathogenic action, ignore much of our recent understanding of the disease process and the data available in this field. Dubos, for example, has emphasized the growing recognition that disease, even infectious disease, does not occur solely, or even most commonly, from exposure to a new pathogenic disease agent. As he states (5):

The sciences concerned with microbial diseases have developed almost exclusively from the study of acute or semi-acute infections caused by virulent micro-organisms acquired through exposure to an exogenous source of infection. In contrast, the microbial diseases most common in our communities today arise from the activities of micro-organisms that are ubiquitous in the environment, persist in the body without causing obvious harm under ordinary circumstances, and exert pathological effects only when the infected person is under conditions of physiological stress. In such a type of microbial disease the event of infection is of less importance than the hidden manifestation of the smoldering infectious process and than the physiological disturbances that convert latent infection into overt systems and pathology.

According to Dubos, then, in a large number of cases clinical manifestations of disease can occur through factors which disturb the balance between the ubiquitous disease agents and the host that is harboring or exposed to them. Ten to fifteen years before Dubos, Wolff was arguing that the action of physicochemical disease agents was different from psychosocial factors in that the former had a direct pathogenic effect by damaging and distorting structure and function, while the latter acted indirectly (or, as he termed it, conditionally) by virtue of their capacity to act as signals or symbols (4). Thus, disease can occur by virtue of a disturbance in the balance between the organism and various disease agents, as maintained by Dubos, and if this balance is mediated largely by the neuroendocrine system, as has been maintained by Cannon (1) and Schoenheimer (6) and widely accepted since, then the mechanism through which the signals and symbols produced by the conditional noxious stimuli work presumably will be by altering neuroendocrine secretions and levels in the body and thus changing the balance. As will be referred to later, there is evidence from both animal and human experiments indicating that variations in the social milieu are indeed associated with profound endocrine changes in the exposed subjects.

Viewed in this light, it is most unlikely that any given psychosocial process or stressor will be etiologically specific for any given disease, at least as currently classified. In other words, it no longer becomes useful to consider a subset of existing clin-

ical entities as "stress" diseases as all diseases can in part be due to these processes. Hinkle (7), arguing from the biologic evidence, supports this point strongly when he states:

> At the present time the "stress" explantion is no longer necessary. It is evident that any disease process, and in fact any process within the living organism, might be influenced by the reaction of the individual to his social environment or to other people.

A more reasonable formulation would hold that psychosocial processes acting as "conditional" stressors will, by altering the endocrine balance in the body, increase the susceptibility of the organism to direct noxious stimuli, i.e. disease agents. The psychosocial processes thus can be envisaged as enhancing susceptibility to disease. The clinical manifestations of this enhanced susceptibility will not be a function of the particular psychosocial stressor, but of the physicochemical or microbiologic disease agents harbored by the organism or to which the organism is exposed. Presumably, the disease manifestations will also be determined by constitutional factors, which in turn are a function of genetic endowment and previous experience.

Some reasonably convincing data exist to support this point of view. For example, one of the striking features of animal studies concerned with demonstrating the health consequences of a changed social environment has been the wide range of diseases that have followed such changes. Alteration of the social environment by varying the size of the group in which animals interact, while keeping all aspects of the physical environment and diet constant, has been reported to lead to the following: a rise in maternal and infant mortality rates; an increase in the incidence of arteriosclerosis; a marked reduction in the resistance to a wide variety of direct noxious stimuli, including drugs, microorganisms, and x-rays; an increased susceptibility to various types of neoplasia; alloxan-produced diabetes; and convulsions (8-16). Thus in animals at least, no specific type of "stress disease" appears in response to changes in the social milieu—changes which have been interpreted as "stressors." Rather, the animals appear to respond with a variety of diseases, the particular manifestation being determined by factors other than the disturbed social process. The evidence from human studies is somewhat less direct but nevertheless still consistent with this idea. A remarkably similar set of social circumstances characterizes people who develop tuberculosis (17) and schizophrenia (18, 19), alcoholics (20), victims of multiple accidents (21), and suicides (22). Common to all these people is a marginal status in society. They are individuals who for a variety of reasons (e.g. ethnic minorities rejected by the dominant majority in their neighborhood; high sustained rates of residential and occupational mobility; broken homes or isolated living circumstances) have been deprived of meaningful social contact. It is perhaps surprising that this wide variety of disease outcomes associated with similar circumstances has generally escaped comment. To a large extent this has probably resulted from each investigator usually being concerned with only one clinical entity so the features common to multiple disease manifestations have tended to be overlooked.

One exception to this has been the study by Christenson and Hinkle (23). In an industrial study in the United States, they have shown that managers in a company who, by virtue of their family background and educational experience were least well prepared for the demands and expectations of industrial life, were at greater risk of disease than age-matched managers who were better prepared. They found that this increased risk included all diseases, major as well as minor, physical as well as mental, long-term as well as short-term. A further example illustrating this point is the health consequences that follow the disruption of important social relationships, particularly death of a spouse. It has been shown that widowers have a death rate three to five times higher than married men of the same age for *every* cause of death (24). It is difficult to conceive of a specific etiologic process responsible for the increased death rate from such diverse conditions as coronary heart disease, cancer, infectious diseases, and peptic ulcer, and it would appear more reasonable to consider the loss of the spouse as increasing the susceptibility of such men to other disease agents.

As will be readily appreciated, subscription to such a formulation of the role of psychosocial factors in disease etiology would have important implications from the point of view of both research and intervention strategies. As far as research is concerned, it would suggest that attempts to document that certain social processes are stressors, capable of producing disease, by examining their relationship only to specific clinical entities (e.g. coronary heart disease, hypertension, or various forms of cancer) or even to subsets of diseases labelled "stress diseases" are unlikely to be very useful. If the formulation is correct, certain people exposed to these stressors will develop the clinical entity under investigation. Others, however, will not, but will develop some other manifestation which will not have been recorded or used as evidence as to the importance of the postulated stressor. A more logical approach would be either to examine all disease outcomes related to exposure to the postulated stressor or stressors or alternatively to identify subsets of the population who by virtue of their personal or environmental characteristics are known to be at high risk of specific clinical manifestations and examine the role of psychosocial stressors in facilitating the appearance of those manifestations. If this latter approach were used, it would imply that instead of examining the role of psychosocial stressors in the genesis of coronary heart disease in a random sample of the population, the study should be restricted to those who by virtue of their elevated risk factors (blood pressure, cholesterol, cigarette smoking) are known to be at high risk to coronary heart disease, and who therefore, if they become ill, are more likely to manifest coronary heart disease than tuberculosis.

Should such a research produce promising results, the implications for preventive intervention strategies would be profound. Before discussing these however, it is necessary to consider a further dilemma, our uncertainty as to the nature and properties of psychosocial stressors. Clarification of the outcomes to be expected from exposure to such stressors unfortunately provides no guide as to what these stressors are, much less how they are to be measured.

One of the unfortunate arguments that has clouded research in this area has been the controversy as to whether such stressors are invariant, affecting all people in a similar manner, or whether they are idiosyncratic, affecting each person differently depending upon his personality, interpretation of the situation, and so forth. The position for the latter point of view (which might be summarized as "what is one man's meat is another's poison") has recently been stated quite succinctly by Hinkle (7):

In view of the fact that people react to their "life situations" or social conditions in terms of the meaning of these situations to them, it is difficult to accept the hypothesis that certain kinds of situations or relationships are inherently stressful and certain others are not.

Others, including perhaps the majority of investigators, have treated these factors not only as if they were invariant but as if they were unidimensional, the presence of the factor being stressful, its absence beneficial.

Quite clearly, if the idiosyncratic point of view is correct, much of the work to identify universal or general stressors will be futile and lead to contradictory and confusing results. But equally clearly, the contrary point of view ignores the proposition that these processes do not have a direct pathogenic action but operate in their capacity as signals or symbols triggering off responses in terms of the information they are perceived to contain. And as this perception will almost certainly be a function of the differing personalities and the salience of the experience to different individuals, it is hard to accept the notion that certain social circumstances will always, or even in the majority of cases, be "stressful." This dilemma can best be resolved, I believe, by two changes in our thinking, changes which appear consistent with most of the data and which conceivably explain some of the existing contradictions. The first of these is that the extent to which the postulated psychosocial processes are generally noxious versus idiosyncratic in their action is largely a function of our level of abstraction. If we can identify the characteristics or properties of those signals or symbols which generally evoke major neuroendocrine changes in the recipients, we will have identified a general class of stressors even if the particular circumstances or relationships creating those types of signals or symbols differ for different people. Furthermore, if we can identify the attributes of this class of stressors, it may well be that the same relationships or social circumstances within a given culture (or, perhaps, subculture) regularly produce such a class of signals. Secondly, the existing data have led me to believe that we should no longer treat psychosocial processes as unidimensional, stressor or not stressor, but rather as two-dimensional, one category being stressors, and another being protective or beneficial.

The evidence supporting these points of view comes from both animal and human research. As has been indicated earlier, altering the social milieu of animals by increasing the number housed together leads to marked changes in health status, even when all relevant aspects of the physical environment and diet are kept constant. The biologic mechanisms through which such changes are produced have also been identified. Changes in group membership and the quality of group relationships in animals have been shown to be accompanied by significant neuroendocrine changes affecting the pituitary, the adrenocortical system, the thyroid, and gonads

(25, 26). These same endocrines are those responsible in large part for maintaining what Schoenheimer (6) has termed the "dynamic steady state" of the organism, and thus, presumably, its ability to withstand changes which would result from the action of disease agents.

The question of concern is what are the properties of the changes in this social milieu and are there analogues in the human social system? The usual notion that the crowding itself (that is, the physical density of the population) is responsible for the deterioration in health status has not been sustained by human studies. Despite the popularity of the belief that crowding is harmful to health, a review of the literature shows that for every study indicating a relationship between crowding and some manifestation of poor health, there is another equally good (or bad) investigation showing either no relationship or even an inverse one (27, 28). Furthermore, Hong Kong, one of the most crowded cities in the world, and Holland, one of the most crowded countries, enjoy some of the highest levels of both physical and mental health in the world (29).

A careful review of the data reported from these animal studies may hold a clue to these puzzles. In animals, an almost inevitable consequence of crowding is the development of a set of disordered relationships among the animals. These, while manifested by a wide variety of bizarre and unusual behaviors, often have in common a failure to elicit anticipated responses from the responding animal to what were previously appropriate cues. Thus, habitual acts of aggression (including "ritualized aggression" in defending the nest), or evidence of acceptance of subordination on the part of one animal, fail to elicit appropriate reciprocal responses on the part of another. In social animals under wild conditions, for example, the occupier of a nest will define a zone around that nest which is "home territory." Invasion of this territory by another animal of the same species will lead to a set of highly ritualized aggressive moves and countermoves, rarely leading to bloodshed, but culminating in one or other animal "signalling" capitulation. Under crowded conditions the defending animal may initiate this ritual "dance," but the invading animal fails to respond in the anticipated fashion. Instead he may lie down, go to sleep, attempt to fornicate, walk away, or do something which for the situation is equally bizarre.

This failure of various forms of behavior to elicit predictable responses leads to one of three types of responses on the part of the animals involved, the most common of which is repetition of the behavioral acts. Such acts are always accompanied by profound neuroendocrinal changes, and presumably their chronic repetition leads eventually to the permanent alterations in the level of the hormones and to the degree of autonomic nervous system arousal reported under conditions of animal crowding. The fact that these behavioral acts are in a sense inappropriate, in that they do not modify the situation, can be expected to enhance such hormonal changes. Under these conditions it is not difficult to envisage the reasons for the increased susceptibility to environmental insults displayed by such animals.

An alternative response on the part of some animals is to withdraw from the field and to remain motionless and isolated for long hours on end. It is not uncommon to observe some mice under crowded conditions crouched in most unusual places, on top of the razor-thin edge of a partition or in the bright light in the center of the enclosure, completely immobile and not interacting with any other animals. Such animals do not exhibit the increased pathology demonstrated by the interacting members (8).

The third alternative is for animals to form their own deviant groups, groups that apparently ignore the mores and codes of behavior of the larger group. Thus, "gangs" of young male rats have been observed invading nests, attacking females (the equivalent of gang rapes has been reported), and indulging in homosexual activities. I am not aware of any data on the health status of the these gang members, but according to this hypothesis they also should not exhibit any increase in pathology.

These observations would suggest that at least one of the properties of stressful social situations might be that in which the actor is not receiving adequate evidence (feedback) that his actions are leading to anticipated consequences. While we do not as yet have the appropriate instruments to measure in any direct fashion the extent to which such a phenomenon is occurring in humans, it is not unreasonable to infer that it is highly likely under certain circumstances. First, it is probable that when individuals are unfamiliar with the cues and expectations of the society in which they live (as in the case of migrants to a new situation, or those individuals involved in a rapid change of social scene, such as the elderly in an ethnic enclave caught up in urban renewal), many of their actions and the responses to these actions would fall into this category and thus, if this suggestion is correct, they should be more susceptible to disease than are those for whom the situation is familiar.

Some circumstantial evidence supporting this point of view exists. Scotch (30, 31) found that blood pressure levels among the Zulu who had recently migrated to a large urban center were higher than both those who had remained in their rural tribal surroundings and those who had lived for over 10 years in the urban setting. In two independent studies, Syme et al. (32-34) have demonstrated that occupationally and residentially mobile people have a higher prevalence of coronary heart disease than stable populations, and that those individuals displaying the greatest discontinuity between childhood and adult situations, as measured by occupation and place of residence, have higher rates than those in which less discontinuity could be determined. Tyroler and Cassel (35) designed a study in which death rates from coronary heart disease, and from all heart disease, could be measured in groups who were themselves stable but around whom the

social situation was changing in varying degree. For this purpose they selected 45- to 54-year-old white male rural residents in various counties of North Carolina and classified those counties by the degree of urbanization occurring in that locality. Death rates for coronary heart disease and all heart disease showed a stepwise increasing gradient with each increase in the index of urbanization of the county.

In a further study, Cassel and Tyroler (36) examined two groups of rural mountaineers working in a factory. The first of these was composed of individuals who were the first of their family to engage in industrial work, while the second comprised workers who were the children of previous workers in this factory. The two groups were drawn from the same mountain coves and doing the same work for the same pay. The underlying hypothesis was that the second group, by virtue of their previous experience, would be better prepared for the expectations and demands of industrial living than the first and would thus exhibit fewer signs of ill health. Health status was measured by responses to the Cornell Medical Index and by various indices of sick absenteeism. As predicted, the first group had higher Cornell Medical Index scores (more symptoms) and higher rates of sick absenteeism after the initial few years of service at each age.

A second set of circumstances in which this lack of feedback might occur would be under conditions of social disorganization. This, while still being far from a precise term which can be measured accurately, has proved to be a useful concept in a number of studies. In the hands of several investigators, for example, various indicators of social or familial disorganization have been related to increased rates of tuberculosis (17), mental disorders (37), deaths from stroke (38), prevalence of hypertension (39), and coronary heart disease (33). In addition, this same property might well explain the stressor role ascribed to status inconsistency (40) and role conflict and ambiguity (41). Thus the human data, while by no means confirming the utility of this postulation, are certainly not inconsistent with it and sufficiently intriguing to warrant further research along these lines.

As indicated earlier, however, a fuller explanation of the potential role of psychosocial factors in the genesis of disease requires the recognition of a second set of processes. These might be envisioned as the protective factors buffering or cushioning the individual from the physiologic or psychologic consequences of exposure to the stressor situation. It is suggested that the property common to these processes is the strength of the social supports provided by the primary groups of most importance to the individual. Again both animal and human studies have provided evidence supporting this point of view. Conger et al. (42), for example, have shown that the efficacy with which an unanticipated series of electric shocks (given to animals previously conditioned to avoid them) can produce peptic ulcers is determined, to a large extent, by whether the animals are shocked in isolation (high ulcer rates) or in the presence of litter mates (low ulcer rates). Henry et al. (43) have been able to produce persistent hypertension in mice by placing the animals in intercommunicating boxes all linked to a common feeding place, thus developing a state of territorial conflict. Hypertension only occurred, however, when the mice were "strangers." Populating the system with litter mates did not produce these effects. Liddell (44) found that a young goat isolated in an experimental chamber and subjected to a monotonous conditioning stimulus will develop traumatic signs of experimental neurosis, while its twin in an adjoining chamber, and subjected to the same stimulus, but with the mother present, will not.

The evidence from human studies is somewhat more conflicting. To a large extent I believe this to be due to a lack of recognition in many investigations that social supports are only likely to be protective *in the presence* of stressful situations. Thus the majority of studies have restricted themselves either to attempts at relating the absence of some form of social support to disease or to the effect of some postulated stressful situation, but have rarely examined the joint effects of a stressful situation together with the presence or absence of social supports. Despite this, there have been some studies which have produced reasonably convincing evidence indicating lack of social supports in disease occurrence. The studies referred to above (17-19, 21, 22), indicating the higher disease rates in people with marginal status, probably fall into this category. Separation from the family and evacuation from London during World War II appeared more deleterious for London children than enduring the blitz with their family (45). Combat studies have suggested the effectiveness of the small group (platoon, bomber crew) in sustaining members under severe battle stress (46). While these latter studies have indeed examined the effect of social supports under some form of presumed stressful situation (the blitz in one instance and combat in the other), the exposure of individual subjects to such stressors was not in fact measured, their existence being implicit rather than explicit.

In one recent study, however, both the stressors and the supports were more directly measured. Nuckolls et al. (47) studied the joint effects of these two processes on the outcome of pregnancy. Complete data were obtained from 170 white married primiparae of similar age and social class, all delivered by the same service. Social stresses were measured by a cumulative life-change score, a method developed by Holmes and Rahe (48) to assess the major life changes to which an individual had had to adapt. Social supports, or, as they were termed, psychosocial assets, were assessed by an instrument developed by the investigator designed to measure the subject's feelings or perceptions of herself (with particular reference to this pregnancy), her relationships with her husband, her extended family, and her immediate community in terms of the support she was receiving or could anticipate receiving. Both instruments were administered to the subjects before the 32nd week of pregnancy. After delivery, the records were reviewed blind for any evidence of complications of pregnancy or delivery. Among these patients 47 per cent had one or more minor or major complication, a rate comparable to the 50 per cent found in a national study using the same criteria.

Neither the life-change score alone nor the psychosocial asset score by itself was related to complications. However, when the relations between a high life-change score and complications of pregnancy were examined in the presence or absence of psychosocial assets, important associations were discovered. Ninety percent of women with high life-change scores, but low asset scores, had one or more complications of pregnancy, whereas only 33 percent of women with equally high life-change scores, but with high asset scores, had any complications. In the absence of high life-change scores, the asset scores were irrelevant.

Taken together, these studies would suggest that at both the human and animal levels the presence of another particular animal of the same species may, under certain circumstances, protect the individual from a variety of stressful stimuli. The mechanism through which such interpersonal relationships may function has largely been a matter of speculation. Theories have, however, been advanced and tested, one of the more attractive ones being that of Bovard (49, 50). He suggests, on the basis of animal studies, that stressful psychologic stimuli are mediated through the posterior and medial hypothalamus leading via the release of a chemotransmitter to the anterior pituitary to a general protein catabolic effect. He further suggests that a second center located in the anterior and lateral hypothalamus when stimulated by an appropriate social stimulus (namely, the availability of a supportive relationship) calls forth in the organism a "competing response" which inhibits, masks, or screens the stress stimulus, such that the latter has a minimal effect.

To test the notions advanced in this paper, further work obviously needs to be done to develop the instruments to measure these categories of psychosocial processes. If such research were to support these ideas, it would suggest a radical change in the strategies used for preventive action. Recognizing that throughout all history, disease, with rare exceptions, has not been prevented by finding and treating sick individuals, but by modifying those environmental factors facilitating its occurrence, thus formulation would suggest that we focus efforts more directly on attempts at further identification and subsequent modification of these categories of psychosocial factors rather than on screening and early detection.

Of the two sets of factors, it would seem more immediately feasible to attempt to improve and strengthen the social supports rather than reduce the exposure to the stressors. A recent example of the successful use of community counselors—women without any specific training but carefully chosen on the basis of high levels of empathy, warmth, and concern—in improving the well-being of children with chronic handicapping conditions (51) would suggest that, even in advance of any further specific knowledge, such modes of intervention could be more widely tested. With advancing knowledge, it is perhaps not too far-reaching to imagine a preventive health service in which professionals are involved largely in the diagnostic aspects—identifying families and groups at high risk by virtue of their lack of fit with their social milieu and determining the particular nature and form of the social supports that can and should be strengthened if such people are to be protected from disease outcomes. The intervention actions then could well be undertaken by nonprofessionals, provided that adequate guidance and specific direction were given. Such an approach would not only be economically feasible, but if the notions expressed in this paper are correct, would do more to prevent a wide variety of diseases than all the efforts currently being made through multiphasic screening and multi-risk-factor cardiovascular intervention attempts.

REFERENCES

1. Cannon, W. B. Stresses and strains of homeostasis. *Am. J. Med. Sci.* 189(1):1-14, 1935.
2. Selye, H. The general adaptation syndrome and diseases of adaptation. *Journal of Clinical Endocrinology* 6(2):117-230, 1946.
3. Wolff, H. G. Life stress and bodily disease. Proceedings of the Association for Research in Nervous and Mental Diseases. *Res. Publ. Assoc. Res. Nerv. Ment. Dis.* 29:3-1135, 1949.
4. Wolff, H. G. Quoted in The concept of "stress" in the biological and social sciences, by L. E. Hinkle. *Science, Medicine and Man* 1:34, 1973.
5. Dubos, R. *Man Adapting,* pp. 164-165, Yale University Press, New Haven, 1965.
6. Schoenheimer, R. *Dynamic Steady State of Body Constituents.* Harvard University Press, Cambridge, 1942.
7. Hinkle, L. E. The concept of "stress" in the biological and social sciences. *Science, Medicine and Man* 1:43, 1973.
8. Calhoun, J. B. Population density and social pathology. *Sci. Am.* 206(2):139-148, 1962.
9. Ratcliffe, H. L., and Cronin, M. T. I. Changing frequency of arteriosclerosis in mammals and birds at the Philadephia Zoological Garden. *Circulation* 18(1):41-52, 1958.
10. Swinyard, E. A., Clark, L. D., Miyahara, J. T., and Wolf, H. H. Studies on the mechanism of amphetamine toxicity in aggregated mice. *J. Pharmacol. Exp. Ther.* 132(1):97-102, 1961.
11. Davis, D. E., and Read, C. P. Effect of behaviour on development of resistance in trichinosis. *Proc. Soc. Exp. Biol. Med.* 99(1):269-272, 1958.
12. Ader, R., and Hahn, E. W. Effects of social environment on mortality to whole-body X-irradiation in the rat. *Psychol. Rep.* 13(1):211-215, 1963.
13. Ader, R., Kreutner, A., and Jacobs, H. L. Social environment, emotionality and alloxan diabetes in the rat. *Psychosom. Med.* 25:60-68, 1963.
14. King, J. T., Lee, Y. C. P., and Vissacher, M. B. Single versus multiple cage occupancy and convulsion frequency in C_3H mice. *Proc. Soc. Exp. Biol. Med.* 88:661-663, 1955.
15. Andervont, H. B. Influence of environment of mammary cancer in mice. *J. Natl. Cancer Inst.* 4(6):579-581, 1944.
16. Christian, J. J., and Williamson, H. O. Effect of crowding on experimental granuloma formation in mice. *Proc. Soc. Exp. Biol. Med.* 99(1):385-387, 1958.
17. Holmes, T. Multidiscipline studies of tuberculosis. In *Personality Stress and Tuberculosis,* edited by P. J. Sparer. International Universities Press, New York, 1956.
18. Dunham, W. H. Social structure and mental disorders: Competing hypotheses of explanation. *Milbank Mem. Fund. Q.* 39(2):259-310, 1961.
19. Mishler, E. G., and Scotch, N. A. Sociocultural factors in the epidemiology of schizophrenia: A review. *Psychiatry* 26:315-351, 1963.
20. Holmes, T. H. Personal communication, 1964.
21. Tillman, W. A., and Hobbs, G. E. The accident-prone automobile driver: A study of the psychiatric and social background. *Am. J. Psychiatry* 106:321, 1949.
22. Durkheim, E. *Suicide.* The Free Press, Glencoe, Ill., 1951.
23. Christenson, W. N., and Hinkle, L. E. Differences in illness and prognostic signs in two groups of young men. *J.A.M.A.* 177(4):247-253, 1961.
24. Kraus, A., and Lilienfeld, A. Some epidemiologic aspects of the high mortality rate in the young widowed group. *J. Chronic Dis.* 10(3):207-217, 1959.
25. Mason, J. W. Psychological influences on the pituitary-adrenal-cortical system. *Recent Prog. Horm. Res.* 15:345-389, 1959.
26. Mason, W., and Brady, J. V. The sensitivity of the psychoendocrine systems to social and physical environment. In *Psychobiological Approaches to Social Behavior,* edited by D. Shapiro. Stanford University Press, Stanford, 1964.
27. Cassel, J. Health consequences of population density and crowding. In *Rapid Population Growth. Consequences and Policy Applications,* pp. 462-478. Johns Hopkins Press, Baltimore, 1971.
28. Cassel, J. The relation of the urban environment to health. *Mt. Sinai J. Med. N.Y.* 40:539-550, 1973.
29. Dubos, R. The human environment in technological societies. *The Rockefeller Reviews,* July-August, 1968.
30. Scotch, N. A. A preliminary report on the relation of sociocultural factors to hypertension among the Zulu. *Ann. N.Y. Acad. Sci.* 84(Art. 17):1000-1009, 1960.
31. Scotch, N. A. Sociocultural factors in the epidemiology of Zulu hypertension. *Am. J. Public Health* 53:1205-1213, 1963.
32. Syme, S. L., Hyman, M. M., and Enterline, P. E. Some social and cultural factors associated with the occurrence of coronary heart disease. *J. Chronic Dis.* 17:277-289, 1964.
33. Syme, S. L., Hyman, M. M., and Enterline, P. E. Cultural mobility and the occurrence of coronary heart disease. *Health and Human Behavior* 6:173-189, 1965.
34. Syme, S. L., Borhani, N. O., and Buechley, R. W. Cultural mobility and coronary heart disease in an urban area. *Am. J. Epidemiol.* 82:334-346, 1965.
35. Tyroler, H. A., and Cassel, J. Health consequences of culture change: II. The effect of urbanization on coronary heart mortality in rural residents. *J. Chronic Dis.* 17:167-177, 1964.
36. Cassel, J., and Tyroler, H. A. Epidemiological studies of culture change: I. Health status and recency of industrialization. *Arch. Environ. Health* 3:25-33, 1961.

37. Leighton, D. C., Harding, J. S., Macklin, D. E., Macmillan, A. M., and Leighton, A. H. *The Character of Danger*. Basic Books, Inc., New York, 1963.

38. Neser, W. B., Tyroler, H. A., and Cassel, J. Stroke Mortality in the Black Population of North Carolina in Relation to Social Factors. Paper presented at the American Heart Association Meeting on Cardiovascular Epidemiology, New Orleans, 1970.

39. Harburg, E., Schull, W. J., Schork, M. A., Wigle, J. B., and Burkhardt, W. R. Stress and Heredity in Negro/White Blood Pressure Differences. Progress Report to National Heart Institute, 1969.

40. Jackson, E. F. Status consistency and symptom of stress. *Am. Sociol. Rev.* 27(4):469-480, 1962.

41. Kahn, R. L., Wolfe, D. M., Quinn, R., et al. *Organizational Stress: Studies in Role Conflict and Ambiguity*. John Wiley & Sons, Inc., New York, 1961.

42. Conger, J. J., Sawrey, W., and Turrell, E. S. The role of social experience in the production of gastric ulcers in hooded rats placed in a conflict situation. *J. Abnorm. Soc. Psychol.* 57(2):214-220, 1958.

43. Henry, J. P., Meehan, J. P., and Stephens, P. M. The use of psycho-social stimuli to induce prolonged hypertension in mice. *Psychosom. Med.* 29:408-432, 1967.

44. Liddell, H. Some specific factors that modify tolerance for environmental stress. In *Life Stress and Bodily Disease*, edited by H. G. Wolff, S. G. Wolf Jr., and C. C. Hare, pp. 155-171. Williams and Wilkins, Baltimore, 1950.

45. Titmuss, R. M. *Problems of Social Policy*. His Majesty's Stationery Office, London, 1950. Quoted by E. W. Bovard in The effects of social stimuli on the response to stress. *Psychol. Rev.* 66(5):267-277, 1959.

46. Mandelbaum, D. G. *Soldier Groups and Negro Soldiers*, pp. 45-48, University of California at Berkeley. Quoted by E. W. Bovard in The effects of social stimuli on the response to stress. *Psychol. Rev.* 66(5):267-277, 1959.

47. Nuckolls, C. B., Cassel, J., and Kaplan, B. H. Psycho-social assets, life crises and the prognosis of pregnancy. *Am. J. Epidemiol.* 95:431-441, 1972.

48. Holmes, T., and Rahe, R. The social readjustment rating scale. *J. Psychosom. Res.* 11:213-218, 1967.

49. Bovard, E. W. The balance between negative and positive brain system activity. *Perspect. Biol. Med.* 6:116-127, 1962.

50. Bovard, E. W. The effects of social stimuli on the response to stress. *Psychol. Rev.* 66(5):267-277, 1959.

51. Pless, I. B. Chronic Illness in Childhood: The Role of Lay Family Counsellors. Paper presented at Health Services Research Conference, Chicago, December 8-10, 1971.

7

Hypertension as a disease of modern society

JOSEPH EYER

About 50 per cent of people in modern societies have blood pressure sufficiently elevated to result in increased mortality. This proportion is much smaller in undisrupted societies of hunter-gatherers. In most cases the elevated blood pressure in modern societies is associated with physiological changes characteristic of chronic stress. The difference between blood pressure in modern populations and that in undisrupted hunter-gatherer societies cannot be accounted for by genetic differences or differences in salt consumption. Two primary features of modern society which contribute to the elevation of blood pressure are community disruption and increased work pressure. Drug therapy and relaxation therapies for hypertension attempt to counteract the physiological effects of social stress. However, it is more appropriate to use the occurrence of hypertension as an indicator of fundamental social problems which need to be solved.

DEFINING HYPERTENSION

Hypertension is defined medically as elevation of blood pressure above a given level, for instance the 140/95 measure commonly used now in community screening. It is also defined as elevation more than a certain amount above the average blood pressure level for the population of a given age. This latter criterion defines a young person as hypertensive at 140/90, but a 70-year-old only at 170/110 (1).

If we define hypertension, not in terms of an arbitrary criterion, but in terms of its consequences as a disease, a very different definition emerges. Hypertension increases the risks of heart attack, stroke, and kidney damage. About 50 per cent of modern men

die of causes of death in one way or another related to elevated blood pressure, by this definition. Prospective studies of representative samples of the American population show that people who maintain their blood pressure around 100/60 throughout their life-span have the lowest death risks. Below this value, people experience problems with fainting and the consequences of circulatory deficiency. For each increment of blood pressure above 100/60, there is a corresponding increase in death risks from heart attack, stroke, and kidney damage. It is clear that we ought to define hypertension as blood pressure above 100/60, if we use death risks to define the problem (2-4).

By this definition, most of the American population is hypertensive. This fact has led many practicing doctors to reject our reasoning. They argue that something this

Reprinted from International Journal of Health Services 5:539-558, 1975.

widespread in the population cannot be considered a disease, since it is rather the normal state of affairs; and, that were such a criterion used, the medical system would be totally overloaded in treating a disease for which it has only just recently discovered any effective means of cure. Since the major curative agents are drugs, it is not surprising to find that the drug companies, on the other hand, are among the strongest advocates of the low criterion for hypertension.[1]

Cross-cultural epidemiology of normal blood pressure and associated pathology reinforces our definition of hypertension. Undisrupted hunter-gatherers have low blood pressure, constant through the life-span. Where studies have been done, they have indicated low atherosclerosis among the population, based on autopsy at a given age, as well as a lack of other consequences of elevated blood pressure. Undisrupted hunter-gatherers are the most primitive social form of humanity, probably the form into which we evolved genetically, the form in which 94 per cent of all humans that have ever lived existed. Though over 99 per cent of the span of existence of the human species has been in hunter-gatherer form, the rise of settled agriculture, class societies (civilization), and particularly modern society, have confined today's hunter-gatherers to extremely marginal environments, such as the desert; today these peoples constitute a small fraction of total world population (2, Chap. 5; 5-17).

Disrupted peasant or pastoral societies, such as the West African tribes from which the American Negro slaves were derived, have average blood pressures which start slightly higher and increase progressively with age at a moderate rate (18-26). Among these populations, it is common to find elevated blood pressure associated with kidney damage, but in these cases the causal relation is opposite to the one characteristic of peoples in modern developed countries. Among peoples in underdeveloped countries, kidney damage most often is the product of infectious disease, such as tuberculosis, and hypertension is a consequence of kidney damage, not its cause (17, 27). In these populations atherosclerosis detected on autopsy at a given age is uncommon, despite the fact that many of these groups consume diets as high in saturated fat and cholesterol as the American diet (2, Chap. 5; 17). Where reliable mortality statistics are available for such populations in underdeveloped countries, the death rates for hypertension-associated disorders, particularly coronary heart disease, are two- to threefold lower than the rates characteristic of developed countries (2, Chap. 5; 28).

The highest average blood pressures, rising most rapidly with age, are found in two social categories: in both urban and rural areas in developed countries, and among populations in less-developed societies which have evolved under especially oppressive conditions, e.g. the Caribbean and South American black former slave areas, or the South African black urban areas (7, 8, 27, 29-44). These are also the societies with the highest death rates for hypertension-related disorders. Diet appears to play a role in *distributing* the deaths into one or another category in this whole system of diseases. Thus in Japan, whose citizens consume relatively little saturated fat and cholesterol, hypertension itself, stroke, and kidney damage are much higher than in America or Finland, but coronary heart disease is lower. In the latter countries, where dietary intake of atherogenic compounds is high, death rates from stroke and hypertension are relatively low, but death rates from coronary heart disease are high (2, 45).

It is hard to look at these data, which have been carefully studied and certified for accuracy for over 20 years, without concluding that they imply a criterion for hypertension identical to the implication or prospective studies within the United States. In a word, the normal state of modern populations is hypertensive, while

---

[1]See in particular Merck, Sharpe and Dohme's advertisements in medical journals in recent years.

that of undisrupted primitive societies is not.

PHYSIOLOGY OF ESSENTIAL HYPERTENSION

Why this difference? A survey of the hypothesized causes of hypertension sheds light on this social differential. Medical science divides hypertension into two broad varieties: types of elevated pressure for which specific cause can be found, and all the rest, termed essential hypertension, for which causation has not yet been fully worked out. Among the populations of present-day developed countries, essential hypertension comprises about 90 per cent of all hypertension. The remaining 10 per cent is attributed to pituitary or adrenal tumors, which can affect hormones such as noradrenalin that elevate blood pressure via constricting the arterioles; or to conditions that result in decreased blood flow through the kidneys, such as kidney damage from tuberculosis or glomerulonephritis (2, 46).

Just as hypertension associated with infectious kidney damage is today a major cause of elevated blood pressure in disrupted underdeveloped countries on the brink of economic development, this was probably also the major type of hypertension during the 19th century among populations of present-day developed countries due to the great rise of tuberculosis and other infectious diseases in early modern development prior to the introduction of public health measures (47). Essential hypertension has increased recently in developed countries as a proportion of total hypertension, as tuberculosis death rates have declined. Although the older historical statistics for death rates from circulatory and kidney disorders in populations of developed countries are subject to many interpretations, it is reasonable to infer from the social cross-sections that, since total hypertension is greater in more-developed countries than in less-developed ones, essential hypertension in particular has increased rapidly with recent modern development.

Quite a bit is known about the physiology of essential hypertension. Young essential hypertensives show elevated blood levels of adrenalin, which has its major cardiovascular effects in an increase of heart rate and output; and of noradrenalin, which has its major effects on peripheral resistance via constriction of the arterioles. Older hypertensives show an elevation of noradrenalin alone. Correspondingly, younger hypertensives show both increased cardiac output and increased peripheral resistance, while older hypertensives have normal or lowered heart output and greatly increased peripheral resistance (46, 48-51). The pattern of constriction of the arterioles involved in increased resistance is that characteristic of chronic stress: vasoconstriction to the gut, kidney, and skin; and relative vasodilation to the muscles (52). This patterned vasoconstriction could be maintained directly by noradrenalin, a hormone secreted in increased amounts in stress, or by the excitation of the sympathetic nervous system, which regulates the arterioles and is activated in stress. This physiology clearly implies that essential hypertension is a disease caused by stress.

Further support for a stress hypothesis emerges from the experience with treatment of essential hypertension. Many different kinds of relaxation techniques are effective in reducing the blood pressure of essential hypertensives. These techniques are most effective with young hypertensives, less so with older ones. Where the follow-up studies have been done, it is found that when the hypertensive leaves the special program environment that reinforces relaxation, and returns to the normal social network of his life, his blood pressure rises back to previous levels. (For an example of one type of relaxation technique, see reference 53.) This latter finding suggests that the social environment has a profound influence on the level of blood pressure in essential hypertensives, a point we will develop in detail later.

The fact that relaxation techniques are more effective with younger than older essential hypertensives suggests that there are certain irreversible changes which accompany the development of the disease. Folkow and Neill (46) have summarized much of the literature in this area. What starts in adolescence as a typical physiological stress response is reinforced by muscular thickening of the arterioles in the circulatory branches subject to vasoconstriction. This results in elevated blood pressure even at normal amounts of sympathetic activation and noradrenal secretion, since the muscles are more strongly reactive to a given nervous or hormonal stimulus, and since the additional thickness constricts the vessel's internal diameter somewhat.

Drug treatment of essential hypertension confirms the stress hypothesis. Drugs are usually administered only in the phase of sustained elevated pressure after age 30. The major categories used are powerful tranquillizers, specific vasodilators, and diuretics (54). That tranquillizers are the most effective antihypertensive drugs in terms of pressure reduction obviously supports the stress-tension hypothesis of the disease. The use of vasodilators is evidently related to the mechanisms we have sketched, and it is interesting to note here that many of the so-called specific vasodilators are also general relaxants.

Concerning the final category of drugs, the diuretics, there is disagreement concerning mode of action. In the short term, they appear to operate by decreasing blood volume via increased elimination of body fluid through the kidneys, sometimes as water alone, in other cases by eliminating both salt and water. The decrease of blood volume, all other things being equal, results in decreased blood pressure. This effect lasts only a few weeks, however; plasma volume, total body sodium, and cardiac output all return to previous levels after this time. The sustained depression of blood pressure that nevertheless occurs appears to be due to a gradual decrease in peripheral resistance from the action of these drugs on the arteriole walls. While it is clear that this vasodilation occurs, its mechanism is not understood (54).

All of the drug mechanisms clearly com-

plement a stress hypothesis for essential hypertension. However, the major American schools of essential hypertension choose to lay emphasis on the possible role of the kidney, and this emphasis also appears prominently in popular literature (55). While the temporary effect of diuretics seems to support this role, the long-term effectiveness does not. Recall also that essential hypertension is defined by eliminating other possible causative disorders, particularly of detectable kidney damage or gross alteration of glands affecting the kidneys.

However, the kidneys may well be *secondarily* involved in essential hypertension of stress origins. Both aldosterone (the adrenal hormone causing salt and water retention by the kidney) and ADH (the pituitary hormone causing water retention) are elevated as an integral part of the stress response (56). The juxtaglomerular apparatus in the kidney, which secretes renin, a hormone which speeds aldosterone release, is activated by sympathetic neurons. Also, the juxtaglomerular apparatus will be activated by anything that reduces kidney blood flow, e.g. vasoconstriction in the arterioles leading into the kidney, such as occurs in stress (57). All of these responses are adaptive as part of a short-term arousal response to a threatening situation, in which there may be blood loss or loss of salt and water through the sweat with strenuous physical exertion. These facts also illuminate Laragh's finding of a significant subgroup of essential hypertensives with elevated renin, as well as excess fluid retention in another large subgroup (58, 59).

SALT CONSUMPTION AND HYPERTENSION

Reading the literature from some of the advocates of kidney and salt mechanisms for essential hypertension, one would think that the major function of aldosterone is to cause inordinate body retention of salt whenever this becomes plentifully available in the diet (55, 60, 61). This unfortunate mishap in mammalian body design must then be treated by drastic sodium restriction in the diet and administration of diuretics. In fact, aldosterone's primary body function is to regulate sodium and potassium ion concentrations within rather narrow limits defined by the optimal levels for the function of nerve and muscle cells (57). Aldosterone is secreted or withheld directly in response to blood levels of sodium and potassium flowing past the adrenal cells. When sodium concentrations rise above the optimal levels, aldosterone secretion drops; and vice versa when sodium levels drop below the optimal levels. In a normal healthy mammal body not disturbed by stress responses or other pathology, the concentration of salt is normally regulated within narrow limits, and increased salt intake is quickly matched by increased salt excretion through the kidneys. Even large doses of salt produce only moderate, transient blood pressure elevations in humans (62).

An increased salt load will be retained, however, if the baseline level of aldosterone is reset upward, as occurs in chronic stress. Reexamining the evidence that has been selected to support the salt-consumption theory of hypertension, it becomes plain that it supports even more a stress/salt-consumption mechanism for blood pressure elevation. When additional evidence, not ordinarily noticed by the advocates of this theory, is brought to bear, however, the relation between salt consumption and blood pressure levels begins to appear more tenuous.

While dietary salt intake by and large increases with modern social development, paralleling the increase of blood pressure trends, there are many examples of societies whose populations salt their food heavily but do not show elevated blood pressure trends. Perhaps the most striking example is the Kung bushmen, who salt their food heavily (63) and have blood pressures constant at low levels throughout their life-span (15). This result would be expected if these groups were also under little social stress, as we shall argue in the section on social stress origins of hypertension.

Widening the view of the epidemiological data a little more, there are many examples of populations under stress which have higher blood pressures than other groups in the same area under less stress, despite similar salt-consumption levels (31, 32, 36, 37). There are also groups widely differing in salt intake with similar blood pressure distributions (16, 30, 31). Looking at all of the available data, the relation between salt-consumption levels and hypertension is much weaker than the advocates of the theory would have us believe (64).

Our stress/salt-consumption hypothesis is also supported by experimental results with normal laboratory rats (62, 65). These rats are typically strangers grouped in a cage for the purpose of experimentation. Male rats show a much greater stress response than do females to such grouping, whatever the density; this is accompanied by an initial period of fighting followed by formation of a dominance hierarchy (65, 66). The process of stranger grouping itself produces blood pressure elevations in rodents (67). In many of the salt-consumption experiments, only males showed the expected elevation of blood pressure with increased dietary salt intake, a finding consistent with diet-stress interaction.

The relative quantitative contribution of stress and diet-stress interaction in the genesis of modern hypertension is not completely determinable from presently available evidence. However, it has been shown that the effect of massive sodium restriction in the diet of modern hypertensives is only a moderate decline in blood pressure (68). Dietary modification is rightly viewed as secondary to drug treatment in the conventional management of essential hypertension (54). These facts imply that salt-consumption level is not responsible for the majority of blood pressure elevation in essential hypertensives. Even for that part in which increased salt retention from the diet does play a role, a reexamination of the evidence suggests a stress mechanism as the cause of the retention.

GENETIC THEORIES OF HYPERTENSION

Among many practicing doctors it is taken as an unquestionable article of faith that essential hypertension is primarily an inherited disorder. This belief is renewed with every family history review on an incoming patient. Aside from the problems of selective recall and suggestion, that are as important in doctors' interviews as in any other kind of retrospective research, quantitative analysis of the inheritance of hypertension does not support this medical prejudice.

Just as the risk of pathology goes up with each increase of blood pressure above 100/60, so also, hypertensives grade evenly into the distribution of pressures for the rest of the population (69-73). There is no easily isolable "hump" at the high end of the distribution, as there is for mongoloid idiocy, for instance, on the IQ distribution curves. This result suggests that hypertension is not inherited as a simple Mendelian trait with fixed phenotypic expression.

The trait must, then, be inherited in a more complex fashion, for which polygenic models, or single gene models with variable penetrance, have been proposed (71). The study of such models is most advanced by the quantitative examination of relatives of differing degrees to the identified hypertensive, including identical and fraternal twins (74-76). As a result of this kind of study, an estimate has been made of the relative contributions of heredity and environment to the phenotypes seen in a large population. This estimate, called the heritability, is about 0.2 for hypertension, which roughly signifies that 20 per cent of the variation in phenotypes in a population can be accounted for by heredity of some sort, the rest by environmental influences or genetic-environment interactions. This percentage is much lower than the corresponding figure for height or hair color and certainly does not support the assertion that inheritance is the *primary* factor in hypertension (72).

For the data we have been reviewing, it would really not matter if hypertension had a much higher heritability and a more respectable pattern of genetic transmission. Tuberculosis, for instance, is 30 per cent heritable by the same criteria, and yet no one today treats tuberculosis as a genetic disorder. The tripling of tuberculosis death rates which occurred in early modern development before the introduction of public health measures was due to large scale deterioration of the environment, including housing, nutrition, and food processing. The reduction of tuberculosis in modern countries to less than one-fiftieth its former height during the 20th century was achieved by a reversal of these conditions, as well as the introduction of pasteurization, dairy herd inspection, quarantine and sanatorium treatment, and modern drugs (47). It is *changes* of this kind that the genetic argument must address.

In particular, the genetic argument must account for the increase in the frequency of hypertension, from less than 5 per cent to over 40 per cent of the population affected, which parallels modernization in the social cross-sections we have discussed. This change from a low to a high blood pressure trend can occur in a population in less than 20 years, as in the migration of Atlas Jews to Israel, or Easter Islanders to the South American mainland (13, 77). The longest period over which this change can have occurred is less than 200 years, since developed societies did not exist before 200 years ago.

The empirical evidence on rates of genetic change in human populations indicates that, even with strong positive selection pressures, a fivefold increase in population gene frequency to 40 per cent of the population requires time spans of 1000 years or more (78). This is an order of magnitude longer than the time spans we are considering; so even with strong positive selection pressure, population genetic change can have made only a very minor contribution to the rise of essential hypertension with modern society. However, the character in question seriously increases mortality risks, and there is evidence that hypertensives also have reduced fertility (79). Hence the frequency of this gene in the population must be decreasing.

Despite this probable decrease in population frequency, there might be an increase of hypertensive phenotypes on a genetic basis because, with changing environmental conditions, the expression of the predisposition to hypertension changes. This predisposition in premodern populations might have been expressed as a particular susceptibility to infectious disease in infancy and childhood; with the lowering of infectious mortality in these age groups with modern public health advances, these genetic defectives now survive long past childhood to develop other premature pathology, for instance hypertension, in adult life (80). Fatal counterexamples for this form of argument appear in the data from premodern populations undergoing public health advance, which show equal proportional reductions in death rates across all age groups. As the children experiencing low mortality under these social conditions reach adulthood, they do not show elevated pathology from other causes (81). Additional counterexamples come from the historical urban and rural vital data for developed countries before public health advance. Urban death rates here were two to three times higher than rural, across all age groups, for both infectious and noninfectious causes (82). The populations that experienced low mortality in infancy (rural undeveloped) again show low mortality at older ages. It is only developed populations which show the peculiar combination of reduced death rates in infancy and childhood with relatively elevated older age death rates, and this only after public health advance; prior to this change, the populations most heavily selected against in youth are the ones with highest adult pathology as well. These data clearly imply that the social change of modernization overrides any shift in expression of the predisposition to hypertension which may have occurred with public health measures.

So far we have established that the genetic component in modern hypertension is small. Changes of the frequency of this predisposition in the population cannot account for observed differences in the prevalence of hypertension. Changes in the expression of this predisposition, whatever

its frequency, also cannot account for the observed data. Therefore a genetic factor in essential hypertension, though clearly definable, plays a minor role in causation. The same conclusion emerges from an examination of the data for negroes and whites.

The inheritance of hypertension is often invoked to account for the higher average blood pressure levels, and the higher frequency of hypertension, among American blacks, compared to whites. However, the average blood pressure trends of blacks in the social groups from which the slaves were drawn, largely in West Africa, are the intermediate, lower blood pressure trends characteristic of disrupted peasants or pastoralists (18, 19). Other African blacks, not demonstrably related to the American, have constant low blood pressures to old age (9, 15). The majority of the world's blacks show blood pressure trends considerably below the white levels in developed countries.

Thus, the elevation of blood pressure among black Americans above that of whites may be of environmental origin. A way of approaching this question is to find whites in socioeconomic circumstances similar to those of blacks, and compare blood pressure of the two groups. This kind of study has proved very difficult to do, since it is hard to find whites who suffer similar social contradictions, such as stigmatization. However, a large study recently completed in Detroit has approximated this matching (83). The major finding is that matched blacks and whites have similar blood pressures. From these data we can conclude that if a genetic factor makes a contribution to the difference in blood pressure between blacks and whites in America, the contribution is rather small.

OTHER FACTORS AND HYPERTENSION

Extensive review of the salt theory and the genetic theory is of great importance because they are the basis of the popular education carried on routinely by doctors in treating hypertensives. Other environmental factors, some of which are correlated with modern development, have also been implicated in hypertension. Ones associated with modern development include obesity, tobacco use, coffee consumption, and changes in the diet other than salt. A noncorrelated variable is the composition of drinking water, specifically calcium and magnesium content.

In the case of obesity, the evidence suggest that only populations of disrupted or modernized societies show the positive correlation between weight at a given age and blood pressure (9, 10), while members of undisrupted primitive societies show no relation between weight and blood pressure (9, 15). This is what one would expect if both obesity and blood pressure were the independent products of some other variable, such as social stress, which was present in disrupted or developed societies, but not in isolated primitive societies. Shah's review (64) demonstrates that the other factors mentioned have no simple relationship to blood pressure in the epidemiological studies. While this does not mean that they have no effect at all, it does signify that these effects are small and that the causal relationships are hard to disentangle.

SOCIAL STRESS CAUSES OF ESSENTIAL HYPERTENSION

We have already cited the data indicating that increasing modern development of a population is accompanied by increasing average blood pressure trends and increasing prevalence of hypertension. Modernization is, of course, a complex, multifaceted social and material transformation. Many studies have been done to try to isolate which particular facets are associated with blood pressure elevation. Literacy, for instance, does not appear to be associated with elevated blood pressure across this social comparison (11).

While this kind of comparative study is still in its infancy, it will clearly be of major importance in the design of future social systems which will have the advantages of modern technical and productive power, but will not suffer the disadvantages evident

in pathologies such as hypertension. Broadly speaking, such disadvantages fall into two large spheres of life: the disruption of social communities, and the rise of hierarchically controlled, time-pressured work. Simon Kuznets' *Modern Economic Growth* (84) and other standard socioeconomic histories make it plain that these stressful features are essential, not accidental, to the modernization process.

The basic move in modernization is the wresting of control over social resources, including raw materials, tools, and labor, from the village communities and craft organizations that previously organized work activity, and placing this control in the hands of a new ruling class, either private or state capitalists, who direct the accumulation of material productive power by society. This transfer of power entails the destruction of the settled rural kin-based extended family and village community, through migration to the city, and the rise of a nuclear family unit, stripped of its unnecessary kin relations and traditional work patterns, delegating socialization and work training to an extracommunal educational system. Such units are capable of migrating wherever the chances of profitability or policy dictate that labor demand will grow or decline.

People who are uprooted from stable communities, thrust into hostile, competitive urban environments in which their normal social institutions and reaction patterns make no sense, experience great elevations of blood pressure associated with this loss of control over the communal aspects of life (13, 35, 40, 77, 85-87). Adoption of social forms which more or less fit in the new environment (such as the nuclear family, fewer children (35)) reduces blood pressure somewhat from this peak, but not nearly back to levels comparable to those in the stable rural social form.

Migration continues in modern society at a much higher rate than in premodern societies, as technical change, uneven patterns of material development, and class struggle over share of the social product produce constant shifts in the profitability pattern. The reason why these migrations are also associated with blood pressure increases may be a large change in the nature of migration, as well as its rate, from premodern to modern society. In premodern social organizations, migration typically occurs in a noncompetitive context. For instance, in hunter-gatherers, it is a means of helping resolve social disputes within a local group. Migration is easy since there is little property to carry along, and the group to which one migrates is usually part of the extended kin or marriage alliance system. Finally, since such groups live amidst resources sufficient to fulfil their culturally determined needs, migrants in particular are not brought into antagonistic competition with people in the group in which they migrate (88). Resource competition within a hierarchical system of opportunities with apparent overall scarcity of desirable goods is, however, the situation confronted by every modern migrant.

Modernization is also characterized by increased breakdown of the nuclear family itself, through separation and divorce. In general, people in modern society who have the fewest close relations and feel most alien from potential intimates have the highest blood pressure (40, 87), a fact in particular true of the divorced and separated compared with those with stable marriages (79).

Mass unemployment is also a modern phenomenon. In the historical statistics, urban rates of unemployment have remained fairly constant over development, while rural rates have risen with the creation of an agricultural labor market; since the population as a whole is urbanized at the same time, the national unemployment rate rises. These data are put into higher relief by the fact that unemployment as we understand it does not exist in premodern social formations. For us, even with unemployment compensation and welfare, unemployment means a substantial reduction in income and disruption of normal social relationships, especially in the partial community on the job, and the one remaining outpost of intimate community, the nuclear family. In premodern societies, when there is less work to do or less social product available, people generally relax and share what they have within the kin network and local community. People who undergo unemployment in the modern economy show a rise of blood pressure which lasts from the initial uncertainty about their future until they are settled into a new job (89).

The continual development of new technology and work organization also sets off modern society from previous social forms. Combined with the accompanying specialization and hierarchical division of labor, this development necessitates multiple work role adjustments during the life-span, and this in turn means that a higher proportion of people experience a lack of fit between their skills and preparation and the work position they find themselves in. To use the language of sociology, modern society is characterized by elevated rates of status incongruity (90). This incongruity tends to be cumulative with age, both at work and in the community, so that old people in modern society, rather than accumulating wisdom from long social experience, become confused and demoralized, out of date. Within the developed economy, people who do not have correct qualifications for their job, or who experience conflicting demands within the job, have higher blood pressures than those who do not (40, 91).

The rate of technical and organizational change, the degree of unemployment, and the amount of migration are all intimately tied into the competition between the rulers of economic units for shares of social surplus and thus social power. When this competition occurs between modern states it frequently results in war, involving universal military service and mass mobilization of both troops and civilians in a total war effort. In recent centuries, this kind of mass mobilization is associated with the rise of the new model national states after the French Revolution, though of course previous civilizations have suffered the same phenomenon during their periods of warring states (92). Among societal types, the frequency and intensity of war is lowest in hunter-gatherers (93, 94). The experience of being in a modern army, whether in combat (95) or merely in training (9), is associated with comparatively elevated blood pressure.

The early period of development of a modern economy has often been characterized by a resurrection of slavery within capitalist market forms, or the special oppression of parts of the peasantry (96-98). Social groups subject to special oppression or disruption within developed societies show relatively greater blood pressure levels than those not subject to these conditions. The blacks in the western hemisphere who trace their origins from enslavement through rural sharecropping to urban slums show the highest average blood pressure trends yet studied (7, 8, 27, 29-44). This is true whether one studies the urban slums (83), or the oppressed rural areas (29, 38, 44). Comparable white groups (e.g. the white small farmers in Georgia (38), or the matched whites in Detroit (83)) show similar blood pressure levels.

However, the relationship between social class and hypertension is complex. Comparing city dwellers within a modern economy with rural inhabitants not yet extensively affected by development, we find that higher income, higher education, and skilled and professional work are associated with higher blood pressure (9, 14, 99). On the other hand, the specially oppressed groups *within* the modern economy have even higher blood pressure, despite their very low income, education, and so forth, especially in the rural areas (29, 44). The time-pressured, externally controlled, punishment reinforced character of work which we will show produces relative blood pressure elevation is an experience shared by blue- and white-collar workers alike. Thus, in the American economy, in which all social sectors have experienced the impact of development, there is no relation between the economic level of the population and rates of death from hypertension (36) or between family income and blood pressure, as shown in a national sample survey (100).

The same analysis applies to urban-rural comparisons. Early in the development process, blood pressure differentials between urban and rural areas are marked (9, 35). When development has extensively affected the rural areas, they show blood pressure trends as high as those in urban areas (29, 36, 44). Needless to say, this means that in modern populations, blood pressure trends are not correlated with population density (36).

The breakup of the rural community and craft guilds makes possible perhaps the most basic feature of modernization, a large increase in time-pressured work. This increase appears whether we study time awareness and time ordering of life (101), the socialization of children to believe that work achievement is the most important value, rather than communal intimacy (102), the adult belief that hard work is the supreme moral value (103), or more concretely, the lengthening of the proportion of the year spent working (104) or the lifetime economic work output of an individual (84).

Lennart Levi and his coworkers (105) have demonstrated that piecework pressure greatly increases noradrenalin and blood pressure; and that sorting ball bearings of closely similar size under time pressure increases blood pressure and blood levels of noradrenalin, free fatty acids, triglycerides, and cholesterol. Tax accountants working under deadline pressure show large increases of serum cholesterol and decreases of blood clotting time (106). Russek and Zohman (107) found that work pressure (long hours, two jobs) was a better predictor of heart attacks in young men than the standard risk factors.

Friedman and Rosenman (108, 109) have identified a behavior pattern which is highly associated with elevated blood pressure and particularly heart attack risks. This "coronary-prone behavior pattern" involves extremes of competitiveness in work, constant posing of new tasks and challenges, fast work pace and sense of time pressure, inability to enjoy the fruits of achievement, and inability to relax either at work or in intimate relationships. In their large controlled prospective study, the coronary-prone behavior pattern overlapped highly with other risk factors, such as smoking. In addition, it predicted the overwhelming majority of heart attacks that occurred, while the standard risks predicted only a minority. The difference in heart attack risk between the coronary-prone and the opposite behavior type (easygoing, sociable) is two- to fivefold, depending on age.

The pattern of emergence of elevated blood pressure with age in modern society suggests that, although early socialization undoubtedly contributes to the development of this behavior pattern, it must be backed up by the structure of adult work situations to have pathological consequences. Blood pressure trends in modern society and primitive tribes are similar until adolescence (5-17). Beyond this age, the modern curves rise sharply and continuously while the primitive remain flat. Likewise, the average blood pressure of whites and blacks is similar before adolescence, diverging only beyond this point (100-113).

A similar conclusion can be drawn from the typical life cycle development of a hypertensive (46). Very few hypertensives had elevated blood pressure before adolescence; however, after about age 30, people who are then hypertensive will mostly remain so for the rest of their life-span (114). Between ages 15 and 30, the person goes through the prehypertensive phase, in which blood pressure is sometimes normal, sometimes very much elevated (115-120). As far as these elevations are understood, they seem to correspond to major life cycle crisis points, involving military service, labor market entry, conflicts around integration into a job or career, migration, unemployment, and family formation and breakdown—all social processes which occur at peak frequency in the population at ages 15-30 (121). Beyond age 30, these sources of elevated blood pressure are replaced by the steady experience of work pressure and conflicting job demands that we have reviewed. The stresses of work may thus be responsible, along with the irreversible physiological changes such as vascular thickening, for the continued rise of blood pressure with age in modern populations.

The cluster of social stresses we have mentioned is not an exhaustive list of possible sources of stress in modern society; they are only the ones studied so far. People do rate breakup of intimate relationships, migration, and unemployment, as well as job pressure as among the most subjectively stressful of experiences (122). The situations studied, however, are weighted toward ones which affect men more than women, since a greater proportion of men work. Yet in undisrupted hunter-gatherer societies both men and women have low blood pressure through the life-span (9, 15). In modern society, between men and women on the average there is very little difference in blood pressure trends—both rise rapidly with age (5). This fact points to the necessity of studying, for instance, the boredom and social isolation of the modern housewife as a possible factor in blood pressure elevation for women.

While this list of social stressors certainly does not exhaust all the characteristics of modern societies, it clearly includes an important core shared by many different nations which have undergone development, including both private market and state planned economies. In the latter, the role of unemployment is replaced by the authority of the party and the occasional use of military repression, but this is clearly not an essential difference. The fact that hypertension-associated death rates are at similar levels in Eastern and Western Europe, or in the Soviet Union and the United States, indicates that the similarities are more important than the differences between these social structures, as far as stresses which produce elevation of blood pressure are concerned.

THE POSSIBILITY OF ADAPTATION TO SOCIAL STRESS

These data imply that major social changes are necessary to prevent modern hypertension. These changes seem to lie in the area of substantial increases in the communal control people can exercise over work, neighborhood and intimate life, and a corresponding decrease in the control over these areas by the ruling class. It is not clear that this shift would mean the abolition of modern worldwide technological organization and power, although there would certainly be major redefinitions of the nature of production and productivity, and major reorganization of lifetime work patterns.

This obvious conclusion is avoided by many investigators of social stress and blood pressure elevation (123). These people carry out a characteristic set of mental reclassifications which allows them to see a possibility of lowering blood pressure while society remains the same. Continual breakdown of community and the increase of alienating, time-pressured work are abstracted to the "necessity to make continual behavioral readjustments." If a way could be found to increase people's ability to make such readjustments, the stressful effects of change could perhaps be reduced.

One suggested method is the use of regularly scheduled relaxation-meditation periods, in which the mind is cleared of the convoluted pressing worries (53). While this method has been shown to lower blood pressure significantly, the method of presentation of the data begs the question. Most people are not in a position to relax more, as is evident from the fact that only a minority of people entering transcendental meditation programs become consistent meditators and experience the physiological benefits.

One needs to recall the experience of college students in the last decade in the United States. In the mid-sixties, everything seemed possible to them, and personal self-liberation became the order of the day. As the labor market for college graduates has steadily deteriorated, the students have gotten their noses back to the grindstone. While it is true that many students who make it into medical school could have worked less as undergraduates, this perception is difficult for any individual to realize

before reaching the goal, especially in a society which systematically rewards overwork and increasingly threatens failure to the larger and larger numbers of marginal students. After 20 years of fairly low unemployment, the same situation is now confronting most people in American society.

Given these realities, the exhortation to relax is likely to be effective only for that minority which has the social space in which to maneuver. For this reason, Friedman and Rosenman, in their popular book (108), direct most of their suggestions about how not to be coronary-prone to professional and managerial people. Similarly, the creativity-increasing benefits of transcendental meditation have only been demonstrated for people high in the work hierarchy, not for the majority of workers. As business failures and reorganizations increase, and as the universities consider abolishing tenure in their financial predicament, even people in these strata are likely to see less room for maneuvering and experience more pressure to fill up time with work.

The exhortation to relax could then become blaming the victim, a widespread stigmatization process in modern society, which only increases stress. One could laugh at the spectacle of well-paid mental health workers telling people to relax and lose out, were it not such a grim, all-pervasive phenomenon.

Another line of approach involves cultural relativism. According to this view, there is nothing intrinsic to cooperative, communal relations among human beings which has universal value; neither is it a value to control one's destiny in intimate and work life. Different social forms have different values, and the only problem is one of transition between social forms. Scotch's treatment of factors associated with hypertension in the rural and urban Zulu falls into this category (11, 35).

This idea stumbles on several difficult facts. First, the forms of modern life are continually changing, even within each generation, so there is no possibility to adopt stably a given new system of values. Second, this suggestion is not new, and has been at the core of educational efforts associated with modernization. What is the emphasis on reason and abstraction, on present abstention and future planning, on an ideology of individualism, but the major attempt at creating a stable value-system for modern society? While people who detach themselves from traditional communal feelings and values, and become more flexible in decision making through reasonable abstraction, probably suffer less stress from having their intimate lives disrupted and their work dictated in nature and pace, than those who do not, nevertheless these people experience significant chronic stress. Grossly speaking, one should expect that the oldest and most highly developed modern countries should show an actual reduction of average blood pressure trends below those developing more recently, but this is nowhere in evidence.

We can term this kind of adaptation the individualistic-purposive-involved adaptation to modern society. There is another kind of adaptation which has been tried on a widespread basis historically in the highly disrupted and oppressive periods of a civilization, which can be termed the Buddhist solution. Transcendental meditation has its origins in this kind of adaptation. Defeated by the accumulated contradictions of one's social nexus, the person withdraws from the world and its attractions, and thus its pains. This step is a prelude to seeing reality in a new way, in which all cultural values, all relationships, all power, everything, including death, are equally meaningful or meaningless.

The meaninglessness of things preserves one's ability to avoid pain. The meaningfulness of these things is conceived as uniformly pacific and pleasurable. Disharmony and exploitation in actual social life are transmuted, for instance, into universal harmony; unnecessary early death from preventable causes into a feature of harmony with which one can have only compassion. In the Zen variant of these ideas, playful

participation in any part of the world is not only possible, but recommended.

It is interesting that the social area (India, Southeast Asia (124-128)) in which these ideals have permeated the population most widely have among the lowest average blood pressure trends for premodern agricultural class societies. Other societies in this same culture area (Taiwan (129); Japan (130, 131)) which have experienced modernization, however, have the characteristic elevated blood pressure trends of modern society. The effect of the Buddhist solution under modern social conditions is thus likely to be marginal.

All of these suggested methods of adaptation have as their goal to reduce the reaction of internal stress physiology to social disruption and oppression. Modern science has by and large pursued the same objective by chemical means. While genetic and dietary explanations of hypertension play a large role in the popular mythology of blood pressure, doctors in fact use drugs to deal with the effects of stress, as we have demonstrated. If Nirvana can be attained with a pill, who needs esoteric training methods which take years to master?

We can conceive of drug therapies as having two broad stages of effectiveness. In the first, an attempt is made to counter in detail all of the primary and secondary physiological changes resulting from stress which lead to pathology: thus, vasodilators are prescribed for stress vasoconstriction, renin inhibitors for deranged renovascular function, and so forth. To be effective, these drugs would have to be appropriately administered to the population. For instance, the vasodilators would be given to a majority of the population starting in adolescence, so as to avoid the damaging effects of the large blood pressure fluctuations of the prehypertensive phase, which begin the positive feedback processes in later pathology.

But even under this phase of drug modification of society one could object that the persons will still experience suffering, anxiety, depression and anger, and the other manifestations of oppression and social disruption subjectively, since these drugs only alter the final peripheral expressions of stress, not its central organization. This objection leads naturally to the second phase, the development of drugs capable of altering the function of stress response systems in the central nervous system. The tranquillizers and antidepressants currently in use are rather primitive attempts at this kind of technology.

The success of this strategy would be a transformation of human values more basic than any which has occurred on a wide scale in all previous history. In Toynbee's terms, we are in the "Time of Troubles" of our civilization, a social phase which, in history, has always evoked a massive disaffection from the dominant values and social forms, a disaffection ultimately leading to the breakup of the civilization and the birth of a new one on different social premises (92). This disaffection has always taken the form of a reassertion of the autonomy of intimate human communities from powerful, disruptive hierarchies, whether it appeared in religious or revolutionary form. What the enthusiasts of technological solutions to stress reactions propose is to eliminate this sociohistorical dynamic through an alteration in the basic nature of man.

The technology that is sought is nothing other than the soma of Huxley's *Brave New World,* by which the population is transformed into so many happy alphas, betas, gammas, and deltas, each carrying out his hierarchically assigned tasks. People thus modified can be endlessly uprooted, overworked, made useless, conformed to any necessary intimacy, or, in a more rational scheme, simply maintained as part of the world's total capital equipment in proportion to their usefulness. The coherence of such a world obviously depends upon a solidified consensus among its rulers, something that does not yet exist in our present world. Once such a consensus is achieved, however, one oppressive hierarchy and one particular culture will be capable of endlessly extending itself, playing out far into the future the themes of western capitalist society.

But are we not impossibly distant from this future? The presently available antistress drugs by and large do not work any better than placebos, and have serious deleterious side effects. Psychosurgery is in its infancy, and is likewise relatively ineffective and damaging. But among the antihypertensives, there is a clear progression toward greater effectiveness and lesser side effects over time. Thus the veratrum alkaloids and rauwolfia derivatives, which can produce respiratory arrest, severe nausea and vomiting, or depression, are replaced by drugs like methyldopa (somnolence, constipation, and cramps) and the benzothiadiazides (elevate plasma uric acid and cause disorders of the blood elements).

It is also true that the majority of patients put on antihypertensive medication fail to take it frequently enough to obtain the benefits, perhaps because of the side effects. This difficulty is also present, however, even for drugs without serious side effects, and illustrates the great difficulty of programming in even small changes in behavior, much less big increases in daily relaxation.

But should we be using or rejecting these drugs solely on the grounds of effectiveness, which has been demonstrated, and side effects, which may improve? Should we be involved in arguments about trading off hypertension for depression or blood dyscrasias, when the only effect of such argument given our present social structure is to stimulate the allocation of more millions to find a better antistress technology? Should we maintain that the technological strategy must flop because no sufficiently powerful means of behavior modification have yet been found to guarantee its widespread application?

Rather, we are confronted with a political choice, a choice which goes down to the very foundations of modern western medicine. Down one path, doctors and the mass media will propagate the myth of the genetic and dietary origins of hypertension, while in fact dealing with the effects of stress with their medications. Technological solutions to pathology created by social disruption and oppression will then appear as fortunate gifts from the gods of science to a confused and bewildered but thankful common man. Down this path, doctors and researchers become more and more a priesthood reinforcing the position of a dominant minority. This is ultimately a social dead end, however glorious and respectable its permanence.

We need to recall that, compared to the massive disruption of their "Time of Troubles," the unified world empires of the past have imposed peace; that they have executed vast accomplishments in urban public health; and that they have by and large pursued a tolerant ideological policy and have sought practical adjustment of social contradictions whenever possible. These achievements have never been sufficient to overcome the fundamental disadvantage of such a society, the rigidity and lack of social creativity in the ruling class.

The other path looks toward aiding people to take control over the fundamental determinants of their own lives in an egalitarian community. This in many ways is a new historical and social project, especially when one contemplates not going backward to primitive social forms, but preserving worldwide technical and organizational integration at the same time. That this path is as yet open-ended, and that we can see only a few steps into its density does not lessen its attractiveness. We must always keep in mind that the alternatives are continued suffering or the withdrawal from basic human values in order to adapt to a particular social hierarchy. The repulsiveness of these choices must make the path toward cooperation and equality worthy of intelligent effort and action.

Note Added in Proof—The leading figure of the salt-consumption school of essential hypertension, Lewis Dahl, along with Richard Friedman, has just published an article entitled "The Effect of Chronic Conflict on Blood Pressure of Rats with a Genetic Susceptibility to Experimental Hypertension" (Friedman and Dahl, *Psychosomatic Medicine,* 37(5): 402-416, 1975). The authors execute four major achievements in this article, all of them moves toward the stress/salt-consumption hypothesis of hypertension suggested in my review.

First, Friedman and Dahl demonstrate that the kind of chronic stress that I showed to be possibly causative of hypertension in humans is reproducible in an animal-experimental paradigm, and produces large, sustained elevations of blood pressure. They also review the other relevant animal experimental literature demonstrating this point. The critical variable emergent in this literature is the ability of the animal to control punishing or disruptive stimuli.

Second, the sustained hypertension developed in their animals persisted only so long as the reinforcement paradigm was present, a finding parallel to our own for the role of social environment in sustained hypertension in humans.

Third, the blood pressure response of the hypertension-susceptible strains was much larger than that of strains not susceptible on a genetic basis. This larger sensitivity was mediated by a hyperresponsiveness of the arterioles of the susceptible strains to the vasopressor agents, noradrenalin and renin. These observations are similar to the finding in humans that people with highly labile blood pressure, due to great vascular reactivity, are at high risk of subsequent development of sustained hypertension.

Fourth, and most significant for a one-factor salt-consumption theory, is the fact that the basis of the ease with which these animals develop hypertension under non-stressed conditions in response to high-salt diets is a genetic alteration resulting in basal blood levels of aldosterone and other mineralocorticoids over twice as high as that found in nonsusceptible strains. This finding is not typical for humans who are not under stress, and genetic inheritance plays a minor role in human essential hypertension, as I have demonstrated.

However, the major group of human essential hypertensives do have elevated renin, with consequent elevations of aldosterone and salt retention from a high-salt diet. Since this group also has elevated noradrenalin and other stress hormones, there is good reason to believe that the renin elevation is due to chronic stress as well, rather than to a genetic alteration, as in the susceptible rodent strains. This possibility is explicitly pursued by Friedman and Dahl in their Discussion, citing the relevant physiological literature demonstrating the role of stress and sympathetic activation in elevating blood levels of renin.

REFERENCES

1. Moser, M., and Goldman, A. *Hypertensive Vascular Disease—Diagnosis and Treatment.* J. B. Lippincott, Philadelphia, 1967.
2. Stamler, J. *Lectures in Preventive Cardiology.* Grune and Stratton, New York, 1968.
3. Moriyama, I. M., Krueger, D., and Stamler, J. *Cardiovascular Diseases in the United States.* Harvard University Press, Cambridge, Mass., 1971.
4. Kannel, W., Wolf, P., Verter, J., and McNamara, P. Epidemiologic assessment of the role of blood pressure in stroke: The Framingham study, *JAMA* 214:301, 1970.
5. Epstein, F., and Eckoff, R. The epidemiology of high blood pressure—Geographic distributions and etiological factors. In *The Epidemiology of Hypertension,* edited by J. Stamler, R. Stamler, and T. Pullman, p. 155. Grune and Stratton, New York, 1967.
6. Bays, R., and Scrimshaw, N. Facts and fallacies regarding the blood pressure of different regional and racial groups. *Circulation* 8:655, 1953.
7. Shaper, A., and Williams, A. Cardiovascular disorders at an African hospital in Uganda. *Trans. R. Soc. Trop. Med. Hyg.* 54:12, 1960.
8. Shaper, A., and Shaper, L. Analysis of medical admissions to Mulago Hospital, *East Afr. Med. J.* 35:648, 1958.
9. Shaper, A. Blood pressure studies in East Africa. In The Epidemiology of Hypertension, edited by J. Stamler, R. Stamler, and T. Pullman. Grune and Stratton, New York, 1967.
10. Miall, W. The epidemiology of essential hypertension. In *W.H.O.—Czechoslovak Cardiological Society Symposium on the Pathogenesis of Essential Hypertension,* edited by J. Cort, V. Fencl, Z. Hejl, and J. Jirka. Macmillan, New York, 1962.
11. Scotch, N., and Geiger, H. The epidemiology of essential hypertension—A review with special attention to psychologic and sociocultural factors. *J. Chronic Dis.* 16:1151, 1963.
12. Henry, J., and Cassel, J. Psychosocial factors in essential hypertension: Recent epidemiologic and animal experimental evidence. *Am. J. Epidemiol.* 90:171, 1969.
13. Cruz-Coke, R., Etcheverry, R., and Nagel, R. Influence of migration on blood pressure of Easter Islanders. *Lancet* 1:697, 1964.
14. Maddocks, J. The influence of standard of living on blood pressure in Fiji. *Circulation* 24:1220, 1961.
15. Kaminer, B., and Lutz, W. Blood pressure in the bushmen of the Kalahari Desert, *Circulation* 22:289, 1960.
16. Whyte, H. Body fat and blood pressure of natives in New Guinea: Reflections on essential hypertension. *Australian Annals of Medicine* 7:36, 1958.
17. White, P. Hypertension and atherosclerosis in the Congo and in the Gabon. In *The Epidemiology of Hypertension,* edited by J. Stamler, R. Stamler, and T. Pullman. Grune and Stratton, New York, 1967.
18. Abrahams, D., Alele, C., and Barnard, G. The systemic blood pressure in a rural West African community. *West Afr. Med. J.* 9:45, 1960.
19. Moser, M., Harris, M., Pugatch, O., Ferber, A., and Gordon, D. Epidemiology of hypertension. II. Studies of blood pressure in Liberia. *Am. J. Cardiol.* 10:424, 1962.
20. Dawber, T., Kannel, W., Kagan, A., Donabedian, R., McNamara, P., and Pearson, G. Environmental factors in hypertension. In *The Epidemiology of Hypertension,* edited by J. Stamler, R. Stamler, and T. Pullman. Grune and Stratton, New York, 1967.
21. Donnison, C. Blood pressure in the African native. *Lancet* 1:6, 1929.
22. Heimann, L., Strachan, A., and Heimann, S. Cardiac disease among South African non-Europeans. *Br. Med. J.* 1:344, 1929.
23. Jex-Blake, A. High blood pressure. *East Afr. Med. J.* 10:286, 1934.
24. Vint, F. Post-mortem findings in the natives of Kenya, *East Afr. Med. J.* 13:332, 1937.
25. Williams, A. Blood pressure of Africans, *East Afr. Med. J.* 18:109, 1941.
26. Williams, A. Heart disease in a native population of Uganda: Hypertensive heart disease. *East Afr. Med. J.* 21:328, 1944.
27. Taylor, C. The racial distribution of nephritis and hypertension in Panama. *Am. J. Pathol.* 21:1031, 1945.
28. Puffer, R., and Griffith, G. *Patterns of Urban Mortality.* Pan American Health Organization, New York, 1967.
29. Miall, W., Kass, E., Ling, J., and Stuart, K. Fac-

tors influencing arterial pressure in the general population in Jamaica. *Br. Med. J.* 2:497, 1962.

30. Schneckloth, R., Stuart, K., Corcoran, A., and Moon, F. Arterial pressure and hypertensive disease in a West Indian negro population. *Am. Heart J.* 63:607, 1962.

31. Johnson, B., and Remington, R. A sampling study of blood pressure in white and negro residents of Nassau, Bahamas, *J. Chronic Dis.* 13:39, 1961.

32. Moser, M. Epidemiology of hypertension with particular reference to the Bahamas. I. Preliminary report of blood pressures and a review of possible etiological factors, *Am. J. Cardiol.* 4:727, 1959.

33. Kean, B. Blood pressure studies on West Indians and Panamanians living on the Isthmus of Panama, *Arch. Intern. Med.* 68:466, 1941.

34. Marvin, H., and Smith, E. Hypertensive cardiovascular disease in Panamanians and West Indians. *Military Surgeon* 91:529, 1942.

35. Scotch, N. Sociocultural factors in the epidemiology of Zulu hypertension. *Am. J. Public Health* 53:1205, 1963.

36. Rose, R. The distribution of mortality from hypertension within the United States. *J. Chronic Dis.* 15:1017, 1962.

37. Comstock, G. An epidemiologic study of blood pressure levels in a biracial community in the southern United States. *American Journal of Hygiene* 65:271, 1957.

38. McDonough, J., Garrison, G., and Hames, C. Blood pressure and hypertensive disease among negroes and whites in Evans County, Georgia. In *The Epidemiology of Hypertension,* edited by J. Stamler, R. Stamler, and T. Pullman. Grune and Stratton, New York, 1967.

39. Boyle, E., Griffey, W., Nichaman, M., and Talbert, C. An epidemiologic study of hypertension among racial groups of Charleston County, South Carolina. In *The Epidemiology of Hypertension,* edited by J. Stamler, R. Stamler, and T. Pullman. Grune and Stratton, New York, 1967.

40. Stamler, J., Stamler, R., Berkson, D., Lindberg, H., Miller, W., and Collette, P. Socioeconomic factors in the epidemiology of hypertensive disease. In *The Epidemiology of Hypertension,* edited by J. Stamler, R. Stamler, and T. Pullman. Grune and Stratton, New York, 1967.

41. Adams, J. Some racial differences in blood pressures and morbidity in groups of white and colored workmen, *Am. J. Med. Sci.* 184:342, 1932.

42. Goldstein, M. Longevity and health status of whites and nonwhites in the United States. *J. Natl. Med. Assoc.* 46:83, 1954.

43. Lennard, H., and Glock, C. Studies in hypertension: Differences in distribution of hypertension in negroes and whites: An appraisal. *J. Chronic Dis.* 5:186, 1957.

44. Langford, H., Watson, R., and Douglas, B. Factors affecting blood pressure in population groups. *Trans. Assoc. Am. Physicians* 81:135, 1968.

45. Fejfar, Z., Burgess, A., and Kagan, A. Arterial hypertension and ischemic heart disease: Comparison in epidemiological studies. *Proceedings of the World Health Oganization,* Geneva, 1963.

46. Folkow, B., and Neill, E. *Circulation.* Oxford University Press, New York, 1971.

47. Rosen, G. *A History of Public Health.* MD Publications, New York, 1958.

48. Eich, R., Cuddy, R., and Smulyan, H. Hemodynamics in labile hypertension. *Circulation* 34:299, 1966.

49. Frolich, E., Tarazi, R., and Dustan, H. Reexamination of the hemodynamics of hypertension. *Am. J. Med. Sci.* 257:9, 1969.

50. Louis, W., Doyle, A., and Anavekar, S. Plasma norepinephrine levels in essential hypertension. *New Engl. J. Med.* 288:599, 1973.

51. Shanberg, S., Stone, R., Kirschner, N., Gunnells, J., and Robinson, R. Plasma dopamine β hydroxylase: A possible aid in the study and evaluation of hypertension. *Science* 183:523, 1974.

52. Brod, J., Frencl, V., and Hejl, Z. General and regional hemodynamic pattern underlying essential hypertension. *Clin. Sci.* 23:339, 1962.

53. Wallace, R. *The Physiological Effects of Transcendental Meditation.* Students International Meditation Society, Los Angeles, 1970.

54. Page, L., and Sidd, J. Medical management of primary hypertension. *New Engl. J. Med.* 287:960, 1018, and 1074 (three parts), 1972.

55. Conquering the quiet killer. *Time,* Jan. 13, 1975.

56. Mason, J. Organization of psychoendocrine mechanisms. *Psychosom. Med.* 30(5): whole issue, 1968.

57. Ganong, W. *Review of Medical Physiology,* Ed. 6, p. 286. Lange Medical Publications, Los Altos, 1973.

58. Laragh, J. Evaluation and care of the hypertensive patient. *Am. J. Med.* 52:565, 1972.

59. Laragh, J. Vasoconstriction-volume analysis for understanding and treating hypertension: The use of renin and aldosterone profiles. *Am. J. Med.* 55:261, 1973.

60. Meneely, G., and Dahl, L. Electrolytes in hypertension: The effects of sodium chloride: The evidence from animal and human studies. *Med. Clin. North Am.* 45:271, 1961.

61. Dahl, L. Salt intake and salt need. *N. Engl. J. Med.* 258:1152 and 1205, 1958.

62. Dahl, L. Possible role of salt intake in the development of essential hypertension. In *Essential Hypertension,* edited by K. Bock and P. Cottier, p. 53. Springer-Verlag, Berlin, 1960.

63. Thomas, E. *The Harmless People.* Vintage, New York, 1959.

64. Shah, V. Environmental factors and hyperten-

sion. In *The Epidemiology of Hypertension,* edited by J. Stamler, R. Stamler, and T. Pullman. Grune and Stratton, New York, 1967.

65. Barnett, S. *The Rat: A Study in Behavior.* Aldine, Chicago, 1963.

66. Barnett, S. Social stress. *Viewpoints in Biology* 3:170, 1964.

67. Henry, J., Meehan, J., and Stephen, P. The use of psychosocial stimuli to induce prolonged systolic hypertension in mice. *Psychosom. Med.* 29:408, 1967.

68. Corcoran, A., Tayler, R., and Page, I. Controlled observations on the effect of low sodium dietotherapy in essential hypertension. *Circulation* 3:1, 1951.

69. Pickering, G. *High Blood Pressure.* Churchill, London, 1968.

70. Pickering, G. The inheritance of arterial pressure. In *The Epidemiology of Hypertension,* edited by J. Stamler, R. Stamler, and T. Pullman. Grune and Stratton, New York, 1967.

71. Pickering, G. Hyperpiesis: High blood pressure without evident cause: Essential hypertension. *Br. Med. J.* 2:959, 1965.

72. Pickering, G. The inheritance of arterial pressure. In *Epidemiology,* edited by J. Pemberton. Oxford University Press, London, 1963.

73. Hamilton, M., Pickering, G., and Roberts, J. The aetiology of essential hypertension. 4. The role of inheritance. *Clin. Sci.* 13:273, 1954.

74. Miall, W., Heneage, P., and Khosla, T. Factors influencing the degree of resemblance in arterial pressure of close relatives. *Clin. Sci.* 33:271, 1967.

75. Vander Molen, R., Brewer, G., and Honeyman, M. A study of hypertension in twins. *Am. Heart J.* 79:454, 1970.

76. Strickberger, M. *Genetics,* p. 181. Macmillan, New York, 1968.

77. Dreyfuss, F., Hamosh, P., Adam, Y., and Kallner, B. Coronary heart disease and hypertension among Jews immigrated to Israel from the Atlas Mountains region of North Africa. *Am. Heart J.* 62:470, 1961.

78. Cavalli-Sforza, L., and Bodmer, W. *Genetics of Human Populations.* W. H. Freeman, San Francisco, 1971.

79. *Mortality from Selected Causes by Marital Status.* U.S. National Center for Health Statistics, Vital and Health Statistics, Series 20, 8a, 8b, 1972.

80. Glazier, W. The task of medicine. *Sci. Am.* 228(4):13, 1973.

81. United Nations. *Demographic Yearbooks,* 1946-1972.

82. Dublin, L., and Lotka, J. *Length of Life.* Ronald Press, New York, 1936.

83. Harburg, E., Erfurt, J., Haunstein, L., Chape, C., Schull, W., and Schork, M. Socio-ecological stress, suppressed hostility, skin color, and black-white male blood pressures: Detroit. *Psychosom. Med.* 35:276, 1973.

84. Kuznets, S. *Modern Economic Growth.* Yale University Press, New Haven, 1966.

85. Cruz-Coke, R. Environmental influences and arterial blood pressure. *Lancet* 2:885, 1960.

86. Syme, S., Hyman, M., and Enterline, P. Some social and cultural factors associated with the occurrence of coronary heart disease. *J. Chronic Dis.* 17:277, 1964.

87. Gampel, M., Slome, C., and Scotch, N. Urbanization and hypertension among Zulu adults. *J. Chronic Dis.* 15:67, 1962.

88. Lee, R., and De Vore, I. *Man The Hunter,* Aldine, Chicago, 1968.

89. Kasl, S., and Cobb, S. Blood pressure changes in men undergoing job loss: A preliminary report. *Psychosom. Med.* 32:19, 1970.

90. Dodge, S., and Martin, W. *Social Stress and Chronic Illness: Mortality Patterns in Industrial Society.* University of Notre Dame Press, London, 1970.

91. Christenson, W., and Hinkel, L. Differences in illness and prognostic signs in two groups of young men. *JAMA* 177:247, 1961.

92. Toynbee, A. *A Study of History.* Oxford University Press, New York, 1946 and 1957.

93. Quincy, W. *A Study of War.* University of Chicago Press, Chicago, 1939.

94. Sorokin, P. *Contemporary Sociological Theories.* Harper and Row, New York, 1928.

95. Graham, J. High blood pressure after battle. *Lancet* 248:239, 1945.

96. Williams, E. *Capitalism and Slavery.* G. P. Putnam & Sons, New York, 1966.

97. Wolf, E. *Peasant Wars of the Twentieth Century.* Harper and Row, New York, 1969.

98. Moore, B. *Social Origins of Dictatorship and Democracy.* Beacon Press, Boston, 1966.

99. Miall, W., and Oldham, P. Factors influencing arterial blood pressure in the general population. *Clin. Sci.* 17:409, 1958.

100. Gordon, T., and Devine, B. Hypertension and Hypertensive Heart Disease in Adults. U.S. National Center for Health Statistics, Vital and Health Statistics, Series 11, No. 13, 1966.

101. Mumford, L. *Technics and Civilization.* Harcourt, Brace, New York, 1934.

102. McClelland, D. *The Achieving Society.* Free Press, New York, 1961.

103. Weber, M. *The Protestant Ethic and the Spirit of Capitalism.* Scribners, New York, 1958.

104. Mandel, E. *Marxist Economic Theory,* Vol. 1, p. 135. Monthly Review Press, New York, 1968.

105. Levi, L. *Stress and Distress in Response to Psychosocial Stimuli.* Pergamon Press, New York, 1972.

106. Friedman, M., Rosenman, R., and Carroll, V. Changes in serum cholesterol and blood clotting

time in men subjected to cyclic variation of occupational stress. *Circulation* 17:852, 1958.

107. Russek, H., and Zohman, B. Relative significance of heredity, diet and occupational stress in coronary heart disease of young adults. *Am. J. Med. Sci.* 235:266, 1958.

108. Friedman, M., and Rosenman, R. *Type A Behavior and Your Heart.* Knopf, New York, 1974.

109. Jenkins, C. Psychologic and social precursors of coronary disease. [Review of Friedman and Rosenman.] *N. Engl. J. Med.* 284:244 and 307, 1971.

110. Diehl, H. Racial differences in blood pressure. *Minn. Med.* 14:726, 1931.

111. Szent-Gyorgi, N. Blood pressure studies among Americans and foreign-born students. *Circulation* 14:17, 1956.

112. Karpinos, B. Blood pressure and its relation to height, weight, race and age. *American Journal of Hygiene* 68:288, 1958.

113. Rose, R. A study of blood pressure among negro schoolchildren. *J. Chronic Dis.* 15:373, 1962.

114. Kannel, W. The origins and evils of essential hypertension. *N. Engl. J. Med.* 284:444, 1971.

115. Thomas, C. B. Observations on some possible precursors of essential hypertension and coronary artery disease. In *The Precursors of Essential Hypertension and Coronary Artery Disease,* edited by C. B. Thomas. Johns Hopkins Press, Baltimore, 1951.

116. Thomas, C. Characteristics of the individual as guideposts to the prevention of heart disease. In *The Precursors of Essential Hypertension and Coronary Artery Disease,* edited by C. Thomas. Johns Hopkins Press, Baltimore, 1957.

117. Stamler, J., Schoenberger, J., Shekelle, R., and Stamler, R. The problem and the challenge. In *The Hypertension Handbook.* Merck, Sharpe and Dohme, West Point, Pa., 1974.

118. Ostfeld, A., and Lebovits, B. Blood pressure liability: A correlative study. *J. Chronic Dis.* 12:428, 1960.

119. Harris, R., Sokolow, M., Carpenter, L., et. al. Response to psychologic stress in persons who are potentially hypertensive. *Circulation* 7:874, 1953.

120. Kalis, B., Harris, R., Bennett, L., et al. Personality and life history factors in persons who are potentially hypertensive. *J. Nerv. Ment. Dis.* 132:457, 1961.

121. Eyer, J. *Stress Related Mortality and Social Organization.* Health-PAC, New York, in press, 1975.

122. Holmes, T., and Rahe, R. The social readjustment rating scale. *J. Psychosom. Res.* 11:213, 1967.

123. Benson, M., and Gutmann, M. The relationship of environmental factors to systemic arterial hypertension. In *Stress and the Heart,* edited by R. Eliott. Futura Publishing Company, New York, 1974.

124. Padmavati, S., and Gupta, S. Blood pressure studies in rural and urban groups in Delhi. *Circulation* 19:395, 1959.

125. Wilson, J. Arterial blood pressures in plantation workers in North East India. *Br. J. Prev. Soc. Med.* 12:204, 1958.

126. *Nutrition Survey of the Armed Forces: A Report by the Interdepartmental Committee on Nutrition for National Defense* [Thailand]. U.S. Government Printing Office, Washington, D.C., 1960.

127. Bibile, S., Cullumbine, H., Kirtisinghe, C., Watson, R., and Wikramanayake, T. Variation with age and sex, of blood pressure and pulse rate, for Ceylonese subjects. *Ceylon Journal of Medical Sciences* 6:79, 1949.

128. *Nutrition Survey of the Armed Forces: A Report by the Interdepartmental Committee on Nutrition for National Defense* [Vietnam]. U.S. Government Printing Office, Washington, D.C., 1959.

129. Liu, T., Hung, T., Chen, C., Hau, T., and Chen, K. A study of normal and elevated blood pressure in a Chinese urban population in Taiwan (Formosa). *Clin. Sci.* 18:301, 1959.

130. Sagan, L., and Seigel, D. Adult Health Study: Clinical and Lab Data, 1958-60. Atomic Bomb Casualty Commission, Japanese National Institute of Health, Technical Report 12-63, Nagasaki.

131. Switzer, S. Hypertension and ischemic heart disease in Hiroshima, Japan. *Circulation* 28:368, 1963.

PART III

New dimensions in the alleviation of stress

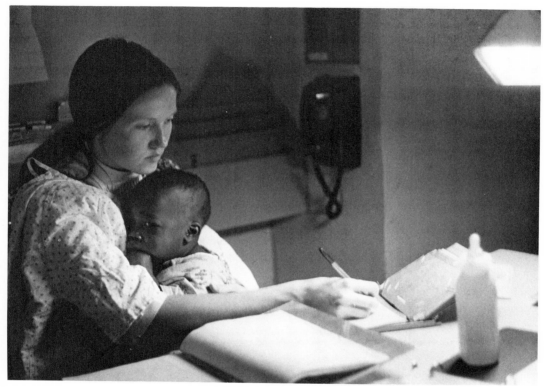

Photo by Helen Nestor

8

Psychotherapy of bodily disease: an overview

JEROME D. FRANK

ABSTRACT—This article reviews clinical and experimental studies of the interaction between psychological states and bodily diseases and considers some implications for the role of psychotherapists in diagnosis, prevention and treatment of these conditions.

The role of psychotherapy in the treatment of bodily diseases obviously depends on how big a part psychological factors play in their etiology and course. This presentation reviews a few recent studies demonstrating the intimate relations of mental states to bodily illnesses, and then considers some possible implications for the role of psychotherapy in their treatment.

First, however, since the term 'psychotherapy' covers a lot of ground, it requires a definition. For the purpose of this paper, psychotherapy includes all systematic interactions between a sufferer and a socially designated healer, both operating in terms of the same belief system, in which the healer undertakes to relieve the suffer's distress by symbolic communications. These are primarily and characteristically words, but can also include administration of placebos—inert substances which serve as tangible manifestations of the therapist's healing power—as well as bodily rituals and exercises believed to have healing effects. Active pharmacological agents may be used

Reprinted from Psychotherapy and Psychosomatics **26:**192-202, 1975.

to facilitate psychotherapy but are not integral to the process itself.

Western healing arts, both psychological and medical, have been dominated by the Cartesian split between mind and matter, with the body being a form of matter. For various reasons, its hold has been so strong as to prevent full acceptance of the implications of the obvious fact that psychological responses and bodily diseases are intimately intertwined. The great eighteenth-century English surgeon *John Hunter,* who suffered from syphilitic heart disease (allegedly contracted experimentally), said, 'My life is in the hands of any rascal who chooses to annoy and tease me,' and indeed dropped dead after an argument. Sir *William Osler* (21), the first professor of medicine at the Johns Hopkins Medical School, wrote eloquently of 'The Faith that Heals' and commented: 'Faith in St. John Hopkins as we used to call him . . . worked just the same sort of cures as did Aesculapius at Epidaurus.' According to a current bestseller in the United States, *Type A Behavior and Your Heart* (12), persons with a type A behavior pattern, described as aggressive involvement in 'a chronic incessant struggle to achieve more and more in less and less time . . . against the opposing effects of other things or persons', are three times as likely to develop coronary disease within 10 years than persons without this pattern. And, of course, the psychosomatic literature burgeons with studies exploring mind —body interactions.

Yet, while paying lip service to the importance of treating the total person rather than his disease, physicians in actual practice seldom do so. Nor does the recognition that psychic and bodily states interact sit comfortably with psychotherapists. Many vigorously maintain that their healing procedures have nothing to do with the 'medical model', which they caricature as the treatment of bodily disease by drugs and operations, and some still resist accepting the etiological and therapeutic importance of genetic and metabolic components of psychoses.

In recent years Westerners have started to pay more attention to the so-called holistic concept of illness and healing held by most of the rest of the world, which views the human as a psychobiological unity integrated within himself and with his environment. Illness is a perturbation of this harmony, and treatment the effort to reinstate it through integrated bodily, psychological and social interventions.

One reason for this new receptivity to the holistic view may be that, after a century in which the West gained ascendancy over the East, we are now seeing the piston reverse itself as the philosophy, art and power of the East begin to penetrate our lives and consciousness (22). Simultaneously, ways are emerging of testing Eastern concepts with Western scientific instruments, thereby making them more palatable to us.

In short, the time is ripe for what has been termed a 'paradigm shift' (15). It is time we freed ourselves from the thrall of Cartesian dualism and learned to adopt the holistic view that illnesses can be arranged in a continuum with respect to the relative importance of bodily and psychological components. The psychological component is

greatest in neuroses and personality and behavior disorders, the bread and butter of psychotherapists. The bodily components of most of these are still obscure, but they will eventually be found. Next are addictions, including alcoholism, and psychoses, which are now recognized to involve genetic vulnerabilities. Next come psychosomatic illnesses, in which there is no question as to the existence of organic pathology but the etiology and course of the disease are clearly affected by psychological states. The finding that these are the only conditions for which psychotherapy is demonstrably more effective than no psychotherapy (18) is especially intriguing. Finally, there are the bona fide organic illnesses, which can presumably be explained without reference to the mind, such as injuries, infections and metabolic or degenerative diseases. This presentation focuses on psychological features of these conditions, which represent the hardest cases for the holistic view.

A major source of psychological responses that interact with illness is the person's psychosocial environment. A recent methodological advance has enabled the application of quantitative methods to analysis of the relationship between life experiences and illnesses. Using the ratio-scaling method devised by *S.S. Stevens* in psychophysics, *Thomas Holmes* and his colleagues (20, 32) have devised highly reliable scales of life experiences on the one hand and illness on the other in terms of degree of severity on a scale of 1—1,000. Life changes range from going on vacation to death of a spouse; illnesses from dandruff and hangnails to leukemia.

A large-scale study of naval crews using these scales found a statistically significant positive relationship between their scores on the scale of life experiences during the 6 months prior to going to sea and their total number of illnesses reported during the cruise period (24). In another study, hospitalized patients were asked to score the life experience scale retrospectively with respect to the preceding 2 years. The correlation of severity of these stresses and seriousness of illness was 0.73 (p = 0.001). This holds for chronic illness only, and the severity of the life experiences did not predict specific illness but only the greater likelihood of becoming ill (32). Apparently efforts to adapt to life changes create physiological strains which increase susceptibility to any chronic illness.

What about circumscribed trauma? Surely the consequences of a blow or a wound would be thought to be fully explained by the bodily damage they cause. All biological organisms respond to noxious agents by bodily changes involving the pituitary and adrenal glands, which *Hans Selye* (26) has termed the general adaptation syndrome. Recent studies suggest that this syndrome is set off only by injuries to a conscious animal or human, not to an unconscious one, raising the possibility that the psychological significance of the injury rather than the bodily damage is the crucial factor (16).

A specific example of the contribution of environmentally caused psychic stress to bodily changes is the syndrome known as psychological dwarfism. This consists of retardation of growth, motor development, IQ and sexual maturation which are promptly reversed if the child is removed from his home (31). The home environments are usually stormy and frightening to the child. Apparently this is the source of the retardation (23). Once out of the home, growth and development immediately resume.

Hospitalized patients provide an especially good opportunity to observe the effects of psychonoxious and psychotherapeutic forces because patients are exposed to them around the clock and because they can be directly observed and modified. A chronic disease hospital, where patients are immersed in an atmosphere of monotony and hopelessness and are more or less abandoned by their families, would be expected to be especially damaging. Fortunately, as a project conducted in a veterans hospital for chronic neurological diseases has shown, this damage is reversible. A rehabilitation

team developed a program to change the emotional atmosphere of the hospital from a warehouse in which patients were expected to remain indefinitely to a rehabilitation center with the goal of discharging patients back into the community. The program fostered this change in several ways. Within the hospital patients were reindividualized, in that each was reexamined and his medications were changed if indicated. Group activities aimed at raising morale and overcoming isolation were instituted. With respect to the relation between the hospital and the community, social workers reestablished links between the patients, their families and prospective employers.

This program was applied to 289 patients who had been hospitalized 3-10 years, some of whom were bedridden, some incontinent, with striking results. In the first series of 80 patients, in 3 months 70% left the hospital. This discharge rate continued over the next 2.5 years. Since this result could conceivably be explained by lowering of the hospital's criteria for discharge and for community acceptance, the crucial finding is that 40% of the discharged patients became self-supporting. The program thus impressively demonstrated the effectiveness of a holistic approach integrating pharmacological, psychological and social interventions in rehabilitating patients regarded as hopeless (29).

Shifting the focus now from the person's milieu to the person himself, the widespread clinical impression that a patient's emotional state may affect the course of illness and healing has received strong support from studies concerning speed of convalescence from infectious disease and speed of healing following an operation. One such study of patients with undulant fever (brucellosis) concerned 24 patients (all male but one), 8 who had recovered in 2-3 months and 16 who still complained of headache, nervousness and vague aches and pains. There were no differences between the two groups in medical findings at onset or at time of reexamination, but 11 of the 16 who were still ill, as compared to none of the 8 who had recovered, had experienced a seriously disturbed life situation within 1 year before or after the acute infection. This finding confirms the results obtained with the life experience scale reported above. All patients were given a morale loss index, consisting of items selected from the MMPI. Scores on this index were significantly higher in the chronic than in the recovered group (14).

An explanation of this finding which cannot be completely excluded is that the low morale of the chronic patients was the result of their delayed convalescence, not the cause of it, although the authors adduce additional evidence that this was unlikely. To be conclusive, the morale loss score would have to be obtained before the patients became ill. Fortunately, the ability to predict influenza epidemics made such a study possible. All personnel at a military installation were given the morale loss index before such an epidemic was due to strike, yielding a sample of 26 who contracted the disease. Of these, 14 recovered after an average duration of 8 days, while 12 continued to complain for more than 3 weeks. The initial severity of the illness was the same for both groups, but the slow recoverers had significantly lower morale before they became ill (7).

Since symptoms of influenza and undulant fever resemble those of depression (lassitude, weakness, vague somatic complaints) and the physicians had to rely on patients' reports, these studies still do not rule out the possiblility that patients and doctors were mistaking depression for delayed convalescence. To be conclusive, a measure of improvement that did not depend on patient's reports would be needed. One study used such a criterion, speed of healing following operation for detached retina. Patients about to undergo this operation were administered a scale of 'acceptance', which included such items as trust in the surgeon, optimism about outcome, and confidence in one's own ability to cope regardless of outcome. The speed of healing was rated independently by the surgeon,

who did not know the patients' scores on the acceptance scale. A correlation of 0.61 was found between acceptance and speed of healing ($p < 0.001$). The authors conclude: '. . . despite the psychological make-up of the person or the intensity of the threat . . . high acceptance and rapid healing occur . . . when the patient has faith in the healer, his methods of healing, and feels that these methods are relevant to the cause of his illness . . . the person seeking to help the slow healer . . . should focus primarily on what variables enhance or destroy the patient's attitude of expectant faith' (19, p. 140).

It must be emphasized that the findings of these three studies are correlational, which leaves open the question of causality. For example, it may be that both the attitude of acceptance and speed of healing are two aspects of a generally high level of vitality. That expectant faith may be causal, however, is suggested by results obtained by procedures which evoke this attitude, of which the most dramatic are those of shrines of religious healing such as Lourdes.

Leaving open the question of the role, if any, of supernatural forces in so-called miracle cures, two points should be stressed. First, since miracle cures are reported by adherents of all religious faiths, their occurrence must depend on the pilgrim's state of mind, not on the validity of the object of his faith. Second, these cures are not miraculous. The consciousness of cure comes instantaneously, but thereafter healing occurs through normal reparative processes which, to be sure, are greatly accelerated (8). No one has grown a new limb or an eye at Lourdes. Furthermore, mysterious cures of organic disease occur in doctors' offices, but since such cases are very rare, no one physician sees enough of them, so they are easily overlooked. If they had occurred at Lourdes, they would have been called miracles. There is no question that religious shrines release powerful healing emotions of hope and exaltation in many persons. While the physician can seldom mobilize expectant faith as powerfully as healing shrines, he can foster this state in many patients directly by his words, or indirectly by medications and operations.

The physician's power comes from two sources. He occupies a social role of respect, power and trustworthiness analogous to that of a parent, so he mobilizes the attitudes of trust and dependency that an infant feels toward a good parent; and his treatment is based on and validates a theory which expresses the world-view of the society in which both he and the patient function. Since a shared world-view both makes sense out of life and reinforces the sense of group belongingness, medical (like psychological) treatment helps to combat the demoralizing sense of isolation that typically accompanies illness.

A tangible symbol of the physician's role which mobilizes patients' expectant faith is medication. The psychological effects of medication have been studied by giving patients placebos. Since the effectiveness of placebos depends entirely on their symbolization of the physician's healing role, their administration is a form of psychotherapy as defined in this paper. The patient's response is termed 'the placebo effect', an unfortunate term on several counts. Placebo is Latin for 'I will please', which implies both deceit by the physician and absence of therapeutic power in the pill. 'Expectant faith effect' would be more appropriate to the placebo's power. In this connection, until this century most medical remedies were either ineffective or harmful, so the physician's reputation depended primarily on the placebo effect.

The determinants of strength of the placebo effect are very complex, and seem to depend on the interaction between the patient's state and aspects of his situation at the time the pill was administered. However, in general a placebo is between 30 and 60% as effective as the active medication with which it is compared, regardless of the power of the medication. For example, as a pain reliever, placebo is 55% as effective as aspirin, a weak analgesic, and 55% as effective as morphine, a powerful analgesic. Apparently the therapist transmits his belief in the active drug's potency to the patient (10).

If medication can have powerful psychological effects, one would expect surgical operations to have even stronger ones. As compared to a person seeking medical treatment, someone about to undergo surgery is more apprehensive and is totally dependent on the surgeon—he literally places his life in the surgeon's hands. Furthermore, the operation is a single dramatic act which is expected to produce a prompt cure. Surgery on the heart, the organ of life itself, is an especially impressive demonstration of the surgeon's power, so it should not come as a surprise that the expectant faith effect of heart surgery for anginal pain accounts for a large part of its effectiveness. This was first demonstrated by study of an operation for relief of angina which consisted of tying off an artery in the chest. The results were spectacular in that 60—90% of the patients experienced marked symptomatic relief. But then someone decided to do a mock operation, i.e., to give the anesthesia and open the skin, but not touch the artery—and it proved to be fully as effective as the real one in reducing patient's pain. Causing them to cut down their use of nitroglycerin tablets and increasing their exercise tolerance (4).

Recently a new operation has become popular, in which diseased portions of coronary arteries are bypassed by segments of veins, in an effort to improve the heart's blood supply. 90% of patients in whom tests subsequent to surgery show increased cardiac circulation improve clinically, but so do 60% in whom the operation left the blood supply unchanged or actually diminished it (2).

Turning at last to psychotherapy, its rituals are unlikely to be able to inspire expectant faith as powerfully as those of the physician or surgeon, but the psychotherapist is able to induce other states of mind which contribute to healing, notably hypnosis and meditation. Through hypnosis the therapist can influence a wide range of the subject's bodily processes including such unlikely ones as changes in chemical constituents of blood and bile (30), but hypnosis has the disadvantage of leaving control in the hands of the hypnotist. Meditation, on the other hand, enables a person to gain conscious control of his own bodily functions, so that he does not have to depend on someone else. The burgeoning interest in meditation is in part attributable to the growing influence of Eastern thought, already mentioned, but also to the emergence of biofeedback, a means of self-regulation of cortical states and thereby bodily ones that depends on equipment and is therefore appealing to Westerners.

Biofeedback studies have demonstrated that thought and behavior continually affect brain activity; for example, whistling or simply imagining the tune of a song produces changes in the right cortex, reciting or imagining its words activates the left. Since we are always controlling our brains, the obvious next step with the sick would be to teach them to exert this control to promote health instead of illness.

It has been shown that normal persons can learn through biofeedback to control many bodily functions (25). Its effectiveness in treating illnesses, however, seems to be less striking. This is to be expected, since conquering a chronic illness requires changes in life-style, not simply learning a technique. So far, the effectiveness of biofeedback training with patients has been clearly demonstrated only in enabling them to gain voluntary control of skeletal muscles that have escaped this control (as in tension headache, nocturnal bruxism and torticollis); to control cardiac arrythmias and other aspects of the circulatory system, for example, skin temperature; and to control fecal incontinence (9). However, with increasing sophistication in its use, there is reason to think that biofeedback training will aid in the treatment of a wider range of conditions.

The gadgetry of biofeedback must not be allowed to disguise the fact that it is essentially a form of psychotherapy in that the therapeutic interaction is transmitted by symbolic communication. It is readily (although perhaps incorrectly) conceptualized as a method of operant conditioning, and experts agree that its successful use depends on a good therapeutic relationship, a high level of motivation and self-discipline in the patient, and considerable clinical sophistication in the therapist (5).

The ultimate aim of biofeedback, furthermore, is to transfer control of his bodily states to the patient. It is essentially an informational aid to him in his effort to achieve self-regulation of his bodily processes through meditation, a state in which virtually unlimited conscious control of bodily organs can be achieved, as the Yogi have shown. Meditation has been receiving increasing attention as an adjunct to psychotherapy (6) and seems a promising aid in the treatment of schizophrenia (13), which, if one chooses to regard it as primarily a bodily disease, comes within our purview.

Since cancer has long been regarded as a bodily disease relatively uninfluenced by mental states, a particularly interesting recent development has been the accumulation of evidence that psychological states may contribute to its causation. This raises the possibility that psychotherapy may have a place in its treatment. Western medicine has conceptualized cancer as an invasion of the body from inside by cells that have gone wild, and treatment consists of an effort to remove or destroy them by surgery, radiation or drugs. The outcome of this struggle is determined by whether the cancer cells or the destructive agents are stronger. The patient is a helpless bystander or, better, the arena in which the battle is fought. This theory cannot explain spontaneous remissions of definitely diagnosed cancer, which sometimes occur. Two surgeons have accumulated 176 examples of such remissions from the literature, but offer no explanation for them (11).

Recently a holistic concept of cancer has emerged, the so-called surveillance theory, which offers a possible explanation for some at least of these spontaneous remissions, and suggests additional therapeutic approaches. According to this theory, cancer cells are formed throughout life but are promptly detected and destroyed by the person's immunity system. Clinical cancer appears when this fails; hence factors which influence its strength, including psychic ones, are relevant to both cancer's emergence and treatment.

What is the evidence in support of the surveillance theory? First, an increasing number of studies have found that persons with a certain personality style are especially prone to cancer. As compared to matched healthy controls or those suffering from other illnesses, they repress or deny unpleasant affects such as depression, anxiety and hostility (3). Under a facade of cheerfulness and self-confidence, they feel isolated and that life is a hard struggle. This attitude is consistent with the finding that cancer patients, more than controls, reported experiences before the age of 7 which led the child to feel that close emotional relationships brought pain and destruction (17).

This finding has recently found unexpected confirmation from a prospective study of medical students (28). 914 male medical students graduating from 1948 to 1964 filled out a questionnaire including a closeness-to-parents scale. By June, 1973, 26 had developed malignant tumors. The 20 on whom complete data were available had scored significantly lower on the closeness-to-parents scale (p = 0.01) than a group matched by age, sex and class who were in good health. This background would not be inconsistent with the finding that cancer-prone persons are especially shaken when someone they have come to trust dies or otherwise withdraws support. In any case, cancer patients were found to have suffered such a loss 6 months to 8 years before the clinical onset of the disease significantly more often than controls (17).

The possibility of training cancer patients to cultivate healing mental states is currently being explored by a radiotherapist and his wife, a psychiatric social worker (27). Based on the surveillance theory, they reason that if depression and similar emotions can facilitate the growth of cancer, contrary emotions could retard it. On the basis of this somewhat shaky rationale, they use group and individual psychotherapy to try to change the belief of the patient and his family that the cancer is incurable to faith that it can be cured. Concurrently they train the patient to enter a state of meditation three times a day in which he visualizes that his white cells are devouring the cancerous ones.

They make no extravagant claims for this approach. The radiotherapist continues to use radiotherapy with patients who can still tolerate it and states that less than a quarter of his patients can muster the necessary self-discipline to participate in the psychotherapeutic program. Nor will he publish results until he can report 5-year follow-ups. He has, however, observed spectacular remissions in some patients with far-advanced disease. At the very least, these therapists have raised the strong possibility that psychotherapy can sometimes beneficially affect the course of cancer.

This survey of selected studies could well lead the reader to exaggerate the effectiveness of psychotherapy for bodily disease. It therefore should be made explicit that, despite striking exceptions, by and large psychotherapy will probably prove to be an adjunct to conventional medical and surgical treatments for such illnesses, rather than a major treatment method. This review does suggest, however, that if psychotherapists can persuade physicians of their usefulness, they can make diagnostic, preventive and therapeutic contributions.

Diagnostically, psychotherapists can bring into the open emotional stresses that may be aggravating the disease process, including those resulting from the treatment itself. For example, a legitimate problem for psychotherapy would be the exploration, and perhaps mitigation, of the severe psychonoxious effects of dialysis for kidney failure, resulting in a suicide rate of patients undergoing this treatment some 400 times that of the general population (1).

As to prevention, in view of the demonstrated close relationship between life stresses and subsequent illness, programs of crisis intervention may already be functioning in this way. With respect to treatment, both group and individual psychotherapy could be used much more than they are at present to overcome the demoralization of patients with chronic disease, which aggravates their distress and disability, and to foster more health-promoting attitudes. Furthermore, since procedures such as autogenic training, biofeedback and meditation are forms of psychotherapy, psychotherapists are better qualified by training than physicians to teach patients how to gain conscious control of involuntary bodily functions as a means of combatting illness and promoting health. We are entering a period in which the holistic conception of illness and healing is gaining ever wider acceptance. As a result, psychotherapists will be collaborating increasingly with physicians in diagnosing, preventing and treating organic disease.

REFERENCES

1. Abrams, H. S.: Suicidal behavior in chronic dialysis patients. Am. J. Psychiat. 127:1194-1204 (1971).
2. Achuff, S. C.; Griffith, L. S. C.; Conti, R. C.; Humphries, J. O.'N.; Brawley, R. K.; Gott, V. L., and Ross, R. S.: The 'angina-producing' myocardial segment. An approach to the interpretation of results of coronary artery bypass surgery. Proc. 22nd Annu. Scient. Session Am. College of Cardiology, San Francisco 1973.
3. Bahnson, M. B. and Bahnson, C. B.: Ego defenses in cancer patients. Ann. N.Y. Acad. Sci. 164:546-557 (1969).
4. Beecher, H. K.: Surgery as placebo. J. Am. med. Ass. 176:1102-1107 (1961).
5. Blanchard, E. B. and Young, L. D.: Clinical application of biofeedback training. Archs gen. Psychiat. 30:573-589 (1974).
6. Carrington, P. and Ephron, H. S.: Meditation as an adjunct to psychotherapy; in Arieti and Chrzanowski: New dimensions in psychiatry: a world view, chap. 12, pp. 262-291 (Wiley, New York 1975).
7. Cluff, L. E.; Canter, A., and Imboden, J.: Asian influenza: infection, disease and psychological factors. Archs intern. Med. 117:159-164 (1966).
8. Cranston, R.: The miracle of Lourdes (McGraw-Hill, New York 1955).
9. Engel, B. G.; Nikovmanesh, P., and Shuster, M. M.: Operant conditioning of rectosphincteric responses in the treatment of fecal incontinence. New Engl. J. Med. 290:646-649 (1974).
10. Evans, F. J.: The placebo response in pain reduction. Advances in neurology, vol. 4, pp. 284-296 (Raven Press, New York 1974).
11. Everson, T. C., and Cole, W. H.: Spontaneous regression of cancer (Saunders, Philadelphia 1966).
12. Friedman, M. and Rosenman, R. H.: Type A behavior and your heart (Knopf, New York 1974).
13. Glueck, B. C. and Stroebel, C. F.: Biofeedback and meditation in the treatment of psychiatric illnesses. Compreh. Psychiat. (in press).
14. Imboden, J. B.; Canter, A.; Cluff, L. E., and Trevor, R. W.: Brucellosis. III. Psychological aspects of delayed convalescence. Archs intern. Med. 103:406-414 (1959).
15. Kuhn, T. S.: The structure of scientific revolutions (University of Chicago Press, Chicago 1962).
16. Lazarus, R. S.: A cognitively oriented psychologist looks at biofeedback. Am. Psychol. 30:555-561 (1975).
17. LeShan, L.: An emotional life history pattern associated with neoplastic disease. Ann. N.Y. Acad. Sci. 125:780-793 (1965/66).
18. Malan, D. H.: The outcome problem in psychotherapy research. Archs gen. Psychiat. 29:719-729 (1973).
19. Mason, R. C.; Clark, G.; Reeves, R. B., and Wagner, B.: Acceptance and healing. J. Relig. Hlth 8:123-142 (1969).
20. Masuda, M. and Holmes, T. H.: Magnitude estimates of social readjustments. J. psychosom. Res. 11:219-225 (1967).
21. Olser, W.: The faith that heals. Br. med. J. 1910: 1471.
22. Parkinson, C. N.: East and West (Houghton Mifflin, Boston 1963).
23. Powell, G. F.; Hopwood, N. J., and Barrett, E. S.: Growth hormone studies before and during catch-up growth in a child with emotional deprivation and short stature. J. clin. Endocr. Metab. 37:674-679 (1973).
24. Rahe, L. H.: Subjects' recent life changes and their illness susceptibility. Adv. psychosom. Med., vol. 8, pp. 2-19 (Karger, Basel 1972).
25. Schwartz, G. E.: Biofeedback as therapy. Am. Psychol. 28:666-673 (1973).
26. Selye, H.: The stress of life (McGraw-Hill, New York 1956).
27. Simonton, O. C.: Management of emotional aspects of malignancy. Proc. Symp. on New Dimensions of Habilitation for the Handicapped, University of Florida, Gainesville 1974.

28. Thomas, C. B. and Duszynski, K. R.: Closeness to parents and the family constellation in a prospective study of five disease states: suicide, mental illness, malignant tumor, hypertension and coronary heart disease. Johns Hopkins med. J. 134: 251-270 (1974).

29. Veterans Administration: Rehabilitation of the chronic neurologic patient. VA pamphlet 10-29 (Veterans Administration, Washington 1949).

30. Wittkower, E.: Studies on the influence of emotions on the functions of organs including observation on normals and neurotics. J. ment. Sci. 81: 533-682 (1935).

31. Wolff, G. and Money, J.: Relationship between sleep and growth in patients with reversible somatotropin deficiency. Psychol. Med. 3:18-27 (1973).

32. Wyler, A. R.; Masuda, M., and Holmes, T. H.: Magnitude of life events and seriousness of illness. Psychosom. Med. 33:115-122 (1971).

9

Adjunctive biofeedback with cancer patients: a case presentation

KENNETH R. PELLETIER

Extensive research literature supports the correlation between stress and psychosocial factors and the incidence of disease in animals and man.[7,8] Many of these premorbid factors may also contribute to the etiology and alleviation of cancer.[3] Based upon these observations, 12 cancer patients have been treated using biofeedback as a stress reduction adjunct to their primary cancer therapy of surgery, chemotherapy, or radiation. One case is presented in detail in order to explicate the procedure of using clinical biofeedback and stress management exercises to help the individual patient adjust to this disease process. A 38-year-old woman was diagnosed with lymphoma by a biopsy of a right axillary node. Following 4 months of clinical biofeedback and stress management, the palpable nodes were reduced in size and abdominal echograms were normal.

The patient was referred by her oncologist for stress management since his diagnosis was that the lymphoma was of the nodular lymphoid type and incurable. Under these circumstances, she was advised to be reevaluated at a later time to determine whether chemotherapy would be appropriate if the disease progressed. During this waiting period, the patient became extremely tense and developed marked anxiety. At the time of the biofeedback

Presented to the Biofeedback Society, Orlando, Florida, March 4-8, 1977.

therapy, the patient was not undergoing any chemotherapy treatment of the lymphoma.

This woman was seen once per week for 15 sessions of 45 minutes in length. For the intake examination she reported compulsive rumination; it was determined that EEG feedback of the alpha rhythm over the left occipital lobe to lessen this anxiety would be used.[6] After five sessions the patient began a series of visualizations of her disease while keeping the alpha tone on. At the termination of therapy she reported less anxiety, and the palpable nodes of the lymphoma were reduced in size according to records obtained from her oncologist. An 11-month follow-up indicates that her condition is stable at the level reached at the end of the fifteenth biofeedback session.

This case presentation is intended to detail the *procedure* used with this patient and other individuals. A primary focus is on (1) pragmatic instructions in the meditation and relaxation posture used in conjunction with EEG feedback and (2) the visualization method employed with these patients. The outcomes of the other 11 patients are difficult to assess, although the intent of the procedure is to improve the quality of the patients' life by helping them to adapt to the psychosocial stress of cancer. All of the patients are alive at this point, although the case described here is the only instance of a remission.[1,2] Treatment is not necessarily oriented toward remission but toward stress management.

MEDITATION AND RELAXATION PROCEDURE*

Each session was structured in the following manner: (1) 10 minutes of assessing the previous week, (2) practice of the meditation exercise for 15 minutes while maintaining an alpha tone set at 8 to 12 Hz above 20 mV according to the Autogen 120 (Autogenic Systems Inc.), (3) 10 minutes of using the visualization method while maintaining alpha, and (4) 10 minutes to discuss outcome and suggest integrating them into the home practice, which consisted of repeating this entire procedure three times per day. Maintaining the alpha actively was intended to allow the patient to acknowledge the disease process while maintaining a state of diminished anxiety.

Details of the content of this particular patient's process are not detailed here. The main focus is on a simple set of instructions to help patients engage in a similar therapeutic procedure. It is written as a set of instructions for a potential patient, and some of the phrasing is deliberately not in complete sentences to convey a sense of the ongoing procedure. This section details a basic meditative posture followed by a visualization exercise that can be used with any physical or mental disorder for the self-regulation of that psychosomatic condition. Clearly the method employed here is similar to autogenic training, and a great deal of the effectiveness of this procedure is because of the clinical facility of autogenic exercises.[4,5] Also the method of maintaining a meditative posture is adapted from a basic Zazen sitting position.

• • •

One way to start the correct physical posture is to sit on the edge of an ordinary straight back chair so that just a small part of your thigh and your buttocks are on the chair. You should be neither too far forward nor slumped back in the chair, but sitting on the edge of the chair. The whole time that this first posture is established, your arms should be hanging straight down by your side.

Your first goal is to establish a balance from your waist down. This can be done most easily by sliding your right foot forward until you feel your weight coming back on your heel. Then slide your foot back toward you until you feel yourself coming up on the ball of your foot. Then just slide it back and forth until you feel a point at which your foot is flat on the floor—just resting very, very comfortably, neither too far forward nor too far back. Then do the same with the left foot. Slide it forward until you feel yourself going back on your heel, and then slide it back toward you until you feel yourself coming up on the ball of your foot. Then slowly move your foot back and forth trying to sense a balance point where your foot is flat on the floor. When you have both of your feet comfortably placed flat on the floor, there should be an angle of approximately 120° under your leg. An angle of 90° is much too acute, an angle greater than 120° tends to be too extended.

Now with your feet in that position and sitting on the edge of the chair, just allow your knees to fall open naturally. They should fall open approximately one foot. If you feel the muscles on the inside or the outside of your thighs straining, it means you are either holding your knees too close together or pushing them too far apart. Just let them fall open naturally and comfortably. At this point you should have established a three-point balance between the bottoms of your feet and your buttocks. It should be a very comfortable position without using any muscles to hold that position since it should be one of balance.

The next set of exercises is to help you balance the upper part of your body from the waist up. Again during this whole exercise your hands are hanging down by your side. You might at this point try closing your eyes. With your eyes closed, hold your back in an upright erect position—not with

*A tape recording of this meditation and visualization procedure is available from Psychology Today Cassettes, Ziff-Davis Publishing Company, One Park Avenue, New York, New York 10016.

the back muscles locked, but not slumped over your diaphragm. Very simply, hold your back firmly in an upright position. Holding your upper trunk and back in that position, with your eyes closed, allow yourself to move forward until you feel your lower back muscles pulling. Then lean back until you feel your abdominal muscles pulling. Very slowly move back and forth until you feel a point of balance at which neither your back muscles nor your abdominal muscles are pulling. That's a point of balance.

Imagine a "bo-bo" doll with a weighted bottom. Whenever you punch it, it comes back to center. Try establishing a kind of rocking and coming back to center. Once you are in that position, you might want to move a little bit forward until you just feel the slightest sense of your lower back muscles pulling. The reason for this is that most of us carry a great deal of tension in our backs and the muscles are likely to be slightly contracted. While we imagine ourselves to be perfectly balanced and upright, we tend to be leaning a little far back; so come a little bit forward.

The next step is to establish a point of balance for your head. Again with your eyes closed, just let your head roll forward until you feel the muscles in the back of your neck pulling. Let your head move back until you feel the muscles in the front of your neck pulling. You might lean your head to the left side and then to the right side. Again, imagine that your head is a ball and that you're trying to balance it at the end of your spinal column. Without holding, without effort, just try to balance it there.

There are two additional ways to help find that point of balance with your head. First, just as with the lower back, allow your head to come forward with your chin slightly tucked until you feel the trapezius muscles in the back of your neck pulling very slightly. Again, the reason for this is that we tend to contract those muscles and carry considerable tension there. Therefore, when we feel that we are balanced, it's very likely that actually we are back too far. Second, make sure to let go of tension in your jaw.

We've all been taught from about age 5 not to look like the "village idiot" with our jaw and mouth hanging open. The problem, though, is that we tend to lock our jaw and to carry a lot of tension in the masseter muscles; so allow your jaw to go limp and loose. A good way of doing this is to feel your tongue becoming very heavy with its weight resting comfortably in the base of your mouth, which allows your mouth to open very slightly. Now with this posture and with your hands down by your side, you should feel very balanced. There should be no effort to maintain this posture. As you practice you will find that you need less and less effort to maintain that position.

The next phase is to imagine a string running from the top of your head to the ceiling. Imagine that that thread is now pulling you straight up. Move your shoulders down, but feel as if your head and spinal column are being pulled straight up out of your body. Straighten and really sense the pulling until you feel a kind of isometric quaking and tension in your muscles. Do that for a few seconds until you really feel the isometric tension, and then imagine that the string is cut and let your head flop down over your chest like a limp doll. It's very important to let your head fall over your spinal column, but do this with a little bit of curvature to the spine. However, be sure not to collapse completely over your diaphragm and inhibit your breathing. This is one of the most difficult parts of the exercise.

There are two checks you can make to determine whether your head falls into the correct position. Just as your head falls forward at the end of its fall, you may feel a little twinge of pain as the muscles in the back of your neck stretch. That should be totally temporary. If it continues, it means that you probably are holding your head down and you should ease those muscles. On the other hand, if you feel an aching sensation as your head rolls forward, it means that you probably are holding on to tension in the neck muscles and what you really need to do is to really let go.

With your head down and with your

breathing very regular, allow your left hand to come up to your lap and flop as though it were a dead weight. Then allow your right hand to come up to your lap and flop as though it were a dead weight and very relaxed.

In this posture, for purposes of deep relaxation, you repeat the following phrase three times to yourself silently: "My left arm is heavy and warm." The rationale for doing this is not that the words themselves are significant, but it is a reminder to you to feel your hand becoming warmer. If you can sense your hand becoming warmer, then you are feeling the subjective component of vascular dilation in the periphery as an aspect of a general relaxation response indicated by an increased blood flow to the periphery. If you sense heaviness with your arms really becoming heavy, then that heavy feeling is the subjective sensation of muscular relaxation. The transition phrase between concentrating on your left arm and your right arm is "My forehead is cool." Repeat that three times as though there were a cool breeze blowing over your face to remind yourself to induce vascular constriction in the region of the head. Then you move the right arm and again repeat the phrase silently to yourself: "My right arm is heavy and warm."

Coming out of this exercise at the end of this procedure is as important as going into it. The way to end the exercise is to take a deep breath, bring your hands up to your chest, exhale, open your eyes, and stretch your legs, your arms, your fingers, your toes, and your face. Just sense how good it is to feel the tingling, the relaxation, and the energized sense of movement. This entire exercise can be repeated three times in succession. Generally it is suggested that this meditation exercise be repeated three times a day, preferably in the morning and in the afternoon.

VISUALIZATION EXERCISE

By using the basic physical posture, which induces a state of relaxation, it is possible to use a visualization method in conjunction with this exercise. After you

have said, "My right hand is heavy and warm," three times and entered the state of relaxation, you can then use a four-stage visualization exercise to engage the psychologic element of the psychosomatic disorder. This basic visualization can be used for any physical or mental disorder. There are just a few suggestions about visualization before starting the exercise.

Many individuals will insist that they close their eyes and don't see anything but black. Some of that phenomenon is the result of a misconception about visualization itself. Although the method is termed visualization, there needn't be an actual visual image with which a person works. Some individuals work with a tactile sensation such as something soft, hard, sticky, or cold. Also they have an olfactory sensation. In other cases they sense an audible tone. For some individuals who are very visual, they see images in color with a definite shape and form.

A second factor of visualization is that it may not involve a total picture but a fragment or a section of a picture. It may involve the hint of a form, like a sphere, or just simply a swatch of color, like red changing to blue. There need not be a total visual image, and that is very important to remember.

A third point is that most individuals, when they close their eyes and begin to visualize, think that immediately they are going to see everything in three dimensions, color, and quadraphonic sound. This is not usually the case, but this misconception prevents many people from working with visual images that in fact are available to them.

One simple exercise can be employed to give a sense of visualization. Just close your eyes and ask yourself how many windows there are in your living room at home. You will probably say some number of windows. Then ask yourself how did you know that number, and you will realize that when you closed your eyes you saw an image of your living room and counted the windows. That degree of vividness of what you saw is all that is required for you to be totally effective in working with the visualization process. There is no need to be any more vivid than that.

A fourth consideration is that what you see is definitely not as important as the fact that you are totally involved in the process. Many individuals who can visualize absolutely perfectly in great detail fail to become well. Other individuals who visualize in very abstract, childlike, or impressionistic ways can do a great deal better. In considering this observation, I have noted that in my clinical practice I find that individuals who know physiology and anatomy, like physicians and physiologists, tend to visualize very abstract or childlike forms. In contrast to this, individuals who are physiologically and anatomically naive tend to want to visualize in very graphic, anatomically precise ways. They want to know precisely what a hip joint, heart, or ulcer looks like. I think it is not so important that either of these modes is correct or that one is more correct than the other; what this observation does indicate is that the person is willing to enter into a different mode of perception from his normal one. It indicates that a patient gives up his normative associative processes and enters into and explores the disease or the disorder in an innovative way that encourages healing to take place.

One last consideration is that, if you are having difficulty visualizing and wish to visualize a little better, there is another very simple exercise you can do. Take any familiar object in your home. Look at that object, close your eyes, and try to see that object. It might be a lamp or a vase. Look at the lamp, close your eyes, and try to see the lamp in your internal visual field. Open your eyes and look at more detail before closing your eyes and trying to enhance the image. Let this go on until you get very familiar with how that lamp looks internally. Then try a lamp that you are not looking at directly but one that is familiar to you. Try to see that image. You might progress from that to making up an abstract lamp. This would enable you to sense *how* to visualize with various degrees of acuity.

Each state of this visualization requires approximately 3 to 4 minutes; so the whole visualization takes 10 to 12 minutes, a very short period of time. Staying in the relaxed meditative physical posture, first imagine yourself being in a place, either real or imaginary, where you feel perfectly safe. Preferably this place should be outdoors. When you get a sense of this place allow it to become vivid in as many sensory modalities as possible. Try to see all around you, 360 degrees. What's in back of you? What are you sitting on? Is it hard or soft? Is it gravel, dirt, or grass? If it's grass, how long is it? Is it dry? Is it green? As you listen, do you hear the trees rustling? Is there a stream nearby? Do you hear the ocean? Are you sitting on sand? What are the smells like? Are there flowers around? What season is it? Is it summer, winter, spring, or fall? Are there birds? Is the sky blue? Are there clouds in the sky? Is there a mountain range in the distance? Anything that you can feel or touch? Try to get a total sense of where you are so that it is as complete and vivid as possible. Once you are in this place, take approximately 2 or 3 minutes to make it very real and then enjoy it.

The second stage is to allow an image of your disorder to spontaneously appear in the gray or black area in front of your eyes. Just ask for it to spontaneously appear. Here is a critical point. If an image appears and you think, ''That's exactly the way I expected it to look,'' it is probably wrong because it has an element that is already familiar. When the unconscious speaks it is not likely to be terribly familiar at first. However, if a very unlikely image, a fragment of a very unlikely image, a sense, a smell, a tactile sensation, or a color appears, it's very likely to be useful. If nothing comes, you see absolutely nothing, and you sense a sort of frustration, then purposefully project an image you feel is representative of your disorder. If it's a headache, you might imagine a red jagged line. Once you project that image then allow it to change. Remember that you have projected that image deliberately and allow it to transform. With that image in mind, look at it with as much detail as possible. Imagine that it is a perfect crystal and that you want to turn it and see all of its facets without fascination or repugnance. You look at that image and feel its weight, color, texture, shape, and size with as much detail as possible. Take 2 or 3 minutes to do that. During this stage it is much more important that you realize that you are fully acknowledging the presence of and implications of your disorder in an anxiety-free state of deep relaxation. That is the critical variable more than what is actually being visualized.

The third stage is similar to the second stage. With that image in mind, transform it in a positive direction. You can tell a great deal in terms of monitoring your own visual images since many variations can occur. The image can change very rapidly, indicating a Pollyannish denial that is more of a wish fullfillment than an actual positive transformation. The image can become worse, indicating that you feel impotent or helpless. In another case, the image may refuse to change in a positive direction and will not be altered. You might experience a feeling of frustration or an inability to adequately adapt to this condition. Usually the image will simply begin to transform. If it is a black sticky viscous substance, the picture may become less sticky and lighter and turn to a gray ash. If the image is a jagged red line, it might become smooth and then become a serene blue color. It is important to allow that image to transform without pushing it. There is no need for it to go to completion. Just let the image evolve as far as is comfortable for approximately 2 or 3 minutes. Again, watch the transformation with as much detail as you watched the disorder.

At this point you are acknowledging an efficacy through an active participation in alleviating your condition. This psychologic factor is perhaps more important than what is being visualized. At the end of this positive transformation, simply allow the visual image to fade back into the gray or black field you sense in front of you.

Stage four involves becoming aware of yourself back in the place where you feel

perfectly safe, comfortable, and quiet. Acknowledge with all the modalities that you can and become aware of the fact that you can return to this place at any time, that it is immediately accessible to you, that this positive transformation has in fact taken place in your disorder, and that you can replicate this phenomenon at any time. Then come back to the physical posture that you maintained and come out of this visualization exercise in the same way that you came out of the meditative exercise, which is to bring your arms up to your chest, take a deep breath, exhale, open your eyes, stretch, and feel how good it is to move about again.

The visualization and meditation processes help treat symptoms, which are messages to you from your body that you have exceeded the level of stress your body can tolerate. A symptom is a perfect commentary on the fact that you are engaging in some activity or behavior that is self-destructive. A headache has a message; the activation of an ulcer has a message; the aggravation of a cancer condition has a specific message that you have exceeded your normal level of activity. The meditation and visualization process is a means of listening to the wisdom of your body and to the wisdom of your psychosomatic balance, and very simply you should ask yourself, "What is my symptom telling me about an aspect of my life that I need to modify and change to reduce excessive and illness-provoking stress, to maintain a higher level of health, and to prevent me from contracting a severe psychosomatic disorder?"

These exercises and visualizations are demonstrably effective when an individual practices in a conscientious manner. There are marked psychophysiologic changes that can take place, constituting a beneficial relaxation response that does occur. It is important to remember that the recreation of the parasympathetic response needs to be practiced like any other skill. The ability to let go of excessive stressful activity is not necessarily an innate endowment and literally needs to be practiced. At one point in our lives we knew how to do this, but for any number of reasons we have gradually learned to not attend to these biological cues because of various social rewards. Soon we loose the ability to enter a relaxed period of parasympathetic rebound. So all of these exercises are not teaching you a trick; they are helping you to relearn a skill that you had and have forgotten. This is a reacquisition, a relearning, of a previous skill. With very little practice it does return and has a lasting effect beyond those few minutes of practice. There is a tendency for the body to normalize and stabilize for increasingly long periods of time following the periods of meditation and relaxation.

SUMMARY

This concludes the instructions that can be used with a patient in applying meditation and visualization procedures for a wide variety of psychosomatic disorders. Results of this case are considered as a detailed example of similar procedures used with 12 cancer patients with a variety of metastatic diseases. Ongoing research is exploring the monitoring of each patient's immunologic response as an empirical index of stress response. Biofeedback and meditative relaxation procedures appear to be a useful adjunct to cancer therapy in helping the patient manage the stress associated with the course of this disease.

REFERENCES

1. Boyd, W.: The spontaneous regression of cancer, Springfield, Ill., 1966, Charles C Thomas, Publisher.
2. Everson, T. C., and Cole, W. H.: Spontaneous regression of cancer, Philadelphia, 1966, W. B. Saunders, Co.
3. Fox, B. H.: Premorbid psychological factors as related to incidence of cancer: Background for prospective grant applicants, Washington, D.C., 1976, National Cancer Institute.
4. Luthe, W., ed.: Autogenic methods, New York, 1969, Grune & Stratton, Inc.
5. Luthe, W., ed.: Autogenic therapy VI, New York, 1973, Grune & Stratton, Inc.
6. Pelletier, K. R.: Diagnostic and treatment protocols for clinical biofeedback, Journal of Biofeedback **2(4):**11-21, 1975.
7. Pelletier, K. R.: Mind as healer, mind as slayer: A holistic approach to preventing stress disorders, New York, 1977, Delacorte Press.
8. Selye, H.: The stress of life, New York, 1956, McGraw-Hill Book Co.

10

Therapeutic touch: the imprimatur of nursing

DOLORES KRIEGER

Therapeutic touch by the laying-on of hands looks absurdly simple but is profoundly complex. The act consists of the simple placing of the hands for about 10 to 15 minutes on or close to the body of an ill person by someone who intends to help or to heal that person. It is an ancient practice, recorded in the hieroglyphics, cuneiform writings, and pictographs of earliest literate cultures, and it persists to this day. However, it continues as it has been throughout the centuries: a little-understood enigma of a signally human interaction.

Touch is probably one of the most primitive sensations. Neurologically, touch and pain—two sensations one is very much involved with when helping ill people—are conducted by the central nervous system fibers that are myelinated earliest in the fetus. One of the first sensations that the newborn baby has, as he descends through the birth canal, is that of cutaneous stimulation. Developmental stages follow which derive their certainty from a whole series of touch experiences that evolve from the first gropings of hand-mouth exploration that tell us of our world, to the complexities of hand-eye coordinations by which we make the world our own. These functions, extending from the far reaches of time, are built into the very fiber of human development throughout life.

It is perhaps because touch is so primitive that it is so powerful a therapeutic tool. For instance, one can hardly imagine the most basic of nursing skills being performed without the act of touch. Indeed, touch is, so to speak, the imprimatur of nursing. Everyone, whether nurse or therapist, family member or friend, can look back on times when touch was extremely meaningful in a personal way. I have on file over 100 first-person accounts from nurses in this country and abroad which tell of the spontaneous use of touch quite unknowingly, or rather unknowledgeably, during acts of nursing intervention which brought therapeutic results so unusual that they frequently came as a surprise. It should be noted, however, that even the most renowned healers (and, I would suspect, nurses) do not claim greater than a 30 percent cure rate (1).

The therapeutic, comforting effects of touch are such common occurrences that most people become all but indifferent to them. Part of the reason for this may lie in the strong personal overlay that surrounds any act of touch, whose subjective nature understandably makes controlled study difficult. This limitation, together with the development of modern medical technologies, has been important in the progressive decline throughout most of the twentieth century in the practice of healing by the laying-on of hands.

EARLY STUDIES

In the early 1960's Bernard Grad, a Canadian biochemist, became interested in this phenomenon. With the cooperation of a renowned healer. Oskar Estebany, he conducted double-blind studies on mice and on barley seeds (2-4). In the former study, Grad selected 300 standardized mice and wounded them all in a specific manner. One third of the mice, used as a control group, were allowed to heal without outside intervention. Another 100 were treated by Estebany with the laying-on of hands. The remainder were held by medical students who did not profess to heal. After two weeks, healing in Estebany's group had accelerated to a degree that could have happened by chance less than once in a thousand times.

In the double-blind study on barley seeds, Grad soaked the seeds in saline solution to simulate a "sick" condition, and then divided them into groups, as in the experiment on mice. The first control group was watered by tap water, the second by water from flasks held by disinterested persons, and the third group (experimental group) was watered from flasks held by Estebany. The seeds which were watered with fluid from the flasks held by Estebany sprouted more quickly, grew taller, and had more chlorophyll than the seeds in the control groups.

In the late 1960's, another biochemist and enzymologist, Sr. M. Justa Smith, did further research on the laying-on of hands. Her basic assumption was that if an energy change occurs during healing, from whatever means, the change should be apparent at the enzymatic level, for it is the enzymes that are crucial to the basal metabolism of the body. She developed a double-blind study using the enzyme trypsin as the test object and Estebany as the healer (5). Trypsin solution was made fresh daily.

After dividing the trypsin solution into four aliquots, she exposed one fraction to high ultraviolet rays to break the bonding sites and thus simulate a "sick" condition. This fraction and a second unaltered fraction were held in flasks by Estebany for 75

minutes a day. A third fraction was kept in its natural state as a control, and the fourth sample was exposed to a high magnetic field. During the first hour of each day of the study, the sample held by Estebany and the sample exposed to the high magnetic field demonstrated similar qualitative and quantitative effects, as demonstrated by graphs of their daily relative percents of activity. Sr. Justa repeated these tests with other healers and also used a variety of other enzymes. Her conclusions were that the healer's ability does not affect all enzymes the same way—in fact, some are not affected at all. However, within the context of what enzymes do in the human body, the substantive effects all seem to contribute to improving or maintaining health (5).

OBSERVATIONS

I became interested in research on the laying-on of hands as a nurse. Both the Grad studies and those of Sr. Justa challenged me as a practitioner, teacher, and nurse researcher. However, because I am a nurse, my concern is with the total human being rather than the dissociated enzyme, or plants, or animals. I have concentrated on human studies to help clarify the underlying bioenergetics in people who were treated by the laying-on of hands.

Over several years I had an opportunity to use my nursing abilities during the few weeks each year that Estebany visited the United States to set up a temporary healing clinic with Dora Kunz, a well-known observer of paranormal healing (6). I took case histories, checked vital signs, and, in general, acted as a nurse as the need arose. Many people came from all over the country as patients. I was able to observe their interactions with the healer quite closely. What I saw was not startling. The atmosphere was friendly and quiet, and conversation, when it occurred, was natural and spontaneous. Estebany's touch was light and relaxed. To a casual observer it might have appeared that nothing was happening. However, a significant number of these patients got better. Most of them had verfied medical histories and had been referred by physcians who, when the patients returned for follow-up examination, confirmed their improvement. Nothing in my previous experience had prepared me for these findings, so I decided to study therapeutic touch in considerable detail.

SEARCHING FOR THE RELATIONSHIP

An extensive search of the literature from Western countries, however, did not yield a clue to the modus operandi of this healing process. I have a considerable background in the study of comparative religions, particularly the Eastern religions, so I reread material I had come upon several years ago for clues that might guide my search.

The East holds different assumptions about man and a different view of the dynamics of human relationships than the West, particularly about the personal interaction that occurs during the laying-on of hands. The basis for this interaction between healer and subject is thought to be a state of matter for which we in the West have neither a word nor a concept. In Sanskrit it is called *prana*. Our nearest translation would be vitality or vigor. Eastern literature states that the healthy person has an over-abundance of prana and that the ill person has a deficit. Indeed, the deficit is the illness(7). Prana can be activated by will and can be transferred to another person if one has the intent to do so. The literature also states that prana is intrinsic in what we would call the oxygen molecule(8).

As I pieced together the literature and previous research findings, I realized that my test object might well be hemoglobin. Hemoglobin is the oxygen-carrying pigment of the red blood cells which transfers oxygen to the tissues. I recalled that Grad's studies on barley seeds showed an increase in the chlorophyll content of the sample that had been irrigated with water that Estebany had held, and that chlorophyll and hemoglobin are tetrapyrroles and have a similar stereochemical structure. Their major differences are that the chlorophyll molecule has magnesium atoms at its center while the hemoglobin molecule centers about iron

atoms, and that there are some differences in the side chains. A second deduction, based on Sr. Justa's findings that enzymes are sensitive to the laying-on of hands, was that hemoglobin, both in its biosynthesis and in its utilization functioning, is involved with several enzyme systems. Therefore, it became apparent that studying hemoglobin would be a valid method to study the bioenergetics underlying the laying-on of hands.

In 1971 I conducted my first pilot study, using 19 ill persons in the experimental group and 9 ill persons in the control group. The ages and sexes of both groups were comparable. Estebany served as the healer(9). My substantive hypotheses were that the mean hemoglobin values of the experimental group after treatment by the laying-on of hands would exceed their before-treatment hemoglobin values, and that the mean hemoglobin values of the control group at comparable times would show no significant difference. My hypotheses were confirmed, the former at the .01 level of confidence. In 1972 I did a full-scale study, using 43 ill persons in the experimental group and 33 ill controls. The groups were comparable in sex and age distribution. Again the hypotheses were confirmed at the .01 level of confidence(10).

In 1973, I replicated my research with 46 subjects in the experimental group and 29 in the control group(11). This time I was able to control for a number of possible intervening variables which might affect hemoglobin values, such as the practice of meditation, breathing exercises by subjects who did yoga or strenuous exercises, biorhythm change, smoking (in reference to its effect on carboxyhemoglobin), diet, and medications. I also used a more rigorous instrument to determine hemoglobin values. My hypotheses were again confirmed at the $p. > .001$ level of confidence in spite of firmer control over the research design.

During these research studies, I became convinced that healing by the laying-on of hands is a natural potential in man, given at least two intervening variables that I think are critical to the process: the intent to help heal another, and a fairly healthy body (which would indicate an overflow of prana).

With the help of doctoral students who observed and took notes of my actions during the practice of therapeutic touch, I tried out these ideas. As a result, I know that when I lay my hands on or near an ill person he has a subjective sense of heat in the area that is ill or diseased, a sense of relaxation and well-being, and his hemoglobin values change following treatment. It can also be stated that faith on the part of the subject does not make a significant difference in the healing effect. Rather, the role of faith seems to be psychological, affecting his acceptance of his illness or consequent recovery and what this means to him. The healer on the other hand, must have some belief system that underlies his actions, if one is to attribute rationality to his behavior. Convinced that the practice of therapeutic touch is a natural potential in physically healthy persons who are strongly motivated to help ill people, and that this potential can be actualized, I conducted another study in 1974.

NURSES AS HEALERS

More than 75 registered nurses in metropolitan New York volunteered to take part in this research as healers. However, be- cause of the control which I thought necessary for the research design, only 32 nurses qualified for inclusion in the study. The more important delimitations were that the participating nurse had to secure the patient's informed consent, and the cooperation and permission of the patient's physician and the health facility's department of nursing. Where there was a board of research review in the health facility, a formal request for approval was presented, including materials on the proposed research and papers describing previous research.

Finally, nurses in the experimental group had to use therapeutic touch on a minimum of two patients. If the nurse was in the control group, she would do the simple touch required in routine nursing procedures but refrain from using the therapeutic touch involved in the laying-on of hands.

All participating nurses were taught methods of therapeutic touch by me or by Kunz, who had been my teacher. As an added precaution, tape recordings of both teaching sessions were compared for similarity.

I believe that there must be a strong motivation in a healthy person to help or to heal in order for therapeutic touch to be effective. Because these qualities are found in Maslow's concept of the self-actualized person, all participating nurses were asked

Mean standard scores of 32 RN's on 6 scales and the support ratio of the personal orientation inventory (POI)[1]

	POI Scales	Experimental (N = 16)	Control (N = 16)
*	Inner directed	54.2	52.1
	Self actualizing value	58.1	53.6
	Spontaneity	57.3	55.9
	Self-regard	55.9	53.1
	Self-acceptance	48.7	47.9
	Capacity for intimate contact	53.7	52.8
	**Support	1:3	1:2.8

*On the adult norms for the POI, the mean standard score for these scales is 50, with a standard deviation of 10.
**The ideal for self-actualizing persons is 1:3.
[1]Adapted from Shostrum, reference 13.

to answer a forced-choice questionnaire by Shostrum which is designed to measure self-actualization(12,13).

As the table shows, the means of both groups exceeded or approached the means for the self-actualized sample on whom the test was standardized. Based on Shostrum's interpretation, therefore, the general characteristics of all nurses participating in this study appeared to be inner directed, independent, self-supportive, freely expressive of feelings, possessing a high sense of self-worth, accepting of themselves in spite of weaknesses, and having a positive capacity for intimate contact. Furthermore, an appropriate proportion of their personal orientation was divided between a sensitivity to the opinions and approval of others and an inner directedness which guided their actions. These qualities, I believe, might well serve as a basic description of the humanistic nurse.

Pretest blood samples were drawn from all patients included in the study. Change in the mean hemoglobin value following treatment by therapeutic touch in the experimental group was chosen as the critical variable that would indicate the difference of this mode of treatment. Hemoglobin values were also determined at comparable times for the patients in the control group so that there were pre- and post-test hemoglobin values available for both groups. The laboratory technicians were not told that a study was going on and did not know that the patients were in any way differentiated from the rest of the health facility's population. A further delimitation was that only blood data analyzed by the same apparatus (Coulter) were included in the study; otherwise there would have been little basis for comparison of the data.

To ensure basic comparability, the pretest blood data of both groups of patients were statistically analyzed. No significant difference was found between the means of the initial hemoglobin values of the experimental and control groups. This comparability also held for the mean age and the proportion of either sex in each group. Both age and sex have important effects on hemoglobin.

The nurse experimental group consisted of 16 registered nurses who included treatment by therapeutic touch while caring for their patients; the control group included 16 registered nurses who gave nursing care to their patients without using therapeutic touch. Each nurse worked on two patients, for a total of 64 patients in the study.

The hypotheses were that following treatment by therapeutic touch the mean hemoglobin values of the patients in the experimental group would change significantly from their pretest value and that there would be no significant difference between the pre- and post-test hemoglobin values of the patients in the control group. These hypotheses were supported by statistical analysis (Fisher's t Test for the Difference Between Correlated Means) at the .001 level of significance. For the control group, the difference between the pre- and post-test means was not statistically significant.

As technology and research grow more sophisticated, research findings of a previous day frequently are seen to be but artifacts of a deeper reality. I well realize that future studies may relegate current research on hemoglobin change as a function of therapeutic touch to that category. Nevertheless, the results of these studies hold many significant inferences for the broad spectrum of nursing. There is need for deeper studies on therapeutic touch and serious discussion of these inferences. I invite the reader to the dialogue.

REFERENCES

1. Harry Edwards, quoted in Hammond, Sally. *We are All Healers*. New York, Harper and Row, 1973, p. 129.
2. Rorvik, D. M. The healing hand of Mr. E. *Esquire* 81:70, 154, 156, 159-160, Feb. 1974.
3. Grad, Bernard, and others. The influence of an unorthodox method of treatment on wound healing in mice. *Int. J. Parapsychol.* 3:5-24, Spring 1961.
4. Grad, Bernard. A telekinetic effect on plant growth. Part 2. Experiments involving treatment of saline in stoppered bottles. *Int. J. Parapsychol.* 6:473-498, Autumn 1964.

5. Smith, Sister M. J. Paranormal effects on enzyme activity. *Hum. Dimensions* 1:15-19, Spring 1972.

6. Karagulla, Shafica. *Breakthrough to Creativity*. Los Angeles, DeVorss and Co., 1967, pp. 123-146.

7. Govinda, A. B. *Foundations of Tibetan Mysticism*. London, Rider and Co., 1969, pp. 122, 137, 148, 150-159.

8. Athawa-Veda, Hymn to Prana. In *Prashnopanishad,* verse XI, line 47.

9. Krieger, Dolores. The response of in-vivo human hemoglobin to an active healing therapy by direct laying-on of hands. *Hum. Dimensions* 1:12-15, Autumn 1972.

10. _____. The relationship of touch, with intent to help or to heal, to subjects' in-vivo hemoglobin values: a study in personalized interaction. In *American Nurses' Association Ninth Nursing Research Conference,* held at San Antonio, Tex., Mar. 21-23, 1973, Kansas City, Mo., Amercian Nurses' Association, 1974, pp. 39-58.

11. _____. Healing by the laying-on of hands as a facilitator of bioenergetic change: the response of in-vivo human hemoglobin. *Psychoenergetic Systems,* Vol. 3, number 3, 1974.

12. Maslow, A. H. *Motivation and Personality*. New York, Harper and Brothers, 1954.

13. Shostrum, E. L. *Personal Orientation Inventory Manual*. San Diego, Calif., Educational and Industrial Testing Service, 1966.

11

Psychobiological aspects of "spontaneous" regressions of cancer

GOTTHARD BOOTH

THE SOMATIC VERSUS THE PSYCHODYNAMIC CONCEPT

Reports of spontaneous regression of cancer have been published from time to time, but isolated cases met with widespread medical scepticism. This attitude cannot be maintained any longer. In 1966, Everson and Cole, two surgeons, reviewed the more than 700 publications which reported the phenomenon since 1900, and documented in detail 176 histologically proven cases. The authors defined "spontaneous" as "regression in absence of any external factor." They hypothesized the agency of any one of several accidental events within the organism, none of which could be substantiated.

The monograph of 560 pages completely ignores the steadily growing number of scientific publications asserting the influence of psychological factors on cancer. They were reviewed in 1959 by LeShan. My own research (1965-1969[1]) led me to the following conclusions.

1. As infants, cancer patients experienced traumatic frustration in their mother relationship. Their personalities bear the imprint of dominant pregenital fixations.

2. The life histories of precancerous indi-

viduals are characterized by a desperate need for control of a specific object which may be a personal relationship, a socioeconomic career, or a vocation in the arts or sciences.

3. The neoplastic process began when the patient experienced the irreparable loss of control over his idiosyncratic object. The loss could be caused by external events, by declining vitality, or by both factors.

4. The neoplastic process is localized in the organ whose function dominated in the genetic make-up of the patient, and consequently determined the nature of the object to be controlled.

5. The tumor represents the internalized lost object in keeping with Freud's (1920) classical description of the psychodynamics of depression.

6. The course of the disease depends upon the balance of power between the unconscious satisfaction derived from the neoplastic process, and the satisfactions derived from the remaining object relationships.

The preceding insights into the dynamics of cancer were gained by applying Freud's method and basic discoveries to the biographies and the Rorschach imagery of 115 patients. The history of Freud's own life, as described by Jones (1953, 1957) and Schur (1972), dramatically illustrates the genesis of his cancer.

The fateful imprint was received when

Reprinted from Journal of the American Academy of Psychoanalysis 1:303-307, 1973. Reprinted by permission of John Wiley & Sons, Inc.

the very intense relationship between Freud's mother and her "golden Sigi" was disturbed by the very early arrival of a brother who died before Freud was two years old.

Jealousy and possessiveness characterized Freud's attitude toward his wife, his followers, and his theories. The early infantile resentment against his mother found expression in the antifeminine dogma that castration fear and penis envy are the "organic rock-bottom of psychoanalysis." On the level of somatic self-expression, Freud was so dependent on heavy cigar smoking that he did not stop even after oral cancer had developed.

The neoplasia of the jaw began when, at the age of 70, Freud faced the impending loss of his most beloved grandson, Heinele. As he wrote in later years, this death affected him more deeply than any other. He was never able to become fond of anyone after that misfortune, and found the blow more unbearable than his cancer. Nevertheless, for 16 years Freud's will to live was maintained by unceasing devotion to his work.

On the last day of his life, Freud read Balzac's *La Peau de Chagrin* and called it a "story of starvation." Both Jones and Schur failed to mention that the actual content of the story expresses the infantile fantasy which, for 82 years, Freud had repressed, but throughout his adult life symbolically expressed by way of compulsive cigar smoking. The protagonist of the philosophical fairy tale finds himself dying, with the power of having one last wish fulfilled. He breaks down the locked door of his mistress and expires *biting her breast*.

Freud certainly knew the content of the story when he selected it as his final reading matter. Dying from cancer of the jaw, he put into concrete form the definition of the death instinct which he (1920) had given three years before the illness: "(his) striving to safeguard (his) own individual path toward death."

I have given the preceding description of the psychodynamics of cancer in some detail because it provides the necessary background for understanding the factors involved in regression of the neoplastic process. Specifically, I hope to clarify that "spontaneous" regression involves the same dynamics which account for the prognosis of cancer in general.

THE DYNAMICS OF CANCER THERAPY

Physicians and laymen are equally aware that the prognosis of an individual cancer patient is unpredictable. To counteract the resulting anxiety, the most *concrete* elements of current therapies have been emphasized: early detection and radical destruction of the tumor. Nevertheless, even under seemingly ideal conditions, some cases end badly, whereas other, apparently hopeless cases completely recover.

Since 1926, when Evans discovered the role of the idiosyncratic object relationship in neoplasis, more and more observers have become aware that the prognosis depends not only upon the perfection of surgery and radiology, but also on *rehabilitation* with respect to the lost object relationship.

Under conditions of conventional therapy this need is frequently satisfied without the conscious help of the physician. Two basic processes are involved.

1. Family and friends frequently respond to the discovery of a malignancy as they would to a suicidal attempt. They understand the evident jeopardy of life as a signal of distress, and rally in efforts to make the sick happy. Although the causal relationship between depression and cancer is not part of contemporary thinking, those close to the cancer patient are apt to know something about his emotional needs.

2. The other factor influencing the social rehabilitation of the cancer patient is his *psychological reaction* to the crisis in his life. His recovery depends on his capacity for replacing the lost object relationship by a new one. This is difficult for these constitutionally rather inflexible characters, but we know from the neurophysiological work of Eccles (1953, 1970) that the experience of a crisis can result in the mobilization of ex-

traordinary psychological resources. Under great stress, the electronic activities in the synapses reach a level which enables the will to steer the configuration of excitation in the neuronic network. To put it less abstractly, in the state of high cortical excitement the opportunity arises for establishing a *new object relationship*. Sargant (1969) describes the same phenomenon as the establishment of a new faith, explaining it in terms of Pavlovian psychology. Although theoretically independent from each other, both Eccles and Sargant confirm the first aphorism of Hippocrates which attributes to the crisis a strategic role in healing (Booth 1969[2], 1973).

The role of the brain in the development of cancer has been clarified by extensive clinical and experimental work of Kavetskii and his school (1960). Specifically, Balitsky (1969), demonstrated that animals as well as human beings respond to the presence of neoplastic tissue in the organism with abnormally heightened cortical activity. When the defenses of the organism fail, cortical activity declines to an abnormally low level. In case the neoplasias are resorbed, the depressed phase does not occur and cortical activity returns to the normal level.

Cases of so-called spontaneous regression of cancer are of great practical importance because they prove that the psychosocial process between patient and environment can cure neoplasia without any physical attack on the tumor itself. Surgical and radiological therapy are methods which can bring about the critical change, but many times nonmedical agencies have the same effect. Several case histories of Everson and Cole (1966) report that the regression of tumors coincided with treatments as diverse as intercessory prayer, conversion to Christian Science, mudpacks, vitamin therapy, and force-feeding. They have only one thing in common, *faith in the procedure*. Unfortunately, the authors were so convinced of the irrelevance of the psyche that the concept occurs only in the last paragraph of the book: "The remote possibility of spontaneous regres-

sion of cancer may be of some psychotherapeutic value in the patient with cancer that is not amenable to surgical or radiation treatment."

Considering the psychosomatic literature and my own observations, I have drawn a more optimistic conclusion from the existence of so-called spontaneous regression: orthodox and unorthodox therapies are effective if, under the impact of the existential crisis, the patient puts faith in the procedure and can use it for his psychosocial rehabilitation. I will come back to this point in a moment, but first I would like to discuss the psychodynamic aspect of surgery and radiation. As I previously stated (1965, 1969[1]), neoplasia develops in the organ that represents the genetically *dominant* function of the individual organism, following the loss of its object. Physical reduction of the overvalued organ, therefore, has symbolic meaning. The sacrifice may give a healthy direction to the post-operative psychological orientation. Unorthodox healing methods, however, prove that *physical* sacrifice is not always necessary for the cure of the neoplastic process. The occasional successes of quacks have been a blessing for the theoretical understanding of the dynamics of cancer therapy, but a great risk for the general public. The latter is easily led to believe that the secret of the success resided in a repeatable act of the healer. This one-sided concept of therapy also bedevils many medical practitioners.

Having outlined my interpretation of surgery and radiology, I wish to qualify my emphasis on the psychological needs of cancer patients. Most of them have made good reality adjustments and are capable of benefiting from support which addresses itself to the overt situation, i.e., they are depressed, seriously ill, and faced with somatic and social uncertainties. They are at a loss in the depersonalized atmosphere of modern hospitals (Booth 1966, 1967). Under these conditions, humane concern with the concrete situation can produce the miracle of seemingly spontaneous regression, for instance:

1. A woman in her sixties was found to have an inoperable cancer of the pancreas. She returned to her home expecting to die. At this point her daughter, a devout Catholic, prayed for the recovery of her mother with whom she had been on bad terms for as long as she could remember. She finally wanted a reconciliation and her mother responded with what seemed to be a complete recovery. After 14 months of a harmonious relationship, the mother's health suddenly declined and a new operation was performed. It was found that the original tumor had regressed so much that it could have been removed if a small part of the tumor had not entered the bile duct (personal observation).

2. At the age of 63, composer Bela Bartok was found to be in what seemed to be the terminal stage of leukemia. He had been very depressed by the lack of response to his work in America. Unexpectedly, Serge Koussevitzky visited him in the hospital and commissioned him to write a work for the Boston Symphony Orchestra. It immediately became apparent that Bartok had taken a new lease on life. He returned to the South and wrote the most successful of his 106 works: the "Concerto for Orchestra" which had its premiere in the following year. He then composed his "Third Piano Concerto" and finished all but the last 17 bars when the final recurrence of leukemia killed him 27 months after the visit of Koussevitzky (Heinsheimer 1968).

3. Before leaving for a vacation, LeShan (1970) had noticed a completely withdrawn terminal case on the ward. When he returned, the old man had been discharged very much improved. Neither the physician nor the nurse had an explanation, only the occupational therapist. She had repeatedly tried to involve the patient in her work, but he had persistently refused. One day she observed the patient's response to the visit of his grandchild, and she suggested that he make a toy for the little girl. To this opportunity for reestablishing a human relationship, the patient responded, and he improved so much that he could return to his family.

These three incidents illustrate the same point I first made in abstract form: that psychological support is effective if the patient *can use it* for his psychosocial rehabilitation. The following case history of Shapiro (1963) makes clear the futility of exploiting the suggestibility of a patient without providing a satisfactory objective for maintaining his improvement. The patient had been hospitalized with multiple, orange-sized sarcomas. After one day of Krebiozen treatment, the tumors shrank to half the original size, the patient returned home and held his own for two months. Then, after reading a critical report on Krebiozen, he suffered a relapse. The physician reassured him and gave him an injection of a saline solution which he represented as "double-strength Krebiozen." Again the patient responded, became ambulatory and symptom-free for more than two months. He suffered a relapse after reading that the American Medical Association had taken a firm stand against the claims of the inventor of Krebiozen. Within a few days he had to return to the hospital where he died on the second day. Since his last improvement had been based upon his faith in the physician, the disease became fatal after discovering that he had been fooled.

Recognition of the decisive role of psychosocial rehabilitation in seemingly spontaneous cases of regression implies that this factor ought to be considered in all orthodox cancer therapy. Whereas Everson and Cole felt that all cases of spontaneous regression were due to mere "coincidence" with unorthodox, physically ineffective treatments, the truth about the successes of orthodox therapies seems to be that they are due to *coincidence* with external and psychological opportunities for social rehabilitation. Such opportunities are easily missed if the patient is told that his salvation depends entirely on somatic procedures. This approach condemns him to passive submission and enhances his original pathogenic experience that he has lost control over the object relationship which had made his life worth living.

Rational cancer therapy requires that the

patient is encouraged to accept responsibility for resolving the existential crisis of which the neoplasia is the somatic expression. From this point of view certain general principles of psychological management follow.

1. The patient must be allowed to know the truth *completely;* not only that he has cancer, but also that his own attitude will influence the prognosis.

2. Since a rational response to the crisis is crucial, the patient's mind should not be manipulated by means of psychotropic drugs. As Sargant (1969) pointed out, their effect reduces the potential for a creative response to the crisis, a point ignored by Mastrovito (1966).

3. The anxieties and guilt feelings of the patient should not be intensified by blaming him for having delayed seeking medical help, or for not having heeded the authoritative warnings against cigarettes.

4. The verdict "inoperable cancer" should be qualified by pointing out that even these cases may regress *if* the patient finds a solution to his pathogenic situation.

5. An attempt should be made to clarify the pathogenic situation.

The therapist who tries to implement the proceeding guide lines is likely to find himself confronted with problems of communication with the patients, particularly in our age of popular faith in the *physical* conquest of nature in general, and of cancer in particular.

COMMUNICATION WITH CANCER PATIENTS

Prior to the present century, it was common medical knowledge that cancer is a symptom of depression (LeShan 1959). Today physicians are discouraged from asking personal questions because they are expected to deal only with the "purely physical" disease. Even if they want to know something about the psychological state of the patient, they are apt to be awkward because they do not wish to appear "nosey."

The problem of the physician is compounded by the fact that cancer patients are very secretive, as Kissen (1963) and I (1965) discovered independently. These patients were born with an above average need for affection and experienced traumatic frustration in their mother relationship. Never having developed Erikson's (1962) "basic trust," they protect themselves throughout life by a possessive attitude concerning all important elements in their personal lives.

Since the tumor represents the lost vital object, it keeps alive the narcissistic injury. At the same time it causes guilt feelings, at the very least, on an unconscious level. Being strongly fixated on the anal level, cancer patients are particularly sensitized to the infantile implication of loss of object control: *soiling.* This moralistic aspect of cancer explains the observation of Goldsen (1957) and Gold (1964) that these patients delay seeing a physician, particularly after ominous symptoms have become manifest.

Feeling personally accepted, the cancer patient often is capable of establishing sound communication with the therapist, but, in an unknown number of cases, the anal object relationship has created conscious, realistic guilt. Such persons rather die than disclose the origin of their guilt feelings, particularly if nothing can be done about the specific predicament. The following two personal observations will illustrate this point.

1. A 36 year old man had been in psychotherapy for one year because of a seemingly endogenous depression which had been steadily deepening. His physical health had been excellent until one day he complained about having caught the flu. Although his cough was slight, I insisted on an x-ray and it proved that he had a very small opacity suggesting an easily operable lung cancer. The patient refused an operation for six weeks, by which time surgery revealed that the tumor had become inoperable. Obviously, I inquired from the moment of the first somatic symptom what had occurred preceding the physical illness. The answer was always "nothing at all." Two years after the death of the patient, a married woman came to see me. I had known that she and my patient had entertained a mocking flirtatious

relationship since their college days. Three days before the "flu" started, my patient disclosed to the woman that he was passionately in love with her, tried to seduce, and finally, to rape her. Finding himself firmly rejected, he felt unbearably humiliated without any hope for his future.

2. A 57 year old business woman came to see me because six months after the death of her husband she had developed metastases of a breast cancer which had been operated on 12 years previous. The metastases were localized in two cervical vertebrae which had partly collapsed and caused excruciating pain in spite of an orthopedic collar. Her response to supportive psychotherapy was nearly instantaneous. Within ten days she discarded her plastic collar, returned to full time work in her office, and for a whole year led a very active social life, although, after six months, symptoms of lung metastases had become manifest. Since she had recovered six years earlier from lung metastases, following radiation and ovariectomy, I tried to find out what had happened at that time. The answer to all questions was "nothing." Eventually she became hospitalized and deteriorated more and more. When I visited her for the last time, she could only talk with great effort, but unexpectedly volunteered information on what had happened at the time of her first pulmonary episode. She was following the coffin of her father to the grave when she complained to her husband about shortness of breath. She had been feeling very guilty at that time because she had kept her father in a cheap nursing home, not wanting to sacrifice her own freedom of enjoying the theater, concerts, and travel. When her husband died very suddenly, she found herself threatened by her father's fate. Because her husband had never made a will, his children from a previous marriage claimed their share of the money which would have secured a comfortable retirement income.

The two preceding cases should make everybody sceptical of claims that neoplasias are purely somatic and require only somatic therapy. At the same time, the cases exemplify the limits which certain life situations set for the physician.

To understand the extraordinary resistance against considering the psychosocial dimension of cancer, one must take in account that industrialized societies depend, to a very large extent, on anal motivations of their members. This situation can exist only at the expense of nonmaterialistic values. Guilt feelings, therefore, are widespread even among the more than 80% of people who are not cancer prone. Then early universal reaction to this guilt is *denial*. The denial is implicit in the dogma that cancer can be cured by the physical sciences. The *intensity* of the guilt is reflected, most tellingly, in the vast amount of money spent in support of this dogma in spite of the lack of results. The acceptance of so many extraordinary measures to prolong life, without concern for its quality, often seems to be explained by guilt.

In the face of this popular prejudice, cures of cancer without scientific blessings are quickly forgotten as if they were nonsense syllables. The story of Sir Francis Chichester provides a fascinating example. From 1960, until his death in 1972, newspapers and magazines have made him a well-known man on account of his numerous exploits as a single-handed sailor. Since newspaper files have an unfailing memory, the public always has been reminded of the fact that Chichester's sailing career had begun after his "spontaneous" recovery from lung cancer at the age of 57. Chichester was sufficiently aware of the psychological background of this experience that, in 1964, he wrote his autobiography, a unique document for anybody interested in understanding the psychodynamics of lung cancer. Nevertheless, as I confirmed in many lectures, nearly everybody seems to have forgotten his lung cancer, even those people who are interested in psychosomatic medicine. Eventually, even Chichester became embarrassed by his unorthodox recovery. Ten years after the event, I asked him whether the cuts of his autobiography, mentioned by the editor, included the part of the manuscript dealing with the cancer episode. He answered: "I am glad that you are interested in my account of my illness, but I regret I do not wish to write anymore about it; in fact, I had hoped not even to think about it anymore after I had written my story."

THE ATTITUDE OF THE MEDICAL PROFESSION

Although many physicians have published observations of seemingly spontaneous regression of cancer, they share the feelings of Sir Francis: they do not wish to think about it any more. Today, however, *thinking* about the phenomenon has become more important than further documentation that it exists.

The fact is that the death toll of neoplastic disease has been steadily rising over the last 120 years although an ever increasing amount of scientific research has been devoted to the problem. Practically all these efforts have been based on molecular and cytological models of the disease. The conclusion ought to be drawn that these models are inadequate, but so far only one leading oncologist, Sir David Smithers (1964) has taken the stand that cancer cells are effects of *organismic disorganization*, "repercussions, not driving forces." The concepts of Smithers cover the dynamics of the so-called spontaneous regressions of neoplastic disease. Systematic biographical studies confirm that neoplasia is the localized symptom of a traumatic interaction between the patient and his human environment. If, intentionally or accidentally, the traumatic interaction ceases, healing can take place.

Although the application of the cytological approach to cancer has failed in practice, the majority of the medical profession continues to cling to it. This can only be understood as the symptom of a collective neurosis. Faced with the threat of a deadly disease which allegedly can strike everybody, modern scientists and laymen are too anxious to think clearly and constructively. The consequence is a regression to pre-

logical faith in magic, based on the spectacular achievements of physics and chemistry: the scientific control of inanimate matter seems to promise the conquest of animate nature. The recent lavish government funding of cancer research was justified by the reasoning that money made the moon shots possible, and would therefore also conquer cancer. This irrational mood ignores the lesson of the ecological crisis, not to mention the many leading scientists who, in the last three decades, have demonstrated the supramolecular dimensions of animate nature; physicists like Schroedinger (1945), biologists like Portmann (1967), physiologists like Eccles (1970) and Selye (1967), physicians like Ellerbroek (1973) and Siirala (1973).

The repression of the psychological dimensions of the cancer problem among oncologists is particularly evident in the fact that nobody seems to have been interested in pursuing the observation of Koroljow (1960) who treated two deeply depressed patients with inoperable cancers by insulin coma. For at least two years the tumors completely regressed and the depressions disappeared. Apparently the connection of cancer and depression aroused too much anxiety among somaticists, although Koroljow interpreted his results on the cytological level. Only Goldfarb (1967), another psychiatrist, tried to follow Koroljow's lead, but his results were less convincing because he combined ECT with conventional methods. Considering the number of inoperable cancer patients, and the availability of insulin and ECT, the lack of interest from cancer institutes is very revealing.

Everson and Cole, by their documentation of the reality of "spontaneous" regressions of cancer, unintentionally strengthened the position of these who hope that more and more physicians will abandon the purely physical approach, and rediscover the potential of medicine as a humanistic art, integrating physical science and psychological understanding. The way back will not be easy, because humanistic therapy presupposes capacity for personal direct relationships. As I pointed out in 1969, this capacity was progressively impaired by the Industrial Revolution and its impact on the first year of life, the undercutting of the roots of basic interpersonal trust by the progressive depersonalization of nursing. The result was the transformation of the tuberculosis epidemic into the cancer epidemic which began in the middle of the last century. It progressed parallel with the scientific depersonalization of infant care, so fully analyzed by Spitz (1965).

Scientific depersonalization of medicine is certainly responsible for the sad state of the cancer problem. As the techniques of diagnosis˙ and therapy became more demanding, correspondingly less time became available for attention to the *human situation* of the patient. During the last ten years, however, there has been a growing number of meetings and papers on psychosomatic cancer research. Should this development persist, we may expect to hear more about regressions of cancer, and fewer physicians may find them mysterious.

SUMMARY

1. Sometimes cancer regresses in the absence of physical manipulation aimed at destroying the cancer cells. Such regressions of cancer are not spontaneous but responses of the organism to a favorable change in the psychosocial situation of the patient.

2. So-called spontaneous cases of regression agree with the concept that cancer is the reaction of a pregenitally fixed personality against the loss of a vitally important object relationship.

3. Healing is mediated by the defense reaction of the cerebral cortex against cancerous tissue. The healing potential can be aided by physicians who utilize the plasticity of the brain function in a state of crisis.

4. The capacity of patients for cooperation with the therapist is limited by their intrinsic secretiveness and guilt feelings, compounded by the pervasive aura of pessimism surrounding cancer. These limitations make the psychotherapeutic approach difficult, but not impossible.

5. Physicians, confronted with these difficult patients, are often reluctant to invest the necessary time in view of the uncertainty of the results. This negative approach is rationalized in terms of the prevailing prejudice that cancer is a disease of cellular origin. This prejudice is based upon the fantasy that animate nature can be manipulated by methods which have proved successful in controlling inanimate matter.

6. The growing evidence of the unpredictable results of purely somatic therapy gives reason for hope that the emphasis of cancer therapy will shift from physical destruction of the tumor to reconstruction of the patient's relationship with his human environment.

REFERENCES

Balitsky, K. P., et al. (1969). Some psychophysiological peculiarities of the nervous system in malignant growth, *Ann, N.Y. Acad. Sci.,* **164**(2), 520-525.

Booth, G. (1965), Irrational complication of the cancer problem, *Amer. J. Psychoanal.* **25**, 41-55.

Booth, G. (1966), The cancer patient and the minister, *Pastoral Psychol.* (Feb.), 15-24.

Booth, G. (1967), Physicians, clergymen and the hospitalized patient, *J. Amer. Med. Ass.,* **200**, 334-335.

Booth, G. (1969[1]), General and organ-specific object relationships in cancer, *Ann. N.Y. Acad. Sci.,* **164**(2), 568-577.

Booth, G. (1969[2]), The auspicious moment in somatic medicine, *Amer. J. Psychoanal.,* **29**, 84-88.

Booth, G. (1973). The auspicious moment in somatic medicine, in *The Auspicious Moment,* H. Kelman (Ed.), to be published, Jason Aronson, New York.

Chichester, F. (1964), *The Lonely Sea and the Sky.* Hodder & Stoughton, London.

Eccles, J. C. (1965), *The Neurophysiological Basis of Mind,* Clarendon, Oxford.

Eccles, J. C. (1970), *Facing Reality.* Springer Verlag, New York.

Ellerbroek, W. C. (1973), Hypotheses toward a unified field theory of human behavior with clinical application to acne vulgaris, *Perspec. Biol. Med.,* **16**, 240-261.

Erikson, E. H. (1962), *Childhood and Society,* Norton, New York.

Evans, E. (1926), *A Psychological Study of Cancer.* Longmans, Green & Co., New York.

Everson, T. C. and W. H. Cole, (1966), *Spontaneous Regression of Cancers,* Saunders, Philadelphia.

Freud, S. (1917), Mourning and melancholia, *Stand. Ed.,* **14,** 237-260.

Freud, S. (1920), Beyond the pleasure principle, *Stand. Ed.* **18,** 3-64.

Freud, S. (1937), Analysis terminable and interminable, *Stand. Ed.,* **23,** 209-253.

Gold, M. A. (1964), Causes of patient's delay in diseases of the breast, *Cancer,* **17,** 564-577.

Goldfarb, C. et al. (1967), Psychophysiologic aspects of malignancy, *Amer. J. Psyciat.* **123,** 1545-1552.

Goldsen, R. K. et al. (1957), Some factors related to the patient delay in seeking diagnosis for cancer symptoms, *Cancer,* **10,** 1-7.

Heinsheimer, H. (1968), *Best Regards to Aida,* Knopf, New York.

Jones, E. (1953, 1957), *Freud Vol. I, III.* Basic Books, New York.

Kavetskii, R. (1960), *The Neoplastic Process and the Nervous System.* Nat. Sci. Found., Washington.

Kissen, D. M. (1963), Personality characteristics in males conducive to lung cancer, *Brit. J. Med. Psychol.,* **36,** 27-36.

Koroljow, S. (1962), Two cases of malignant tumors with metastases apparently treated successfully with hypoglycemic coma, *Psychiat. Quart.,* **36,** 1-10.

LeShan, L. L. and Worthington, R. E. (1956), Some recurrent life history patterns observed in patients with malignant diseases, *J. Nerv. Ment. Dis.,* **124,** 460-465.

LeShan, L. L. (1959), Cancer and personality: A critical review, *J. Nat. Cancer Inst.,* **22,** 1-18.

LeShan, L. L. (1970), private communication.

Mastrovito, R. C. (1966), Acute psychiatric problems and the use of psychotropic medication in the treatment of the cancer patient, *Am. N.Y. Acad. Sci.,* **125**(3), 1006-1010.

Portmann, A. (1967), *Animal Forms and Patterns.* Schocken, New York.

Sargant, W. (1969), The physiology of faith, *Brit. J. Psychiat.,* **115,** 505-518.

Schroedinger, E. (1945), *What is Life?* Macmillan, New York.

Schur, M. (1972), *Freud Living and Dying.* International Universities Press, New York.

Selye, H. (1967), *In Vivo (The Case for Supramolecular Biology).* Liveright, New York.

Shapiro, A. K. (1963), Psychological aspects of medication, in *Psychological Basis of Medical Practice,* H. I. Leif, V. F. Lief, and N. R. Lief (Eds.), Hoeber, New York, 163-178.

Sürala, M. (1969), *Medicine in Metamorphosis: Speech, Presence and Integration.* Tavistock Publications, London.

Smithers, D. W. (1964), *On the Nature of Neoplasia in Man.* Livingstone, Edinburgh.

Spitz, R. (1965), *The First Year of Life.* International Universities Press, New York.

PART IV

Emotional impact on health professional and patient

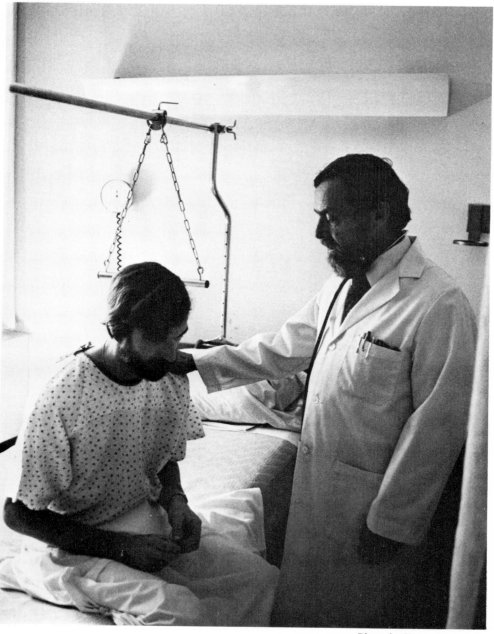

Photo by Katrin P. Achelis

12

The burn-out syndrome and patient care

CHRISTINA MASLACH

The Physician's Game: Mr. Oldman is dying but I must be careful not to let him know this. He asks too many questions. I wouldn't want him jumping out of the window if he found out the truth. Besides, I can't be absolutely sure myself; there *are* miracles in this business. It's not likely in his case, of course; a man eighty-three with cancer and a bad heart doesn't recover. Besides, he's comfortable. The drugs keep him drowsy most of the time. And none of us are going to live forever, are we? It's when he's awake that he gets curious about himself. If he would just leave the treatment to me. He's a child, really, someone you have to pamper. Why do you think I run all these tests? Mr. Oldman is fascinated with tests. They keep him busy, keep him from worrying about himself . . . They don't tell us anything but they do keep his hopes up. I'm not going to let him fall into a depression.

But those questions! I really dread calling on Mr. Oldman. Why do I swing my stethoscope when I go in his room? It distracts him. As I say, he's like a child. But I don't lie to him outright; the words I use, like eschemia and pancreatic tumor, don't seem to mean much to him. And the words he does understand, like inflammation, are quite appropriate to explain his pain . . . It may sound odd for a doctor to say, but death frightens me. I suppose I see too much of it. And

if it frightens me, what does it do to others? No, Mr. Oldman must not find out that he is dying. If he keeps up those questions, I'll order a suction tube for him. That way he can't talk. And what with the tests and maybe an operation, he'll be too preoccupied to care. There's no reason why his last days shouldn't be as comfortable as possible. Thank God, I'm being paged; I can leave now. Remind me to ask the chaplain to look in on Mr. Oldman more often.

The Nurse's Game: Mrs. Oldwoman keeps asking me why she doesn't get better. Even if I knew, I don't think I'd tell her. Dr. Busy doesn't tell me anything either; besides, I think the patient knows more than she lets on. It's hell on the geriatric ward. You can't really make contact with these people. They're like little children. You know they're going to die, so why bother? Oh, I feel sorry for them all right; I do my best to take care of them—that's my job. But that call light is always blinking, and you just can't stop what you're doing and run in every ten minutes, especially when you know they've got about three days to go. Mrs. Oldwoman doesn't need those tubes anyway; she's just hanging on.

Do you want to know what I think? I think she's taking too long to die. We need her bed. I just hope to God the doctor doesn't expect me to pull the plug—that's his job.*

Although these examples of the thoughts and feelings of health care staff are hypothetic, they illustrate the psychologic pro-

The research on which this chapter is based was supported by Biomedical Sciences Support Grant 3-S05-RR-07006-08S1. Parts of this chapter were first presented in an address entitled ''Physician 'burn-out' and prolonged care of the dying,'' at the Second National Training Conference for Physicians on Psychosocial Care of the Dying Patient, Berkeley, California, June, 1977.

*From Dempsey, D.: The way we die, New York, 1975, Macmillan Publishing Co., Inc. Copyright© 1975 by David Dempsey.

cess by which health professionals often keep themselves at a distance from their patients. In maintaining a psychologic distance, they may behave in ways that typify the most frequent patient complaints about health care personnel: They are too impersonal and too busy; they fail to give adequate explanations; they lack personal respect or care for the patient; and they treat the patient more as an object than as a human being. Such behavior, when it occurs, falls far short of the ideal established for health care practitioners, and therefore it may be hard for nurses and physicians to ever admit that they sometimes act in this detached or even dehumanized manner. Although the frequency of their detached behavior may vary widely among individual practitioners, the underlying feelings that give rise to such behavior are common to everyone and can be considered normal emotional responses to the stresses of the health care situation. However, the failure of the health professions to recognize, acknowledge, and understand these feelings makes it especially difficult for them to cope with their emotions successfully in ways that are not detrimental to both self and others. To the extent that this happens, the overall quality of health care declines.

Why should this distance between health care staff and patients occur? What are the sources of the negative thoughts and feelings physicians and nurses sometimes have? One answer lies in the unique challenges and stresses of health care professions.

Health workers must make many difficult decisions, and they must make some of them quickly under pressure. The information on which they base these decisions is not always sufficiently clear-cut. The great deal of uncertainty in medical and psychosocial evidence is further compounded by conflicting opinions between peers. All of these factors make health care a highly demanding occupation, both physically and psychologically, and the attendant feelings of frustration, exhaustion, and anxiety could conceivably find expression in negative attitudes towards those who require

care and treatment (because, in a sense, they are the source of "the problem").

However, I believe that the negative feelings about patients stem directly from the emotionally stressful aspects of patient care. Just as patients have complaints about the behavior of physicians and nurses, so do physicians and nurses have complaints about them. Most commonly these complaints are that patients are demanding and unreasonable, fail to follow instructions, are impatient regarding treatment, waste too much of the physician's or nurse's time in excessive complaints or discussion of other personal problems, are not appreciative, and sometimes have obnoxious or upsetting personality traits. Moreover patients may get emotionally distraught at times, and some of them may suffer from illnesses that are especially difficult to look at or deal with (for example, facial cancer).

To the extent that patients have these characteristics, contact with them can be an unpleasant and even upsetting daily experience. Health care staff often cope with this emotional stress by reducing their contact with such patients and/or removing themselves, both psychologically and physically, from them. This often results in poorer health care for those patients that the health care practitioner dislikes or is uncomfortable with, even though he or she is supposedly obligated to provide good medical care for all who need it regardless of personal preference or moralistic judgment.[11]

The emotional stress of patient care is even greater when the patient is dying. If nurses or physicians should start to develop negative feelings about a patient for any of the reasons listed, it is likely that they will also experience guilt (because of these feelings). At times this guilt will be followed by anger at the patient for causing the person to feel guilty. All of this places an extra emotional burden on the health care practitioner. Additional stress arises from the fact that a patient's dying has a greater personal relevance for physicians or nurses than a patient's illness. Whereas they know that the particular illness may not be one that they will ever personally experience, they realize that they (and their family) will eventually die, and thus the patient's response to death may arouse strong fears and anxieties in them. Furthermore, since health care personnel are trained to see death as an adversary to be fought and overcome, the dying patient may represent a failure or even a betrayal, and this perception will further arouse negative feelings toward the patient.

To perform efficiently and effectively in stressful interactions with patients, health care staff often defend against disruptive emotions through techniques of detachment. Ideally, they gain objectivity and distance from the situation without losing concern for the patient. However, in all too many cases they are unable to cope with the continual emotional stress, and eventually the burn-out syndrome sets in.

THE BURN-OUT PROCESS

Burn-out involves the loss of concern for the people with whom one is working. In addition to physical exhaustion (and sometimes even illness), burn-out is characterized by an emotional exhaustion in which the professional person no longer has any positive feelings, sympathy, or respect for patients or clients. The health worker experiencing burn-out often develops a very cynical and dehumanized perception of these people, labeling them in derogatory ways and treating them accordingly. As a result of this dehumanizing process, the health care professional views his or her patients or clients as somehow deserving of their plight and blames them for their current problems. Burn-out is not an isolated phenomenon attributable to just a limited number of individuals. Rather it afflicts a variety of people within many different health and social service professions. Though practitioners in these professions vary considerably in the type of contact they have with patients or clients, they show a remarkably similar pattern of response to emotional stress originating in their work.

Burn-out plays a primary role in the poor delivery of health and social services to people in need of them. People wait longer to receive less attention and get less care. As a result, burn-out may well be implicated in the increasing number of malpractice suits and thus the soaring costs of insurance for physicians. It also appears to be a major factor in low worker morale, impaired performance, absenteeism, and high job turnover. A common response to burn-out is to quit and get out, either by changing jobs, moving into administrative work (and away from direct contact with patients or clients), or even leaving the profession.

Furthermore, burn-out correlates with other indices of personal stress. Professionals experiencing burn-out often increase their use (and abuse) of alcohol and drugs as a way of reducing their tension and blotting out their strong emotional feelings. They report more mental illness, saying that they have become "bad people" who are cold and callous, and some of them seek counseling or psychiatric treatment for what they believe to be their personal failings. If emotional stress cannot be resolved while on the job, then it is often resurrected at home. Sometimes the professional misattributes the increased fighting and irritability to something that has gone wrong in the family relationship ("I guess we don't love each other anymore"), failing to see that the major source of stress is the job. Many times, after an emotionally trying day with patients or clients, the professional simply wants to get away from all people for a while, but this desire for solitude often comes at the expense of family and friends.

Until recently no research had been done on this important social problem; indeed, it was almost a taboo topic within health and social service professions. Although there has been some investigation of nurses in high-stress jobs,[5] no comparable research has been done with physicians. The pioneering work on the burn-out syndrome has been done by myself and my colleagues[7-9,12] as well as by H. J. Freudenberger.[3,4] Our goal has been to discover the social and psychologic dimensions of the burn-out syndrome. We have tried to identify what inter-personal stresses health care professionals face, what (if any) preparation they have had for coping with those stresses, what specific techniques they use to distance themselves from their patients or clients, and the effects of using such techniques. In addition to making field observations of professionals at work, we conducted extensive questionnaire studies followed by interviews with smaller groups of people. Our initial samples consisted of practitioners in a wide variety of helping professions, ranging from physicians and psychiatrists to social welfare workers and child care staff. However, the findings to be discussed in this chapter are those of relevance to health care personnel. Moreover the emphasis in the discussion will be on the care of the dying patient, although the principles hold for patient care in general.

COPING WITH BURN-OUT

What can be done to prevent the destructive process of burn-out? At the moment we cannot present a total solution to this problem, but our work thus far has pointed to a number of factors that could reduce the harm done by burn-out or prevent its occurrence altogether. These factors include training in interpersonal skills, social-professional support systems, use of humor, variation of amount and type of patient contact, separation between work and home, and maintenance of physical health.

Training in interpersonal skills

Physicians and nurses need to have special training and preparation for working with patients. Although they are usually well trained in medical skills, they are often not well equipped to handle the repeated, intense, emotional interactions with patients that are part of their job. This lack of expertise can be related to two aspects of current medical training: the development of a dehumanized view of patients and the relative lack of attention to emotional factors in the practice of medicine.

In spite of a growing trend toward holistic philosophy in health care, in which attention is given to the entire human being and not just a part, medical training implicitly encourages a fragmented, disease-oriented, nonhuman perception of the patient. The emphasis is on treating an illness rather than on interacting with a person, and so the focus is on symptoms instead of people. This is reflected in the tendency for hospital staff to refer to patients by their immediate medical problems (for example, "the coronary" or "the CBS") instead of by their names. Many specialists do not meet their patients until they are quite seriously ill; as a result, there is little to prevent the specialist from viewing each patient as a case rather than as an individual. This orientation utilizes intellectualization; the practitioner deals with the abstract characteristics of the patient and not with those that are more personal and potentially more emotionally arousing. To the extent that health care practitioners relate to patients more as objects than as humans, they will interact with them in more detached and unfeeling ways.

Medical training also dehumanizes professional perceptions of patients by building in expectations of passive and dependent patient behaviors. Medical students first work with cadavers and experimental animals and may begin to develop a pattern of actively manipulating a nonresisting "patient." Later physicians may continue this pattern with human patients who have learned to be passive and unmoving during physical examinations, to follow the physician's directions, and to speak only in response to the physician's questions. This generally passive stance of patients, combined with physicians' active control of the situation, encourages physicians to perceive patients as objects rather than as people. Even when a patient does behave more actively and thereby makes the situation a stressful one (for example, by asking difficult questions or getting upset), the physician usually has enough control of the situation to deflect the emotional arousal rather than to deal with it directly. For example, the physician may reduce the amount of time he or she talks with the patient, give out termination cues (for example, keeping one's hand on the doorknob during a patient interview), or communicate with the patient in more impersonal ways such as superficial generalities and stereotyped responses:

Physicians sometimes use reassurance for protecting themselves, not the patient, from talking about painful topics in full and emotion-arousing detail. The ready smile and the too quickly given statement, ''I'm sure everything will be just fine,'' frequently amount only to an unrecognized but socially acceptable means of telling the patient that one is really not concerned with him as a human being in pain and difficulty. The ''friendly and reassuring'' pat on the back may also be employed as a polite means of pushing the patient out of the office.[13]

Emotional factors are virtually ignored in medical training, and so health care students are not at all prepared to deal with the strong emotional stress of caring for patients. They are not alerted to the sorts of things that could cause them to feel anxious or upset, nor are they told how to cope with these feelings. The implicit philosophy appears to be one of ''sink or swim''—those who figure out on their own how to handle their emotions under pressure will be the strong ones who survive training and go on to practice medicine successfully. This philosophy rests on several faulty assumptions, one being that people who need help to learn how to cope with emotional stress will not be good health care practitioners. More important, it is erroneous to assume that the solutions people arrive at by themselves are necessarily successful ones either for themselves or for their patients. Withdrawing from upsetting contact with patients or using drugs or alcohol may be effective in reducing experienced stress, but the personal and social costs associated with such responses are considerable.

In general the most guidance that student nurses and physicians receive with regard to their own emotions is the warning to ''be professional.'' What is meant by ''profes-sional'' is rarely made explicit, but the clear implication is that any strong emotions must be kept under wraps because the professional must remain cool and objective *at all costs.* Such a directive is of no help when students face a stressful situation for the first time, since strong emotions inevitably occur.

For example, most students' first contact with death is a very distressing experience, that arouses feelings of fear and personal inadequacy. Knowing that they should be calm and in control of their feelings only makes it worse when the strong emotions erupt, because the students are more likely to interpret those feelings as a sign of personal weakness and professional failure. If they had known earlier that these were normal feelings, common to all ''first-timers,'' they would probably be less devastated by them and more able to cope with them effectively. However, it is usually true that a student learns nothing prior to the event that would prepare them for their emotional responses. A common complaint of medical and nursing students is, ''How come nobody told me it was going to be like this?'' More experienced health care people are surprisingly silent on this topic and do not share their own experiences with younger colleagues, which suggests that the prevailing philosophy is one of ''paying your dues.''

The lack of attention to the feelings of the practitioner may reflect a denial of the emotions involved. Thus the lack of preparation may indicate a reluctance to come to grips with the problem, rather than an oversight. Displays of emotions, especially in men, are often viewed as a sign of weakness and irrationality in our society; this may lead people to avoid acknowledging the presence of any emotion. The lack of preparation for emotional reactions may also result from a lack of knowledge about successful coping techniques and how to teach them.

The achievement of ''detached concern,'' in which the health care practitioner provides sensitive, understanding care by being sufficiently detached to make objective, rational decisions, has been discussed as an ideal of the health professions.[6] However, this ideal is very difficult to achieve. Much like oil and water, detachment and concern do not mix easily. The attitudes and behaviors emanating from these two concepts often conflict, and the best route to reconciliation is not yet known.

Nevertheless some training in interpersonal skills would be a valuable first step in preventing or reducing the occurrence of burn-out. Such training should focus on the emotional stresses inherent in a health care career: What are the sources of such stresses? Which coping techniques are constructive and which are ineffective? What possible changes in attitudes and feelings toward patients may occur? Moreover student physicians and nurses should understand their own motivations for entering a medical career and recognize what they expect to gain from their work with patients. Although many of the health care workers we interviewed stated that they wished they had had prior preparation in interpersonal skills, some reported that there was no time for it in their already packed curriculum. Others felt that such preparation was not an essential part of medical training but was simply an "extra" that would help them make small talk with their patients. In others words, they considered the acquisition of interpersonal skills pleasant but basically unimportant training. In my opinion, such a viewpoint is sadly in error, for it trivializes a critical aspect of the health care worker-patient relationship and fails to recognize that both the health professional and the patient are human beings whose personal feelings can affect not only the delivery but also the acceptance of health care. Therefore I believe that training in interpersonal coping skills should be a basic part of medical and nursing school curricula.

Analysis of personal feelings

Since the arousal of strong emotions is a common feature of health care work, efforts must be made to deal with those emotions constructively and to prevent the emotional exhaustion of burn-out. Surprisingly many of the health care staff we interviewed did not know that other people were experiencing the same changes in attitudes and emotions that they were. Each of them thought that their personal reaction was unique, an abberration rather than a normal experience. This illusion was maintained by their tendency to conceal their feelings from their colleagues and to deny that they were experiencing any anxiety:

The disturbing aspects of this behavior include the blandness of the denial. The blandness makes it difficult for other (physicians) to express themselves, although they vaguely recognize that such flagrant denial might well be used to mask a serious problem in a fellow physician, and are troubled by the implicit accusation that anyone who would admit to being made anxious in his work must be abnormal indeed.[1]

By misattributing the emotional stress they experience to assumed personal problems or inadequacies, health personnel fail to see that situational factors are the major cause of their reactions. On the basis of my research, I would argue that burn-out is not a function of "bad" people who are unfeeling and brutal. Rather it is a function of "bad" situations, ones that are difficult and distressing, in which originally idealistic people must operate. However, by assuming personal causes health care professionals look to personal solutions instead of situational ones, and these solutions may not always provide the most appropriate way of dealing with burn-out. Trying to change oneself to become a "better person" may not result in much improvement unless one can also change the work situation or one's manner of coping with it. Only by sharing one's experiences with fellow staff and seeing what is common to all, can one get a better perspective on the situational sources of emotional stress.

My research findings show that burn-out rates are lower for health care practitioners who actively express, analyze, and share their personal feelings with their colleagues.

Not only do they consciously get things off their chest, but they have an opportunity to get constructive feedback from other people and to develop new perspectives and an understanding of their relationship with their patients. This process is greatly enhanced if the relevant institution, such as the hospital, establishes an appropriate, routine mechanism for feedback. Social-professional support groups, special staff meetings, or workshop group sessions could satisfy this purpose.

Social-professional support system

The availability of formal or informal programs, in which health care staff can get together to discuss problems and receive support, is of critical importance in helping them to cope successfully with the stress of patient care. It allows them to solicit advice and comfort from other staff members after withdrawing from an upsetting situation. Such social support can ease the stress and pain, as well as foster a sense of distance from the situation. By talking to their colleagues, health professionals can get a fresh perspective on how to deal with particularly troublesome patients and a sense of shared responsibility for difficult decisions. As one nurse reported, "When we get together, we bitch a lot to each other. We hash things out. We laugh at it sometimes. We talk about it a lot and try new ways. It helps to talk about it, and if you can't see it another way then somebody else might be able to." The weekly small group discussions utilized by the Shanti Project (see Chapter 40) are an excellent example of this kind of support system in action.

Social-professional support groups are not yet widely recognized as important and necessary for the psychologic well-being of health care personnel. Indeed, some skeptical traditional physicians stated that such a system would only provide nurses with another opportunity to "chit-chat" instead of work. However, my research found that burn-out rates were lower for those health care practitioners who had access to such a system, especially if it was well developed and supported by the parent institution. Some physicians reported that they had participated in a social-professional support group while they were doing their residency. The group would meet regularly so that residents could discuss problems they were having with their patients, vent frustrations, and report their successes. After entering private practice, the former residents found that the lack of such a group was a serious unanticipated loss to them. Sometimes they even made efforts to rejoin the residents' meetings, although not always successfully. Private practice often means isolated practice.

Use of humor

Getting together with one's peers also helps one to use humor as a coping technique. Being able to laugh and joke during or after a stressful event is one way to reduce the tension and anxiety that the health care practitioner might feel. It also serves to make the situation less serious, less frightening, less overwhelming. The battlefield surgeons in M*A*S*H who make "sick" jokes and flirt with the nurses while they perform grave operations are a particularly apt example of this technique at work. It should be noted here that a constructive use of humor does not include humor that is derogatory of patients, that is, jokes that are funny at their expense. Such cruel humor dehumanizes both the object and the author of the joke and can only accentuate any negative feelings health care practitioners might have toward their patients.

Humor can also be used very effectively with patients, as well as with other health care staff. It can lighten a grim situation and make the practitioner-patient relationship more pleasant and less strained on both sides. This is true even when the patient is dying, although this is usually a time when most people avoid humor because it seems inappropriate. However, I would argue that humor represents the life force and can reaffirm one's humanity in the face of death. A judicious use of humor can make the dying patient feel that his or her "old self" is still there, a welcome ally in the face of impending death.

Amount and variety of patient contact

Just as humor can be used to introduce some positive notes into the contact between patient and health care practitioner, so other techniques can be used to ease the emotional strain of such prolonged contact. One approach is to vary the practitioner's patient load so that he or she is not always working in high-stress situations. To be dealing constantly with dying patients and their families is an extremely heavy burden that is very difficult to bear. However, if a person spends only some of his or her time with dying patients and the rest with patients who have a good prognosis and/or are easier to work with, then he or she can balance the more stressful patient contact within a more appropriate scale of life and death. Alternatively, the amount of stressful patient contact can be reduced by providing the physician or nurse with regular breaks from this type of patient care, as well as opportunties for temporary withdrawals when needed. Although people often turn to others for help in coping with emotional stress (as in a social support group), at times they need to get away from all people for a while to unwind from the pain and tension. This need for withdrawal has been recognized in the architectural plan for the New Haven Hospice, which includes a small glass-domed, carpeted, soundproof meditation or ''screaming'' room that will serve as a retreat for staff.

The type of withdrawal available to medical personnel may spell the difference between burn-out and successful coping. The most positive form of withdrawal observed during our research was what I have called a sanctioned ''time-out.'' Time-outs are not merely short breaks from work, such as rest periods or coffee breaks, but rather they are opportunities for the person to voluntarily choose to do some other, less stressful work while other staff take over patient responsibilities. For example, in one of the hospital wards we studied the nurses

knew that, if they were having a particularly rough day, they could arrange to do something else than work directly with patients. They could ask to get assigned to medications (where they would only see patients when calling on them for medicines), or they could do paper work in the office, attend meetings, etc. In this system, when one nurse took a time-out, the other nurses would cover for her and continue to provide adequate patient care.

In contrast to sanctioned time-outs there were the negative withdrawals, or ''escapes.'' In this instance the nurse's or physician's decision to take a break from work always came at the expense of patients because there were no other staff members to take over. These people were more likely to feel trapped by their total responsibility for patients; they could not withdraw temporarily without feeling some guilt. When guilt was heaped upon the already heavy emotional burden they tenuously carried, the load often became too much to bear.

The use of sanctioned time-outs or guilt-arousing escapes seemed to be primarily determined by the structure of the work setting. Time-outs were possible in well-staffed institutions that had shared work responsibilities, flexible work policies, and a variety of job tasks for each person rather than just a single one. When institutional policies prevented the use of voluntary time-outs, there was lower staff morale, greater emotional stress, and more dissatisfied patients frustrated at not getting the care they needed.

Separation between work and home

Many health care practitioners make a sharp distinction between their job and their personal life. They often do not discuss their family or personal affairs with their colleagues, and they rarely tell their spouses and friends about what goes on at work. By leaving their work at the hospital or office and not reliving it at home, they confine the emotional stress associated with that work to a smaller part of their life. Rules forbidding staff to socialize with their patients outside the job setting also encourage this distinction between work and home.

It is critical for the health care practitioner's psychologic and physical well-being that a significant portion of his or her life be reserved for activities that are not job related. That is, a person needs regular free time to spend with family or friends, engage in sports, read or pursue hobbies, or simply rest and relax. The more that work cuts into this private time, the greater the risk of burn-out. Because it is so easy for a professional person's work to take over more and more of his or her home life, it requires real effort to keep the two separate. Parts of one's private life succumb to the job every time one brings home work to do in the evening or on the weekends, brings home unresolved negative emotions that are taken out on the family, puts in overtime, is "on call" (and thus never able to really relax at home), spends little time with family or friends because of a need to be away from people, and so forth.

To the extent that one can change some of these factors and set up boundaries for one's personal time, it becomes possible to prevent the emotional stress of the job from spreading and having detrimental effects on other aspects of one's life. Many people achieve this by having a "decompression routine" between job and home, in which they engage in some activity (such as physical exercise or a hobby) that allows them to unwind from the stress and tension of the job, to stop thinking about the day's problems, and to arrive home relaxed and ready to be with family and friends.

Physical health

A common correlate of burn-out is the deterioration of physical well-being. The person becomes exhausted and run down, is frequently sick, suffers from insomnia, and is often prone to ulcers and severe headaches, as well as more serious illnesses. These physical problems may be caused by the emotional stress of work, or they may be caused by other factors but

intensified by the stress of work. Sometimes the pressures of work lead a person to be less careful about getting enough sleep at night or eating properly (for example, meals are skipped and more coffee is consumed).

To cope with these physical problems, the health care practitioner may turn to tranquilizers, drugs, or alcohol—"solutions" that are often abused. Better measures include regular vacations (where one can rest completely and "recharge one's batteries") and physical exercise. In his 1975 booklet on burn-out Freudenberger[4] suggests:

Encourage your staff and yourself to exercise physically. If you want to run, do it. Play tennis, dance, swim, bicycle, exhaust yourself on the drums. Engage in any activity that will make you physically tired. Many times the exhaustion of burn-out is an emotional and mental one that will not let you sleep.

CONCLUSION

In an increasingly mobile and impersonal society in which the ties to an extended family or immediate community are greatly reduced, people are more likely to turn to formal helping professionals for aid with their personal problems. The number of social workers, lawyers, doctors, and other helpers has grown to a staggering size, thus constituting a service industry of major proportions. However, people go most often to physicians for help, not only for their physical ailments but also for various psychosocial problems and general problems in living. The reason for this preference is that the characteristics of the doctor-patient relationship provide a legitimate way for expressing intimacy and asking for help.[10] Moreover physicians are generally held in very high esteem by the public, and thus it is not surprising that they are viewed as the leading authority and healer to whom people can entrust all of their problems.

While creating the special status and prestige accorded most physicians, this fact also places a special burden on them. They are called on to deal with the hopes, fears, angers, and frustrations of their patients;

the required treatment for these problems often lies in the physician's interpersonal skills rather than in his or her technical ones. As stated in an aphorism attributed to Oliver Wendell Holmes, "The physician's task is to cure rarely, relieve often, and comfort always." The health care worker's ability to comfort and to show genuine caring and interest is as highly valued by patients as his or her medical skills; and it is this ability that patients can evaluate most easily. When the medical skills are of less consequence, as in the case of the dying patient, then the nature of the interpersonal contact between practitioner and patient becomes the basis for judging the quality of health care service. Thus the ability of nurses and physicians to cope successfully with the enormous emotional strains of their work can improve the quality of patient care. Moreover it can also improve the quality of practitioner care and prevent the devastating personal and social consequences of burn-out.

REFERENCES

1. Artiss, K. L., and Levine, A. S.: Doctor-patient relation in severe illness, New England Journal of Medicine **288:**1210-1214, 1973.
2. Dempsey, D.: The way we die, New York, 1975, Macmillan, Inc.
3. Freudenberger, H. J.: Staff burn-out, Journal of Social Issues **30:**159-165, 1974.
4. Freudenberger, H. J.: The staff burn-out syndrome, Washington, D.C., 1975, The Drug Abuse Council.
5. Hay, D., and Oken, D.: Psychological stresses of ICU nursing, Psychosomatic Medicine **34:**109-118, 1972.
6. Lief, H. I., and Fox, R. C.: Training for "detached concern" in medical students. In Lief, H. I., Lief, V. F., and Lief, N. R., eds.: The psychological basis of medical practice, New York, 1963, Harper & Row, Publishers.
7. Maslach, C.: "Detached concern" in health and social service professions. Paper presented at annual convention of the American Psychological Association, Montreal, August, 1973.
8. Maslach, C.: Burned-out, Human Behavior **5:**16-22, 1976.
9. Maslach, C., and Pines, A.: The burn-out syndrome in the day care setting, Child Care Quarterly, Summer, 1977.
10. Mechanic, D.: Public expectations and health care, New York, 1972, John Wiley & Sons, Inc.
11. Pattison, E. M.: Psychosocial and religious aspects of medical ethics. In Williams, R. H., ed.: To live and to die: when, why and how, New York, 1974, Springer-Verlag, Inc.
12. Pines, A., and Maslach, C.: "Detached concern" in mental health institutions. Paper presented at Annual Conference on Child Abuse, Houston, April, 1977.
13. Sheppe, W. M. Jr., and Stevenson, I.: Techniques of interviewing. In Lief, H. I., Lief, V. F., and Lief, N. R., eds.: The psychological basis of medical practice, New York, 1963, Harper & Row, Publishers.

13

The psychological stresses of intensive care unit nursing

DONALD HAY and DONALD OKEN

Much has been written about the stressful psychological experience of being a patient in an Intensive Care (ICU) or other special care unit.[1-5] Less well recognized, however, are the problems posed for those who work in an ICU that provides the complex nursing care required by critically ill, often dying, patients. Notable exceptions include the contributions of Vreeland and Ellis[6] and of Gardam.[7]

The quality of a patient's care, and, hence, outcome, depends greatly upon the people providing that care, and the effectiveness of the latter is a function of their psychological state no less than of their technical expertise. This has special meaning for the ICU patient, whose very life hangs upon the care provided by the nursing staff. Yet, in this special environment, the psychological burdens imposed upon the nurse are extraordinary. Her situation resembles, in many ways, that of the soldier serving with an elite combat group.

Our understanding derives from the experience of one of us (DH) working directly as a member of the nursing staff of a 10-bed university hospital ICU over a period of approximately one year, plus multiple interviews and informal contacts with ICU nurses.* From these observations, we have developed some insights into the nature of the nurses' experience and the methods they develop to handle it. These, we believe, provide useful clues for lessening the stressful nature of the experience, and hence benefit the nurses and (through them) their patients.

THE ICU ENVIRONMENT

A stranger entering an ICU is at once bombarded with a massive array of sensory stimuli,[3] some emotionally neutral but many highly charged. Initially, the great impact comes from the intricate machinery, with its flashing lights, buzzing and beeping monitors, gurgling suction pumps, and whooshing respirators. Simultaneously, one sees many people rushing around busily performing lifesaving tasks. The atmosphere is not unlike that of the tension-charged strategic war bunker. With time, habituation occurs, but the ever-continuing stimuli decrease the overload threshold and contribute to stress at times of crisis.

As the newness and strangeness of the

---

*While our detailed observations were made on a single ICU, superficial contact with several other such units, which have many features in common, leads us to believe that our conclusions have significant generalizability. However, there may be some significant differences from other types of specialized units such as coronary care units, neurosurgical ICUs, transplant and dialysis units, etc.

Reprinted from Psychosomatic Medicine **34**(2): 109-118, 1972.

unit wears off, one increasingly becomes aware of a host of perceptions with specific stressful emotional significance. Desperately ill, sick, and injured human beings are hooked up to that machinery. And, in addition to mechanical stimuli, one can discern moaning, crying, screaming, and the last gasps of life. Sights of blood, vomitus and excreta, exposed genitalia, mutilated wasting bodies, and unconscious and helpless people assault the sensibilities. Unceasingly, the ICU nurse must face these affect-laden stimuli with all the distress and conflict that they engender. As part of her daily routine, the nurse must reassure and comfort the man who is dying of cancer; she must change the dressings of a decomposing, gangrenous limb; she must calm the awakening disturbed "overdose" patient; she must bathe the genitalia of the helpless and comatose; she must wipe away the bloody stool of the gastrointestinal bleeder; she must comfort the anguished young wife who knows her husband is dying. It is hard to imagine any other situation that involves such intimacy with the frightening, repulsive, and forbidden. Stimuli are present to mobilize literally every conflictual area at every psychological developmental level.

But there is more: There is something uncanny about the picture the patients present. Many are neither alive or dead. Most have "tubes in every orifice." Their sounds and actions (or inaction) are almost nonhuman. Bodily areas and organs, ordinarily unseen, are openly exposed or deformed by bandages. All of this directly challenges the definition of being human, one's most fundamental sense of ego integrity, for nurse as well as patient. Though consciously the nurse quickly learns to accept this surrealism, she is unremittingly exposed to these multiple threats to the stability of her body boundaries, her sense of self, and her feelings of humanity and reality.

To all this is added a repetitive contact with death. And, if exposure to death is merely frequent, that to dying is constant. The ICU nurse thus quickly becomes adept at identifying the signs and symptoms that

foretell a downhill trend for her patient. This becomes an awesome addition to the burden of the nurse who has been caring for the patient and must *continue* to do so, knowing his outcome.

THE WORK LOAD AND ITS DEMANDS

If the sense of drama and frightfulness is what most forcefully strikes the outsider, what the experienced nurse points to, paradoxically, is the incessant repetitive routine. For each patient, vital signs must be monitored, commonly at 15-minute intervals, sometimes more often. Central venous pressures must be measured, tracheas suctioned, urimeters emptied and measured, intravenous infusions changed, EKG monitor patterns interpreted, respirators checked, hypothermia blankets adjusted, etc., etc. And, every step must be charted. The nurse begins to feel like a hamster on a treadmill: She finishes the required tasks on one patient just in time to start them on another; and when these are completed she is already behind in doing the same tasks all over again on the first, constantly aware of her race with the clock. A paradox soon becomes apparent. Nowhere more than in the ICU is a *good* nurse expected to make observations about her patient's condition, to interpret subtle changes and use judgment to take appropriate action. But often, the ICU nurse is so unremittingly involved in collecting and charting information that she has little time to interpret it adequately.

The work load is formidable—even in periods of relative calm. Many tasks, which elsewhere would be performed by nurse's aides, require special care in the ICU and become the lot of the ICU nurse. Changing a bed in an ICU may require moving a desperately ill, comatose patient while watching EKG leads, respirator hoses, urinary and intravenous catheters, etc. Moreover, the nurse must maintain detailed records.

Night shifts, weekends, and holidays all mean less work on other floors. Only urgent or fundamental procedures are performed. But, in an ICU, emergency is routine: There is no surcease—no holidays. In fact, the regular recovery room in our hospital shuts down on weekends and holidays so that patients must be sent to the ICU after emergency surgery. It is not rare, on a weekend, to see several stretchers with these patients interposed between the fully occupied beds of the ICU, leaving the nurses with barely time enough to suction patients and keep them alive.

The quantity and variety of complex technical equipment poses tremendous demands on the knowledge and expertise of the nurse.[6,7] Because of this and the nature of her tasks, temporarily floating in nurses from elsewhere when staff is short provides little in the way of help; indeed, this may even prove a hindrance. Yet, ICU nurses are fully able to fill in elsewhere when staff shortages occur; and they are not infrequently asked to do so, leaving the ICU understaffed.

The emergency situation provides added work. Although an ICU's routine is another floor's emergency, obviously there are frequent situations of acute crisis, such as cardiac arrest. These require the nurse's full attention and prevent her from continuing her regular tasks on her other patients. A few remaining nurses must watch and calm all other patients, complete as many of their regular observations and treatments as possible, and prevent other emergencies. Meanwhile, the nurses assisting at the emergency are called upon not only to do things rapidly but to make immediate and accurate decisions that oftentimes include determining the priority of several emergencies.[6]

Habituation is both inevitable and necessary if the nurse is not to work in an exhausted state of chronic crisis. Yet, she must maintain an underlying alertness to discern and respond to cues which have special meaning. This is like the mother who hears the faint cry of her baby over the commotion of a party.

Nor is the work without its physical dangers, and the nurses know this. It is impossible to take fully adequate isolation precautions against infections because of time pressures and the bodily intimacy required to provide the needed level of care. Portable X rays are sometimes taken with inadequately shielded nurses holding immobile patients in proper positioning. Heavy comatose patients must be lifted. Sharp needles, scalpels, etc., must be handled rapidly. Electric equipment must be moved, adjusted, and attached. Physical assaults on nurses by a delirious patient, though infrequent, can and do occur.

There are occasions also when distraught relatives misinterpret a situation, feel that their loved one is getting inadequate care and become verbally—and sometimes physically—abusive. The roots of these more dramatic misunderstandings lie in more general problems about visitors. On other floors, visiting hours occur daily at specified times, but in the ICU there can be no such routinized schedule. Close relatives are allowed to see the patient at any time of the day or night. Though restricted to a brief (commonly 5-minute) period, their presence soon becomes a burden. In his constant inquiries about the patient's condition and prognosis, the relative is asking for more than information. He is seeking reassurance and support.[6,8] The nurse may wish to respond at this deeper level, but usually she cannot, because she has tasks that require more immediate attention. The relative, feeling rebuffed, begins to critically scrutinize the nurse's every action. With so much to be upset about, he is prone to jump to unwarranted conclusions. While many visitors see the nurses as "angels of mercy," others develop a projection of their worst fears. Seeing a nurse spend more time with another patient, he may feel his loved one is not getting adequate attention. Or, he may see blood, vomitus, or excreta soiling the patient's bed and misinterpret this as an indication of poor care, not appreciating the nurse's preoccupation with lifesaving activities. Moreover the nurse has little escape from hovering relatives: She has "no place to hide."

DOCTORS AND ADMINISTRATORS

Visitors are not the only ones who cause problems. Some of the very people who might be expected to provide substantial support add to the stresses on the nurse. The potentially fatal outcome in the gravely ill ICU patients tends to stimulate feelings of frustration, self-doubt, and guilt in their physicians. The ways he deals with these may have major consequences for the nurse. He may, for example, use projection and behave in a surly, querulous manner. He may bolster his self-esteem by becoming imperious and demand that the nurses "wait on" him.* He may also rely on avoidance as a way of distancing himself from his feelings about his seeming failure as a life-saver. Though the nurse must remain on the unit for almost her entire shift, the physician can make good use of his prerogatives to move about freely. Especially at the time of a patient's death, the physician seems to have a way of not being present; the full burden of breaking the news and supporting the family through the acute grief reaction is left to the nurse to handle as best she can. Conversely, compensatory overzealousness may occur, and unnecessary heroic gestures be made to save someone beyond recovery. The physician may order special treatments and an unrealistic frequency of monitoring. The not uncommon incongruity of orders is especially revealing about this. A patient on "q15 minute" vital signs will have nothing done—and correctly so—when these deteriorate. Or, the physician will recognize the inappropriateness of frequent monitoring, yet insist on fruitless *emergency* attempts at resuscitation (e.g., a pacemaker) when death supervenes. This not only increases the nurse's work load but adds to her frustration by diverting her energies from patients who could be saved.

_____

*Another factor in this overdemanding behavior may be his sense of inadequacy and self-doubt if he is unfamiliar with the unit and its highly organized functions.[9] This may culminate in his issuing dictatorial orders and commands that are not commensurate with the realities of the situation.

The physician's immediate availability is essential to the nurse. He is needed not merely for emergencies but for frequently updated changes in treatment orders, for advice—and for reassurance. Thus, whether his absence arises as a consequence of defenses, competing demands for his time, or merely ignorance of the need, the nurse suffers. This is especially prone to happen in situations where medical responsibility for each patient rests with the staff of a specialty service (e.g., medicine, surgery) headquartered elsewhere.

Similarly, the nurses often feel that they do not get much support from their administrative superiors who, they believe, fail to appreciate the realities of the ICU situation. ICUs and similar special facilities have come into their own only in the past decade, and, as Gardam has pointed out,[7] a generation gap exists between ICU staff nurses and senior nurse administrators. As a consequence, nursing administrators find it difficult to recognize the unique characteristics of the ICU, and tend to consider it merely a slightly busier and more acute service whose needs can be met simply by a numerically larger staff. Often they seem to regard the complaints of a dissatisfied or battle-weary ICU nurse as a sign of emotional unfitness rather than as a basis for changes in policy or procedure.

Some of the anger felt toward these superiors is, certainly, scapegoating. This is particularly likely in regard to the ICU head nurse or nursing supervisor-instructor. Nurses in these positions are intrinsically in a difficult bind. While they may be arguing valiantly for the ICU in the front office, on the unit they must conscientiously implement the orders of their superiors. They become enmeshed in an assignment to two simultaneous, incompatible roles: the tough top sergeant and the loving mother. These dual roles resonate, in turn, with the ambivalent attitude of staff nurses (who, as predominantly young, single, incompletely emancipated women, are prone to develop a strongly ambivalent maternal transference to female supervisors). They are, moreover, readily available and sufficiently close in age and status to temper the transference and become permissible targets for hostility.

THE PSYCHOLOGICAL EXPERIENCE

We will now shift from a situational frame of reference to a psychological one and take a closer look at the concerns and feelings of ICU nurses. We will also examine the adaptive devices, individual and group, which they use to cope with their situation.

The work load, so great in its sheer quantity, is unusual also in its variety and the intricacy of its tasks as well as in the rapidity with which these must be performed. Great flexibility is required (which may partly explain why ICU nurses are predominantly in their early 20s).

Mistakes are, of course, inevitable. But, when every procedure is potentially lifesaving, any error may be life-endangering. Hence the ICU nurse lives chronically under a cloud of latent anxiety. The new nurse, particularly, begins to view the never-ending life-dependent tasks as a specter of potential mistakes and their imagined dreadful sequelae. Some, of course, cannot shake this and soon arrange a transfer. The experienced nurse achieves a more realistic perspective, but a degree of residual uncertainty always remains, given the complexity of machines and procedures. Especially at times of stress, she too may become anxious. When this anxiety exceeds minimal levels, it reduces efficiency and decision-making capacity, inviting additional mistakes—the classic vicious circle.

When the inevitable error does occur, the nurse is in a dilemma. To make it public is likely to enhance her guilt and invite criticism. Moreover, it leads to the need to fill out an incident report, a further drain on her time and a potential blot on her record. Yet to fail to do so may compound the error by blocking corrective treatment. The experienced nurse develops a subtle adaptive compromise, reporting serious mistakes but fudging over inconsequential ones. In either case, she must live with her guilt.

The ICU nurse has much in which she can take great pride. Yet her self-esteem takes an awful beating in many ways. Her awareness of her mistakes, both real and exaggerated, is one such factor. Another is her repeated "failure." The ultimate goal of the health professions is to save lives; yet, frequently, her patients die. Nor do the dying patients or mourning relatives provide much source of gratification, as do patients on other floors who go home well. (Even the ICU major successes are usually still seriously ill and are merely transferred.) On the bulletin boards of other units there are warm, sentimental cards and notes of appreciation. In the ICU, the cards are of a different and macabre quality. They say: "Thank you. You did all you could."

Further, the deaths provide a situation of repetitive object-loss, the intensity of which parallels the degree to which the nurse has cathected her patient. The intimacy afforded by the amount and frequency of direct personal contact, involving some of the most private aspects of life, promotes this attachment. This is further enhanced when the patient is conscious and verbal, since he is then so obviously human. Young patients are easily identified with friends and spouses—or with the self, stimulating anxiety about one's own vulnerability. In this country, with its cultural premium on youth, the death of a young patient tends to be regarded as inherently more tragic. Older patients may become transference objects of parental or grandparental figures.

All these warm personal attachments obviously provide great comfort for patients and family and make the job worthwhile. But they expose the nurse to a sense of loss when the patient dies. The balance is a delicate one. With comatose patients, it is easy to limit emotional involvement and subsequent grief. But here, paradoxically, one often sees the nurse project vital qualities into her patient.*

---

*Sometimes this mechanism backfires in an interesting way. The nurse begins to project specific attributes onto the comatose patient. When he recovers and asserts his real personality, especially if this has unpleasant characteristics, she feels a sense of disappointment and betrayal.

The threat of object-loss is pervasive. The nurse simply must protect herself —from grief, anxiety, guilt, rage, exhausted overcommitment, overstimulation, and all the rest. She has no physical escape. But she can avoid, or at least attenuate, the meaning and emotional impact of her work.[10] For example, she may relate more to the machines than to the patient. And, it comes as a surprise to an outsider to observe routinely some of the nurses in the ICU joking and laughing. Even whistling and singing may be observed, phenomena which are inexplicable and unforgivable to distraught relatives. Some of this ebullience arises as a natural product of the friendly behavior of young people working closely together. But a major aspect is gross denial as a defense against their stressful situation. Schizoid withdrawal or a no-nonsense, businesslike manner (isolation) also are used, but cheerful denial is more common. The defensive and, at times, brittle nature of this response is especially evident at times of crisis. At a lull in procedures after a cardiac arrest, for example, giggling and outrageous joking of near hysterical proportion suddenly may supervene. Sometimes the blowup is in the form of anger. But, there are great constraints placed upon the expression of anger by the situation and the group.

THE GROUP

The new ICU nurse experiences the trials of her early days on the job as a *rite de passage*. Some do not make it through. Those who do, learn that they have become members of a special, tightly knit group.* Naturally, they work together on a common job, sharing common experiences. But, there is far more to it than this. Most have volunteered. They have one of the most difficult jobs in the hospital. Nowhere else does a nurse so often literally save lives by her own direct actions. It stands to reason

that nurses who operate special machines and perform special procedures for special patients must be special too! Rightfully, they take pride in their abilities and accomplishments. The very stressfulness of the job is a further source of pride, albeit with masochistic overtones. Like commandos or Green Berets, they have the toughest, dirtiest, most dangerous assignment; and they "accomplish the impossible."

Further cementing group ties are the conditions of the work. They carry on their duties in a common area, using common equipment.[6] In emergency situations particularly, they share the responsibility for each other's patients. Even in nonemergency situations there is a general factor of enforced interdependency. Routinely, for example, one girl must ask another to cover her patients when she goes for a meal. Here an unspoken but potent group norm becomes manifest. Refusal is impossible. Cooperation is absolutely essential for unit function. When a nurse returns from an absence, she may well find that only the most minimal monitoring has been carried out on her patient. No matter how justified its basis, she is likely to be irritated. Yet, group pressures for cooperation and the very fact that there is no time for anger on the job make it imperative to suppress or repress the hostility. These same forces inhibit the expressions of anger that arise inevitably during the course of everyday work when people are in regular close contact. In the total context, this ambivalent hostility serves to bind the group ties with still more intensity.

At the end of a shift of constant work and emotional turmoil, it is near impossible for the nurse to "turn it off" and return to normal pursuits. She needs to unwind. To do so requires the understanding ear of someone who knows what she has been through. Who, then, is a more logical choice of an off-duty companion than another ICU nurse? Thus, one finds much group social activity: parties, showers and just informal off-duty get-togethers. While these might provide an opportunity to express interper-

---

*We have seen similar, though usually less intense, group formation among psychiatric nursing personnel, for some of the same reasons.

sonal hostility, they more often result in "bull sessions" of shared experiences and problems. Similar discussions take place at lunch or coffee breaks, to which they go preferentially with co-workers. These shared feelings feed back to enhance group ties further.

External forces further define the group. The ICU is typically located in an area away from other nursing units. Frequently ICU nurses wear scrub gowns or other protective devices to decrease contamination and soiling; thus they have a distinctive uniform. Very significant is the attitude of other nurses throughout the hospital. Many tend to regard ICU nurses with considerable ambivalence in which envy and projection play a part, and react to being treated as outsiders by retaliatory disregard, isolating the group further.

Group cohesiveness is a logical solution to the multiple practical problems on the job and provides essential emotional support. Being a part of a special group is a major advantage in bolstering the nurse's pride and strength. However, there are not so desirable consequences. The force of the group and the extent of its activities can become all-encompassing, taking over the roles of family and friends. Thus, it can interfere with personal autonomy and outside social relationships. The pressures of the job and group activities may limit healthy introspection. (This may have temporary adaptive value for the girl beset with life problems, or tangled in inner conflict, allowing her to retrench while thus losing herself. But obviously, this can be seriously maladaptive if pursued as a long-term escape.) Absence from the group due to a concurrent social activity may be seen unconsciously as disloyal by both the nurse and the group, though inevitably the familial and social aspect of the group will wear thin for the girl who has achieved maturity and seeks a life of her own. Yet the nurse who fails to use the group may find herself taking out the tensions of work on her family. She may let off steam to a boyfriend, a roommate, or a husband. But

soon, she learns that this can strain the relationship since the person on the receiving end cannot know what it is like to work in the ICU.

Group loyalty reinforces work pressure in stimulating guilt about any absence. The nurse with a minor illness (or one suffering from "combat exhaustion") cannot, in good conscience, stay away as she should. This would increase the work load for her peers. If she does stay home, she cannot "rest easy." Nor, as described above, can she say no to a request to cover another girl's patients, even if she is already working at peak load. This would violate the group norms and threaten the shared fantasy of omnipotence linked to the concept of being special and to the defensive denial of anxiety about mistakes.

This same mechanism can work also to the collective detriment of the group. Like the individual nurse, the group self-destructively cannot say no to situations where its total work load is unrealistic. Paradoxically, the individual almost never can get the group to support protest about realistic problems or unfair exploitation so that changes can be made. Intragroup competitiveness and rivalry may play a part in this. The nurse who will not submerge constructive criticism to the group norm finds she must leave. Since many such nurses will be thoughtful, aggressive people with good ideas, leadership potential is drained away. The whole situation lends itself to perpetuating the status quo and to no recourse but permanent flight (i.e., resignation) when the pressures on an individual build to the point of intolerability.

SOME POSSIBLE SOLUTIONS

From the foregoing, it seems obvious that a constructive approach will capitalize on the many positive aspects of the group process, while attenuating its pathological features. One excellent way to accomplish this is through regular group meetings devoted to exploring the work experience, especially its stressful aspects.[9] These discussions can provide: (a) an avenue for ventilating suppressed intragroup hostilities as well as shared gripes; (b) a recognition that fears, doubts, guilt, and uncertainty are shared, acceptable feelings; (c) the abreaction and working through of feelings aroused at times of stress but which cannot be expressed due to work demands; (d) the sharing of innovative ad hoc techniques which individuals have found helpful in dealing with problems arising on the job; (e) recognition of realistic superior abilities and their delineation from masochistic fantasies of omipotence; (f) a realization that minor mistakes are ubiquitous and inevitable, leading to the detoxification of guilt and shame; and (g) the development of constructive solutions for problems and effective suggestions for communication to administration.

The person who leads these sessions must be experienced and psychologically sophisticated. Communication must be continually focused on the ICU situation rather than expending into more general self-exploration; the interchange cannot be allowed to transcend limits that prevent comfortable working together between sessions. The leader cannot be a member of the ICU administrative hierarchy, nor of the staff group itself, yet he must have a genuine understanding of the work. In fact, he must spend some time regularly on the unit to retain his awareness of the ongoing situation and, thereby, be able to spot sources and signs of sudden increases in stress. Such a role may be filled by a "liaison psychiatrist," who can serve also as a consultant on individual patient management.[14] But it might appropriately be a selected nurse, now that there is a growing cadre within the profession of clinical specialists and others who have had advanced training in group and individual psychology. Or, such a nurse might serve as a co-leader, thereby helping to broaden perspectives and improve doctor–nurse relationships.

While this group process can enhance the appropriate sense of pride and "specialness," more can be done to bolster self-esteem. Here, we have something to learn from studies of morale in combat troups.[11] A distinctive uniform or an identifying patch may be helpful. A small pay differential, like that paid for special shifts, "hazardous duty pay," is an indication of special regard as well as a material reward. Periodic, brief, extra vacations (R and R—Rest and Recreation Leave) will do the same. Such periods might involve work on other nursing units rather than a true vacation, thereby providing education and communication for both staffs. One might consider also whether there should be a finite tour of duty on the ICU, with an enforced interval before a second tour. At the least, transfer to another unit should be made accessible and free from stigma; our experience suggests that often ICU nurses work past the point of "combat exhaustion" and then resign, sometimes with a sense of failure.

Another alternative might be to create a Unit Coordinator position through which the ICU nurses would periodically rotate. Freed from the regular nursing role and its duties, she could fulfill a number of important functions. In an emergency, she could help the head nurse organize the situation or provide an often crucial extra pair of hands. She could help orient new personnel. When consulting physicians arrive on the unit, she could familiarize them with its facilities and routine, thereby reducing their need for direct nursing assistance. She could serve as a major communication link with visitors, providing them with crucial emotional support, and keeping them "out of the hair" of others.

Competitive selection of nurses with superior skills appropriate for the job also will add to pride. In addition to technical expertise, applicants should be screened for psychological aptitude, perhaps by the liaison psychiatrist. In any event, an initial period of training and orientation[12] is essential, and should focus on job characteristics specific to the ICU. The group leader(s) should play a major role in this, so that the psychological aspects of the job experience are fully considered.

A sufficiently large nursing staff is necessary to allow coverage for vacations, weekends, and holidays without the use of outside "floating" assignees. The special characteristics of the unit should also be reflected in the assignment of other personnel. Insofar as the acuteness of its patients and the difficulty of their care are concerned, the ICU is highly specialized. In another sense, however, it is general: It provides care for almost every type of disease process. To provide the full range of treatment required, and to do so on a 24-hour, everyday basis, means that the ICU must be "a hospital within a hospital." Thus representatives of all relevant hospital services always must be at hand. Given a unit of sufficient size, a permanent pharmacist, inhalation therapist, X-ray technician, etc., may become a necessity as part of the regular ICU staff. At the very least, the person "on call" in each of these fields should be given the ICU as his regular assignment to ensure familiarity with the unit.

A *full-time* physician is an especial necessity, constantly and immediately available to examine patients, and as a source of information, advice, and support.[13] Whether a member of the attending or house staff, he must be delegated sufficient authority to be able to write new "orders" whenever indicated by the constantly changing condition of the patients, without necessarily consulting senior physicians of the specialty services to which the patients may be administratively assigned.

All must be familiar not only with their ICU and its patients, but with one another. Whatever their specialized delineation of function, all should act as, and identify themselves as, members of a single unified team. The group meeting, described earlier, should include all,[14] and efforts should be taken to ensure that difference of status and role are not allowed to block effective and open interchange.

The physical design of the ICU also deserves some comment. Consideration should be given to attenuation of the noise and visual bombardment, and some possibility for staff privacy. One potentially use-ful model is the circular one, in which patients occupy "spokes of a wheel."[15] (Each is separated by dividers providing some privacy, stimulus attenuation, and a barrier to contagion, while all remain in view of a central "hub" nursing station.) A nursing station enclosed in glass can permit the exchange of the "unthinkable" out of earshot of visitors and patients. A completely private lounge is also desirable. This can be used for breaks (which would have to be built into the work schedule—otherwise they would never occur!)[9] Also, there are times when the nurses may need the privacy to work out a dispute, to recover emotional stability connected with death, to "escape" from inescapable relatives, etc.

CONCLUSION

Perhaps it will seem as if we have been overly dramatic in our descriptions of the ICU as being so stressful. Most such units function very well. Other parts of the hospital (e.g., emergency and operating rooms) share many of the same stresses, and each deserves examination to understand its particular features. Moreover, nurses who work in the ICU do so by choice, suggesting that, for them, other assignments might be less gratifying or even more stressful. Yet, we believe that the seeming dramatization is, on careful scrutiny, an accurate portrayal and that the intensity and variety of the sources of stress in the ICU is unique. In any event, stress is there. Doubtless it is useful to an extent, enabling the nurses to maintain their critical alertness and ability to respond effectively to the needs of their patients. Yet there are many signs that its intensity goes well beyond this adaptive level. And since there are approaches to deal with this, it behooves us to utilize these for the benefit of both staff and patients.

ACKNOWLEDGEMENT

The authors thank Mary Toomey, R.N., B.S.; Herbert Taylor, R.N., M.S.; David Robinson, M.D.; and Thomas Szasz, M.D., for their assistance and advice.

REFERENCES

1. Abram, H. S. Adaptation to open heart surgery: A psychiatric study of responses to the threat of death. *American Journal of Psychiatry* **122:**659-667, 1965.
2. Bishop, L. F., & Reichert, P. The psychological impact of the coronary care unit. *Psychosomatics* **10:**189-92, 1969.
3. DeMeyer, J. The environment of the intensive care unit. *Nursing Forum* **6:**262-272, 1967.
4. Hackett, T. P., et al. Detection and treatment of anxiety in the coronary care unit. *Amercian Heart Journal* **78:**727-730, 1969.
5. Margolis, G. J. Postoperative psychosis on the intensive care unit. *Comprehensive Psychiatry* **8:**227-232, 1967.
6. Vreeland, R., & Ellis, G. Stresses on the nurse in an intensive-care unit. *JAMA* **208:**332-334, 1969.
7. Gardam, J. F. Nursing stresses in the intensive care unit (Letters to the editor). *JAMA* **208:**2337-2338, 1969.
8. Salter, M. Nursing in an intensive therapy unit. *Nursing Times* **66:**486-487, 1970.
9. Kornfeld, D. S. Psychiatric view of the intensive care unit. *British Medical Journal* **1:**108-110, 1969.
10. Rome, H. The irony of the ICU. *Psychiatry Digest* **30:**10-14, 1969.
11. Grinker, R. R., & Spiegel, J. P. *Men under stress.* Philadelphia: Blakiston, 1945.
12. Boklage, M. G. ICU training program. *Hospitals* **44:**78-80, 1970.
13. Kornfeld, D. S. Psychiatric aspects of patient care in the operating suite and special areas. *Anesthesiology* **31:**166-171, 1969.
14. Koumans, A. J. Psychiatric consultation in an intensive care unit. *JAMA* **194:**633-637, 1965.
15. Armstrong, R. C. "Special care" unit for all intensive care needs. *Hospital Progress* **51:**40-42, 1970.

14

Cancer, emotions, and nurses

SAMUEL C. KLAGSBRUN

The small cancer research unit in a major East Coast university hospital was unique in many ways. It was tucked away in a corner off a main corridor and was screened in by a glass partition that architecturally demonstrated its separateness. It was the only service to which no house staff was assigned. It was funded in a different way from all the other services. And it was the only service in the hospital that had little hope for success in its struggle to ward off death.

The patient population was selected for research purposes. If a patient experienced a remission, he was discharged to the outpatient clinic and followed by the same medical and nursing staff that worked on the inpatient unit. The entire staff got to know the patients, their families, and their friends on an intimate basis.

The psychiatric consultation service of the hospital had been called in from time to time by the cancer research unit to help in the management of difficult patients. We became aware of the tremendous strain the patients placed on the medical and nursing staff. To a great extent the staff saw these patients as walking dead; and since "one should not speak ill of the dead," the staff felt constrained to keep their feelings about the patients to themselves.

But the angry feelings—and guilt at having those feelings—did exist and were very evident in the approach of the staff toward the patients. There was covert rejection of the patients' emotional needs, especially in the face of terminal illness. Numerous struggles between patients and staff took place over such medical issues as the side effects of some of the experimental drugs being used. The patients complained of being used as guinea pigs. "Uncaring doctors" and "unavailable nurses" were phrases that were often repeated to anyone who would listen.

This was the setting, then, in which the following pilot project was attempted.

The psychiatric consultation service assigned me to work as the cancer unit's own psychiatrist in an attempt to analyze and develop a workable approach to the problem of patient management of a cancer unit. I decided that the best approach was to try to alter the ward culture as a whole rather than to deal separately with each patient management problem. The assumption was that the patients' morale and behavior could be improved greatly if they could continue to see themselves as functioning and productive human beings. Meeting these goals would require the creation of an antiregressive atmosphere. And the creation of such an atmosphere would depend largely on the nursing staff. The nurses spent much more time with the patients than anyone else; therefore, their impact was likely to be more pervasive than anyone else's influence on the patients.

MEETINGS WITH THE NURSES

My first job was to make the nurses aware of the importance of their role. After receiving clearance from the medical staff, I began to hold weekly meetings with the nursing staff. The initial object of the one-hour-a-week meeting was to discuss patient management problems. No hint or suggestion was made to indicate that the ultimate object was to deal with the ward culture or with the nursing staff's feelings toward the patients. The reaction of the staff to the appearance of a psychiatrist in their midst was a mixed one. They were gratified to have this effort made on their behalf by a medical service of the hospital, but they also felt self-conscious and somewhat threatened. An initiation phase began. Problems of an emotional nature were not brought up at all. Instead, matters pertaining to drug dosage, organic illness, or the care of weeping sores on the buttocks of patients sent in from other units rose to the surface. My medical competence was thoroughly tested during this period, and only when it became obvious that I was comfortable as well as interested in these aspects of a patient's care were the nurses willing to accept me as a member of the staff.

The head nurse, an extremely competent and perceptive person, broke the ice one day by saying, "Now look, ladies, this is a psychiatrist. Why don't we tell him things he's supposed to know about?"

With that, a flood of feelings began to come out. Many of these were directed not toward the patients, as might have been expected, but toward the medical staff in charge of the unit. What the nurses complained about most bitterly was the lack of emotional backing by the medical staff, rather than the demands of the patients or the depressing nature of their work.

The following incident exemplified their feelings: A middle-aged woman, well known to the staff, had died a few days prior to our weekly meeting, and the mood of the unit was still low. The nurses spoke of their sense of despair and frustration. At one point, a member of the staff turned toward a large, bulky brown bag sitting on the floor in the corner of our room. "Those are her clothes," she said. " I haven't called the family to pick them up."

"This patient was different," another nurse said. "She tried so hard. She was always cheerful, and when she was sent home last time to continue her treatment in the clinic she was so happy."

"And yet other patients have gone through the same thing." I commented. "There must be something different about her."

"It's the way we feel about what the doctors did on the night she died. We saw she was going, and we called the family in to be with her. We also notified the doctor on call, who knew there was nothing he could do. We had earlier decided not to use any heroic measures since there was no way for her to continue her life. The doctor said that we should help the family accept the inevitable and to let him know when she had died. That was it. I was so angry at his coldness I could have cried. But what can you do? I had to control myself because the family was there and there were other patients to take care of."

"What happened when she died?" I asked.

"The family kept asking, 'Is the doctor coming?' It was terrible. I told them that he had left all the necessary orders, but they kept on asking when he would be coming. Finally, they left after she died. We all cried and they thanked us for what we had done. We felt terrible."

"And the clothes?"

"I guess we just don't want to face them. . . . The doctors never come in when there's a situation like this. It's as though the research drug is the most important thing. If it can't be used anymore, they just lose interest. Oh, I guess that's not true, but it's not fair for them to leave this stuff to us to handle."

The meeting continued and cooled down as the nurses spoke up, with less and less anger being directed at the doctors. Finally, at the end, one of the nurses volunteered to call the family to pick up the brown bag of clothes.

The following week the nurses seemed more guarded and distant, as though they had revealed too much in the previous session. In order to let them deal with their feelings about their doctors with some degree of safety and distance, I decided to use another hospital setting as an example of the problem they had raised. I described a meeting the psychiatric consultation service had held with the surgical, medical, social service, and psychiatric staff of a major hospital devoted exclusively to cancer research. We were interested in exploring the emotional effects of some of their radical work on cancer patients. The medical staff had been placing patients in "life islands" for the purpose of keeping them in a sterile atmosphere during periods of low white counts while they were under antimetabolite treatment. They hoped thereby to prevent infections. These patients lived for weeks in a plastic bubble with ultraviolet light shining constantly. The hospital had also been doing hemicorporectomies on patients in the hope of eliminating extension of the disease. In response to some of our questions, one surgeon had summed up his feelings very clearly when he said, "If I thought about what I was doing to the person, I couldn't do it. But I don't think that that is my job."

I asked the nurses for their reaction. After talking about how gruesome they thought these research procedures were, they moved on to discuss the purpose of the procedures. Finally they came around to appreciating the truth and honesty of the surgeon's remarks. As one nurse put it, "If our doctors had to worry about all the nausea and vomiting a drug caused, they probably would feel terrible about prescribing it. I guess that puts us right in the middle. We'll have to handle the patients."

"They give the drug and we stand there with the emesis basin," another added.

RECOGNITION OF DOCTORS' FEELINGS

What emerged from that meeting was a much clearer recognition and understanding of the doctors' need for distance as well as the nurses' own central role in the care of the patient. The exciting part of the meeting was that for the first time the nurses seemed able to accept the emotional burden of the patients without expecting to be supported by the doctors. What was left unsaid was that, given the backing of a psychiatrist, they were able to free their doctors from answering their needs and thereby allow the doctors to spend more time in the labs.

Once the nurses' role was clarified, they began to look at their patients in a more critical way. They became less frightened of being put upon and therefore more open to learning. The methods patients used to express their needs were recognized more quickly. Management problems were analyzed from the point of view of "What is the patient really asking for?" The nurses became sophisticated in recognizing subterfuges for the expression of anxiety. The number of complaints—calling for nurses, turning of nighttime into daytime, repeated questions about what is really in the I.V. bottle—all these were now understood as expressions of fear, and the nurses became quite free in calling the shots as they saw them.

"Let's talk, Mrs. Jones. You really don't need the bedpan again, do you?"

"I know you didn't call, Mr. Brown, but you look sad. Anything I can do?"

The nurses were encouraged to seek out contact before the patients created a crisis situation that required their presence. They now understood that symptoms were often communications on a nonverbal level. In addition, my willingness to use more tranquilizers and antidepressants gave them a sense of confidence. They knew that methods of control were readily available in case of severe agitation and depression that they felt unable to handle. They experienced a marvelous new sense of freedom and openness. "When I told Mr. Smith that if I were in his shoes, I'd be asking many more questions than he was asking," reported one nurse, "I could actually see the tension coming out of his face."

This free and easy approach, however, soon led to complications. Patients were now communicating their worries to the nurses, and many of them asked fairly direct questions about their prognoses. The nurses felt comfortable in talking openly to the patients about anxiety or depression, but they felt they were overstepping their boundaries when patients started asking them about diagnoses, prognoses, and medications. The most frequent question raised was what to tell the patient in response to the question, "Am I going to die?"

The experienced nurses, who really understood their patients and the patients' families, could judge what answer was expected of them.

One example was that of a husband who had refused to bring his sick wife to the hospital because he was sure that the staff would tell her her diagnosis, and he was convinced that she would not be able to tolerate the truth. His wife, on the other hand, asked the nurses not to tell the husband that she had cancer because she was sure he needed to protect her from the truth, since that helped his manly image. But she also knew he would probably be unable to keep it to himself and would feel terrible if he blurted it out to her. She was trying to protect him. The nurses had no difficulty in refraining from talking to him about her illness while listening and talking to the patient about how she was doing.

A second example of courage coupled with wisdom was one reported by a nurse the day after a sad experience. An old woman who was failing rapidly called in one of the nurses and said simply, "I am dying. I feel it is the end, isn't it?" The nurse looked at her and said quietly, "Yes." The nurse sat down next to the old woman, took her hand and held it. "I don't want to die alone," the woman said. "I'll stay with you. You won't be alone," the nurse answered. The woman said, "That's good." And she died in ten minutes, with the nurse holding her hand.

As the nurses got to know their patients better, they realized that the patients were not dead yet and that even those who seemed to see themselves as dead could emerge from the grave in response to crises

in their families or to important external events.

EXPERIMENT IN SELF-CARE

Now everybody was ready for the next step: a radical experiment in self-care. Many of the patients who were in bed did not really need to be there for medical reasons; they simply retired to their beds as part of their withdrawal. The nurses had come to understand that. They began reorganizing the unit. They urged patients to take passes and to leave the ward. They made demands on the patients by asking them to get involved in such projects as sewing and art work. As much as they could, they pushed the patients into activity.

The patients' reaction to the new hustle-bustle varied. Those patients who saw themselves as terminally ill at first resented the expectation that they could take care of themselves. They saw it as further evidence that they were being abandoned by the world. On the other hand, those who found themselves grasping for any bit of evidence that proved they were not sick—or at least not dying—quickly latched on to the new idea that they were still responsible, functioning, and productive people. This group, in fact, began edging the nurses out of jobs and taking over some of the nursing tasks.

For example, one of the first changes made in the ward was to have the patients fix their own beds. Next they were to get their own water and ice. The nurses were a bit fearful of this revolutionary step, and they were upset when the sick patients saw it as a rejection of their needs. But the patient-activists on the ward surprised everybody. They began taking the water and ice to the patients who were too sick to care for their own needs. Then they took over the linen closet and made up beds for the very sick patients. They began eyeing the desk jobs. They wanted to answer the phone and type the admission forms. Finally, they took over the responsibility of running errands to other parts of the hospital. The "revolution" reached the point where the nurses were able to have each new admission oriented to the ward by a welcoming group of the older patients.

The ward acquired a new culture. As the weeks went on, the activists took over the ward, and it was quite common to see a patient get up in the morning with an I.V. drip going into one arm, make his bed with the other, then carry trays of food to the bedridden and explain the new system to the practical nurses who were occasionally assigned to the ward.

The most important step taken, however, was the communal dining room. We decided that providing a nucleus for socialization would add to the atmosphere of liveliness and stimulate the patients further. The dieticians, who took part in all our meetings, arranged for food trays to be brought to a separate room where the patients would gather to eat. This was a major breakthrough that allowed lonely and isolated patients to talk to fellow patients. Now the patients discovered new communal strength that came from shared experience. Patients began organizing evening activities, with the inevitable showing of slides of the latest European trip. Afternoon snacks were delivered to the dining area, and an accumulation of puzzles, cards, and books found its way there. Life was suddenly being lived.

As the experience continued, some of the patients who had had remissions and had gone home began coming back when their illnesses progressed. A common reaction was a sense of relief at returning to a culture that treated them as though something was still expected of them. Some patients had visibly regressed at home, but under the competitive spirit of the ward they too returned to greater activity. Their demands for nursing attention diminished, and they appeared happier.

The self-care atmosphere periodically broke down in the face of actual death and the overwhelming illness of patients, and the nurses learned that in order to maintain this culture they had to nourish and support it. A change in the patient population had to be countered with a renewed nursing effort to teach the new admissions about the ward culture. If the old-time patients of the ward outnumbered the new ones, the culture was protected. Otherwise the authority of the nurses had to be brought into play to back self-care until the new patients could be acculturated.

EFFECT ON MEDICAL STAFF

The impact on the medical staff of the changing culture was interesting. In the beginning they continued to maintain their distance from the patients. But as the ward atmosphere changed more and more, they began asking about the new regulations being instituted. The influence of the ward upon the medical staff was felt to be complete when one of the nurses reported the newest order she had received. The doctor had written, "Patient must eat lunch in communal dining room." The doctor explained that he had noticed that the patient was slipping into a depression and was beginning to regress. He felt that a medical order pushing her into the ward atmosphere would be helpful. This gave us a clue to something we had not been aware of before—namely, that the medical staff had not necessarily ignored the emotional aspects of patient care; they had simply felt they had little to offer. Once it became obvious that there was something that could be done, they turned to it as much as everyone else did.

The increased level of activity of the patients as well as the high level of psychological sophistication of the nursing staff were proven beyond a shadow of a doubt in one incident. A 39-year-old man with cancer had been admitted, and his sexy young wife was a constant visitor. He caught on to the spirit of self-care to such an extent that he decided that he was going to live as normally as possible while he had to be on the unit. The nurse who barged in and found him in bed one day with his wife walked out without another word. At our next meeting, after the giggling died down, the nurses discussed the man's need for denial. They had some serious doubts about whether to forbid this unusual activity on the unit. The final consensus was that it was too much of a radical departure for the ward to handle, and they should not allow it to continue. The fact that they saw it first in terms of patient need and second in terms of ward management showed that the conversion had been accomplished.

In a summary session that was taped, the staff reviewed the history of the experiment after 18 months. The unanimous conclusion was that the changes in the ward were of major importance to the patients. The nurses spoke of the increased will to live that they had noted. They pointed out that patient care was more efficient. And most of all, from an administrative point of view they realized that the turnover rate of nurses, which had been very high, had decreased markedly. Now nurses wanted to work on the unit.

What are the psychological implications of this experience? Certainly the work of some of the investigators reported[1,3-6] shows some correlation between the onset of cancer and the experience of an emotional loss. The implication that such a connection exists in the onset of illness suggests that its remission, or at least its management, may be equally influenced by emotional factors of a positive nature. The effect of a positive ward culture must therefore be considered worthy of research.

Aside from considering the course of the illness, we can think about the quality of life that the patient lives. Palliation need not only be thought of in terms of physical pain; it can also be seen as a legitimate goal to achieve on an emotional level. The response of the patients to the idea that they were expected to function on an adult level decreased their anxiety, dependency, and feelings of being a burden and thereby added to their well-being. the quality of their remaining life was improved.

One of the reactions we frequently see in sick patients is that of shrinking horizons over a period of time. The patient loses interest in the world outside the hospital, then in the life affairs of friends and family, and finally in the ward. At the end, he becomes focused on his own life functions. Maintaining his interest in the surrounding world as long as possible and making him feel responsible for it retards this process and keeps him feeling fulfilled for a longer time.

CONCLUSION

This clinical report suggests an approach quite different from that implied by Kurt Eissler in his famous book.[2] Eissler encouraged the patient's defense mechanism of denial by allowing the patient to imbue his therapist with magical qualities. The therapist enhanced this image by showing concern, bringing gifts, and behaving in a protective way toward the patient. The method implied was "I will take care of you." In contrast, the experience of our cancer unit led us to feel that we could successfully support a patient's denial by using an antiregressive approach.

It might be valuable to test these different approaches in a research project. We certainly do not have the complete answer yet. Our experience indicated that many of our patients did well clinically in the atmosphere we had created. However, I am not convinced that this approach works well during the period just before death. This period is still an unknown entity from a psychological point of view.

There were two main "make-or-break" points in our pilot project when things could have gone very differently from the way they did. The first took place at the initial meeting with the nurses. By focusing the goals of this meeting on patient management rather than anything more radical, I made the road easier for myself. The nurses were able to get to know me without feeling threatened. I could then suggest more significant changes, knowing that I had a comfortable relationship with the staff.

The second point occurred when the nurses decided that they were ready to take a chance and run the ward differently. Without making a major issue of it, I spoke to the medical staff individually and encouraged them to show interest in and appreciation for the project. I pointed out that the more responsible the nurses were made to feel in their involvement with the ward, the less they would burden the medical staff with minor problems. As it turned out, the medical staff became fascinated with the project and invited us to report on it at one of their scientific research conferences.

In any attempt to change a ward culture, as we did, a good deal of groundwork with key people on an informal level becomes necessary. We prepared the medical staff and made sure to discuss all changes with the head nurse, the nursing supervisor, the dietician, and the hospital administration.

Finally, I would like to offer one more observation—the importance of sharing. We all realized that our ability to talk about death and cancer with the patients and to bear their needs without closing ourselves off from them grew in direct proportion to our ability to share our own anxieties at our group meetings. The more we talked together, the more easily we could listen to our patients. As a side note, I was able to serve as a sounding board for the patients and the nurses because I was able to unburden myself at psychiatric consultation service rounds. It seems that if the system works, it does so on all levels.

The implications of this project apply to the hospital as a whole. From a financial point of view the program offers the possibility of reducing costs in that patients may need fewer aides. From a personal point of view it suggests greater stability of staff by decreasing turnover rate. And from a humane point of view, it offers dignity.

REFERENCES

1. Greene, W. A. The psycho-social setting of the development of leukemia and lymphoria. *Annals of the New York Academy of Sciences* **125**:794-801, 1966.
2. Eissler, K. *The psychiatrist and the dying patient.* New York: International Universities Press, 1955.
3. LeShan, L. An emotional life-history pattern associated with neoplastic disease. *Annals of the New York Academy of Sciences* **125**:780-793, 1966.
4. Muslimm, H.L., Gyarfas, K., & Pieper, W. J. Separation experience and cancer of the breast. *Annals of the New York Academy of Sciences* **125**:802-806, 1966.
5. Paloucek, F. P., & Graham, J. B. The influence of psycho-social factors on the prognosis of cancer of the cervix. *Annals of the New York Academy of Sciences* **125**:814-816, 1966.
6. Schmale, A., & Iker, H. The psychological setting of uterine cervical cancer. *Annals of the New York Academy of Sciences* **125**:807-813, 1966.

15

Emotions: their presence and impact upon the helping role

LARRY A. BUGEN

To document the emotional realities of *helpers* who *interact with* persons needing services, I will explore the impact of emotions on caregivers working with people forced to confront a life-threatening illness. Two points should be made clear at the outset. First, a *helper* is a nurse, psychologist, physician, social worker, health educator, member of the clergy, or any other professional whose function it is to promote the health and well-being of people requesting aid. Second, to understand the impact of emotions on the helping role, it is necessary to view the professional not alone, but in interaction with persons needing help.

In most helper-patient relationships, each person values the other person in the interaction. A patient certainly values the training and expertise of the professional, whereas the professional values the health of the patient. They may differ, however, in the extent to which they value various issues related to health care. Dr. Sanchez, for instance, may value a bone marrow transplant, whereas Mrs. Clifton may not. Or, Mrs. Clifton may desire to have her fears and emotional needs regarding treatment alleviated, whereas Dr. Sanchez may be either unable or reluctant to do so.

We can see that a triangular "network" is formed in these situations, consisting of (1) the professional, (2) the patient/client, and (3) some issue related to patient care. When a patient with emotional needs interacts with a professional who does not choose to

acknowledge them, their network is out of balance.[1] In the case cited Mrs. Clifton is likely to experience additional stress and frustration as a result of her physician's failure to meet her needs. Since this particular network is out of balance, Mrs. Clifton will need to cope by (1) modifying her physician's willingness and/or ability to deal with emotions, (2) modifying her own need for emotional expression, or (3) meeting her needs in another network.

People who work with persons facing a life-threatening illness are quite aware of the presence of emotions. How do we as professionals cope with patient/client emotional expression or lack of it? Which emotions are most difficult to respond to? If a helper does have difficulty responding to someone with emotional needs, what resources are available to facilitate the process? When we work with the terminally ill, are we aware of how we feel during the moments we are with them? To whom can we turn when we have difficulty handling our own feelings? Can your emotional reaction to a person with a life-threatening illness affect your perception and treatment of that person?

To summarize:

1. All patients or clients have significant emotional needs that they must cope with to make successful progress.
2. All professionals have significant emotional needs that they must cope with to ensure successful intervention.

3. The helping network established by patients and professionals will not function well unless all of these emotional needs are faced.
4. Emotions, particularly anxiety, can affect professional perceptions, diagnosis, and even treatment of patients.

EMOTIONAL STATES OF PATIENTS

The emotional states of a person facing a life-threatening illness have received much attention in this volume and elsewhere; I will therefore discuss them only briefly. Three models for viewing the dying person exist: (1) the *stage model* proposed by E. Kubler-Ross,[12] (2) the *hive of affect model* proposed by E. Shneidman,[17] and (3) the *stereotyped model* suggested by A. Hutschnecker[8] and O. C. Simonton and S. S. Simonton.[18]

Kubler-Ross suggests that a person facing a life-threatening illness progresses through five relatively predictable stages: denial, anger, bargaining, depression, and acceptance. When first confronting the realization of death, people refuse to believe such a calamity could happen to them. They then become angry about the possibility of dying and may even demand to know "Why me?" Since hope is a powerful dynamic force throughout the dying process, they eventually attempt to make bargains with significant others such as physicians, nurses, or even God. "If I take my medication 'religiously,' Doctor, can you promise that I will have another year?" When their futuristic hopes no longer appear viable, a depression sets in but it does not remain indefinitely. Finally the dying person begins to accept his or her lot and feel at peace both within and with the world around. It is at this time that he or she is ready to die.

The second view, proposed by Shneidman, suggests that a dying person manifests a "hive of affect" in which any one of a number of emotional states may emerge for a while. The dying person wavers between denial and acceptance, between disbelief and hope. One day the person may be ready for last rites and the next day be planning a trip to San Francisco. The extent of pain and the presence of symptoms are certainly powerful forces determining the vicissitudes of rage and envy alternating with acquiescence.

The third view of the dying person, provided by Hutschnecker and the Simontons, holds that the dying patient, even in the face of death, remains true to his or her personality. In addition it is possible to distinguish cardiac patients from cancer patients and cancer patients from one another—all on the basis of personality or emotional expression. For instance, Hutschnecker classifies cancer patients as emotionally passive, dependent, and regressive. In contrast, cardiac patients are characterized as striving for success, aggressive, and rebellious.

The three approaches described have come under close scrutiny. Bugen,[2] for instance, has questioned the validity of the need for distinct stages as proposed by Kubler-Ross. It is nevertheless safe to conclude that there is some truth in each of the models. One important element common to all three is the recognition that persons facing a life-threatening process all experience powerful emotions. However, professionals must understand that diversity, rather than sameness, is the rule. They must also be available or make resources available to promote sharing, talking, crying, or screaming if necessary. This kind of interaction may be mandatory if patients are to reach what Kubler-Ross has described as a calm acceptance of death.

EMOTIONAL STATES OF CAREGIVERS

Interaction with seriously ill people is of course a two-way street. Not only are the progress and welfare of the patient dependent on the attitudes and behaviors of the caregiver; the reverse appears to be true too: The emotional status of caregivers seems to be affected by interaction with persons suffering from life-threatening illnesses. What is the evidence for this contention? Reviews of the clinical literature by both Shady[16] and Schulz and Aderman[15] reach the same conclusion that caregivers must deal with their own feelings about death in order to effectively and comfortably deal with a person facing death. Without self-awareness, persons in a helping role are vulnerable to a wide variety of unpleasant, negative manifestations of anxiety. These aversive states include anger, guilt, helplessness, frustration, and feelings of inadequacy. If you are a caregiver, you might take a moment to reflect on whether you have experienced any of the above emotional states. Or perhaps the more relevant questions are ''When was the last time?'' and ''How did you manage your feelings that time?''

In considering the impact of emotions on caregivers, a more detailed look at the literature seems appropriate. Most of the investigations on the helping role refer primarily to nurses. This is probably so because nurses are more willing to assume daily responsibility for seriously ill persons than other professionals. This is a testimonial to both the nurses' dedication to service and the need for making solid training in this area available to other health care professionals.

Research shows that many hospital staff members typically avoid dying persons. In one study, Waechter[19] found that nurse contacts with fatally ill children decreased as the condition worsened. The nurses both visited the children less often and spent less time with them per visit. Feelings of helplessness combined with increased anxiety are possible explanations for this kind of behavior.

We might think that, the more experience a caregiver has with dying persons, the more manageable his or her feelings and behaviors would become. However, a study by Pearlman and others[14] refutes this belief. In their examination of nursing personnel in a variety of institutions—from state hospitals to nursing homes—they found that those nurses who had more experience with dying persons were *more* likely to avoid the dying and felt more uneasy about discussing death. In fact, 77 percent

reported ''having difficulty'' or avoided discussing matters related to death. Another study by LeShan[11] also documents nurses' avoidance of terminal patients. Using a stopwatch, LeShan recorded how long it took nurses to respond to bedside buzzer calls. He found that it took them significantly more time to respond to terminally ill patients than to less seriously ill persons. These studies suggest that all caregivers, especially experienced ones, avoid contact with patients who are dying.

One explanation for this avoidance is that the medical staff members harbor great anxiety about death and as a result tend to avoid discussions of the subject as well as interactions with patients who are dying. Feifel[4] has reported that physicians are more concerned about death and more afraid of dying than medical students and control groups. A number of observers have noted that, because of this high level of anxiety, physicians, like nurses, avoid a patient once he or she begins to die.[6,12,13]

A study conducted by Kastenbaum[10] pinpointed the strong impact of emotions on the behaviors of caregivers. Kastenbaum was interested in how 200 nurses attendants might respond to a dying person who says, ''I think I'm going to die soon'' or ''I wish I could just end it all.'' Five general categories of responses were established:

1. Reassurance: ''You're doing so well now. You don't have to feel this way.''
2. Denial: ''You don't really mean that. . . . You're not going to die.''
3. Changing the subject: ''Let's think of something more cheerful.''
4. Fatalism: ''When God wants you, He will take you.''
5. Discussion: ''What makes you feel that way today? Is it something that happened, something somebody said?''

Most of the actual responses fell into the categories of denial, changing the subject, and fatalism. You will note that all three of these categories are a form of avoidance. Only 18 percent of the total group of 200 responded by opening up a discussion. As Kastenbaum points out, the "clear tendency was to 'turn off' the patient as quickly and deftly as possible." He offered two reasons for this reaction. First, the nurses wanted to make the patients happy and believed that the best way to accomplish this was to change the subject. Second, most nurses felt very uncomfortable and wanted to protect themselves.

ANXIETY EFFECTS ON PERCEPTION

The foregoing discussion indicates that aversive *emotional states* can affect the *behaviors* of caregivers in very significant ways. A helper who feels anxious being around persons with life-threatening illnesses will tend to avoid or verbally turn off those patients. The implication is that emotions directly affect behavior. However, the relationship between the two may not be so clear-cut.

I have found that emotional states directly affect *perception,* which in turn may affect behavior.[3] In other words, perception may be a key mediating factor in understanding caregiver behaviors. As part of this study, I invited a guest with acute leukemia to speak to a seminar on death and dying composed of 31 students. The topic for that day was "the realities of having a life-threatening illness." Just before the guest speaker arrived all of the students completed Spielberger's (1967) State Anxiety measure; this questionnaire assesses how anxious people feel at the moment, rather than in general.

One might think that anxiety would not be a very vivid emotion during this experience since participants were asked only to listen to the guest speaker and ask questions they wished. I found, however, that the range of anxiety among the participants was quite great: Some persons reported very high anxiety, whereas others reported almost none.

When the guest speaker arrived, she discussed a variety of issues and emotional processes typifying her illness and style of coping. She spoke of the effects of chemotherapy, fears of dying, the importance of having good friends and available resources, and ethical/legal issues relating to the "right to die." She openly and candidly answered the numerous questions asked throughout the presentation.

Once the 45-minute presentation had been completed, the guest speaker departed and all the participants were asked to rate her in the following manner: "To what extent do you believe the following characterizes this person's response to dying?"

	Definitely not true				Definitely true
Denial	1	2	3	4	5
Anger	1	2	3	4	5
Bargaining	1	2	3	4	5
Depressions	1	2	3	4	5
Acceptance	1	2	3	4	5
Hope	1	2	3	4	5

Note that the first five characteristics are the stages of dying described by Kubler-Ross. Since I was interested in the effects of anxiety on the perception of dying stages, the ratings of the 10 most anxious persons were compared to the ratings of the 10 least anxious persons. Significant statistic differences were found. (For a complete statistical report, see reference 3.) The most anxious participants rated this dying person as significantly: (1) *more* denying, (2) *more* angry, (3) *less* accepting, and (4) *less* hopeful. Even though all of the participants observed the same person, at the same time, in the same place, their perceptions of this person varied with their own emotional response, that is, their own anxiety.

This study raises some extremely important questions, particularly for helpers involved in the care of persons with life-threatening illness. As a caregiver are you likely to respond differently to someone you perceive is denying death, compared to someone you perceive is not? For instance, are you more willing to avoid discussing death-related matters in order to "respect the patient's denial?" Similarly are you more likely to avoid persons you perceive to be more angry, less accepting, and less hopeful? Are you more likely to prescribe different medications for such persons? For instance, you may choose to prescribe a tranquilizer to deal with the perceived anger or perhaps a mood elevator to combat the perceived lack of acceptance and hope. To what extent would your behavior as a caregiver affect your patients' responses for coping with death and the progress of the disease process itself?

These questions become vital issues when we stop to realize that our perceptions and our behavior toward persons with a life-threatening illness may well reflect our own discomfort and not theirs. The possibility that we may be projecting our own anxieties onto the dying in ways that affect the course of their treatment mandates that caregivers, as well as caretakers, receive help in coping with their emotions.

MANAGING THE EMOTIONAL RESPONSES OF CAREGIVERS

This chapter has revealed that it is necessary for helpers to be aware of their emotional state while working with patients suffering from life-threatening illness. The emotional realities of such work can be staggering. ICU nurses, for instance, must deal with the constant threat and frequent reality of death, the repetitive routine of close observation (for example, checking vital signs every 15 minutes), complex life-support machinery, frequent acute emergencies, distraught families, frightened patients, and a sometimes unobliging or unsupportive staff. How can they possibly cope in such a situation.

In order for caregivers to manage their emotional responses, two kinds of resources are need.[1] *Internal* resources are those abilities, attitudes, values, beliefs, or techniques that help people handle difficult moments or periods of time. These resources enable them to develop problem-solving strategies that hopefully move them through crises. *External* resources are those people, agencies, customs, or environmental characteristics that facilitate the handling of stressful situations. A friend next door, a counselor, a local widow-to-widow program, and a neighborhood crisis center can all be effective external resources. The Table below lists both internal and external resources that may be helpful in dealing with life-threatening illness. It is important to remember that coping involves two tasks: handling the demands of the external situation and controlling the internal emotional response to it.

As the table points out under internal resources, effective caregivers must do the following:

1. Give up idealism and perfectionist goals. While working with the terminally ill or other populations, it is essential to distinguish between process and outcome. Is it possible to invest totally in the process of helping without expecting some guaranteed outcome such as regeneration of nerve tissue or even life itself? Health care workers certainly cannot save the life of every person with a life-threatening illness. They can, however, help those people live as satisfying a life as possible.

2. Accept feelings. Health professionals

Managing the emotional responses of caregivers

Internal resources	*External resources*
1. Give up idealism and perfectionist goals.	1. Actively invoke help from others.
2. Accept feelings.	2. Find group support.
3. Analyze the problem.	3. Secure a full-time physician or psychologic ombudsman.
4. Maintain self-trust.	4. Carefully design the physical work setting.
5. Focus selectively.	5. Reschedule time commitments.
	6. Maintain inservice training.

are bound to have strong emotional reactions to their work regardless of whether they are therapists interacting with an aggressive client, physicians sharing a dismal prognosis, or nurses working in an ICU. They may at times feel angry, frustrated, depressed, or joyful. Such emotions are the by-products of healthy, caring involvement. Once caregivers can accept the fact that they have these feelings, they can begin the process of sharing them with others.

3. Analyze the problem. Helpers who are reluctant to face their emotions squarely think certain feelings are unacceptable, believe they are unable to handle certain emotions, find that the work setting does not sanction the expression of feelings, or perhaps do not have a support group or person to whom they can turn. As caregivers, we should ask "When do I feel this way? How often? What alternatives are available? Which one should I attempt first? How will I know if it is effective?" This kind of active exploration of reality will encourage us to solve problems rather than hide them.

4. Maintain self-trust. Persons who cope well in a variety of situations have a robust self-esteem. They generally like themselves and what they do. They believe in themselves and rely on this foundation of trust to work through the feelings or difficult moments that inevitably arise.

5. Focus selectively. La Rochefoucould has said that we can't stare directly at the sun or death for any length of time. Helpers who find themselves dwelling excessively on death or other aversive qualities of their work may need to concentrate selectively on the satisfactions of the job or the assets of their patients. Such a constructive use of denial may have the added benefit of focusing attention on the problems of living rather than on those of dying. Caregivers who use this tactic may be able to confront situations in which they can effect change rather than being blocked with feelings of helplessness.

In addition to perfecting these techniques, caregivers can utilize external resources:

1. Actively invoke help from others. Anyone in the helping professions is aware that each individual usually believes he or she is unique in having a particular feeling or a concern. Caregivers involved with life-threatening illness are no different. Social workers, physicians, nurses, or orderlies may consider their feelings of helplessness or depression unusual without checking the validity of this belief with others. Just as helpers interact with their patients, they must also interact with each other to maintain a dynamic and effective problem-solving system.

2. Find group support. If finding help from colleagues can be useful, organizing for such help is also a good idea. The deliberate creation of a supportive structure has been suggested by Kastenbaum,[9] who believes that "a mutual support network should exist among the staff, encompassing both the technical and the socioemotional dimensions of working with the terminally ill." It is not necessary to have the participation of everyone to organize an effective support group. Even a few like-minded people can be effective. They should try to get block time and administrative approval for the group. The success of the group may well depend on the consistency with which all members use one another as resources. Ideally membership in such a group will not come from any single discipline but will offer an opportunity for all persons with an emotional stake in life-threatening illness to give and take.

3. Secure a full-time physician or psychologic ombudsman. The decision-making that is constantly required in the care of the terminally ill can be quite stressful to caregivers, especially if knowledgeable authorities are not available to examine patients and provide information, advice, and support. This is particularly true in hospital settings such as the ICU. The presence of a full-time physician could ease the burdens of the immediate tasks at hand. The availability of a full-time psychologist, social

worker, or psychiatrist with expertise in emotional responses to terminal illness would be an additional, valuable resource in hospital and clinical settings.

4. Carefully design the physical setting. Staff members should have a place to go that ensures privacy and a break from routines. The use of a lounge should be built into work schedules; otherwise such an area may never be used at all. The unpredictable nature of emotions will also require the unscheduled use of such a facility in intervening with grieving relatives or in recovering emotional stability after the death of a patient.

5. Reschedule time commitments. *Burnout* is a phenomenon common to all helping disciplines. It occurs when demands and emotional pressures of work cause staff to become so calloused, frustrated, or anguished that they are forced to change jobs. One way to prevent burn-out while maintaining vitality within a work setting is to schedule shorter rotations for shifts on which intense and emotionally draining interaction is the rule rather than the exception.

6. Maintain inservice training. The need for staff members to assimilate new information and upgrade their skills is constant in organizations that are vital and changing. Caregivers working with the terminally ill may have special needs in understanding loss and grief, learning techniques of bereavement intervention, and exploring the emotional response of helpers. Internal consultants from the work agency itself or external consultants from neighboring facilities should be a component of any health care delivery system. A useful examination of the emotional needs of staff members who interact with persons facing life-threatening illness may require an experiential workshop format. The appropriateness of such methods will become clearer once the goals for inservice training have been elaborated.

It seems best to conclude this discussion by distinguishing between the *role of saving* and the *role of helping*. A helper who takes on the role of saving has an emotional investment in those persons with whom he or she interacts. Such a helper believes that his or her efforts determine the consequences for the patient or client. The logical extension of this attitude is that, the more the caregiver does, the more likely he or she will prolong or even save a life. Health workers who subscribe to the saving role may find themselves the victims of a double-edged sword. The more involved they get in their efforts to save, the more likely they will experience the feelings of failure. It is perhaps these feelings of failure —a concomitant of the role of saving—that account for so much of the avoidance behavior discussed earlier in this chapter.

The role of helping is an alternative to the dilemma. Like the role of saving, the role of helping stresses the need for emotional investment in seriously ill patients and their families. However, helpers do not believe that their efforts are *necessary* to achieve certain desired outcomes. They do not come to work thinking that they have a life to prolong or save. Instead, they believe in a present-oriented involvement by which they give as much of themselves *now* as they possibly can. A patient's welfare at the present time is what matters. If a person's physical, emotional, or spiritual health can be enhanced in any way, a helper will find the means to do so. In contrast to people who take on the role of saving, helpers do not experience a double-edged sword. The more involved they get, the more successful they feel, since the criterion for success is the process of giving and *not* the product of saving.

I believe that caregivers who take on the role of helping are (1) less likely to avoid the emotional needs of those they serve, (2) more likely to be aware of their own emotional responses, (3) less likely to misperceive the needs of their patients/clients, and (4) more likely to utilize the internal and external resources. The task of accepting major responsibility for caring for another person's physical needs and investing energy in the emotional and psychologic welfare of another *is* involvement. There is no way to avoid involvement as a helper. There are ways, however, to nurture it and make it flourish through the process of interaction.

REFERENCES

1. Bugen, L. A.: Fundamental of bereavement intervention. In Bugen, L. A., ed.: Death and dying: theory, research and practice, Dubuque, 1978, William C. Brown Co., Publishers.
2. Bugen, L. A.: Human grief: a model for prediction and intervention, American Journal of Orthopsychiatry **47**:2, 1977.
3. Bugen, L. A.: State anxiety effects upon perceptions of dying stages, Unpublished manuscript, University of Texas, Austin, 1977.
4. Feifel, H., Hanson, S., and Jones, R.: Physicians consider death, Proceedings of the 75th Annual Convention of the American Psychological Association, **2**:201-202, 1967.
5. Friedman, M., and Rosenman, R. H.: Type A behavior and your heart, New York, 1974, Alfred A. Knopf, Inc.
6. Glaser, B., and Strauss, A.: Awareness of dying, Chicago, 1965, Aldine Publishing Co.
7. Heider, R.: The psychology of interpersonal relations. New York, 1958, John Wiley & Sons, Publishers.
8. Hutschnecker, A.: Personality factors in dying patients. In Feifel, H., ed.: The meaning of death, New York, 1959, McGraw-Hill Book Co.
9. Kastenbaum, R.: Death, society, and human experience, St. Louis, 1977, The C. V. Mosby Co.
10. Kastenbaum, R.: Multiple perspectives on a geriatric "death valley," Community Mental Health Journal **3**:21-29, 1967.
11. Kastenbaum, R., and Aisenberg, R.: The psychology of death, New York, 1972, Springer-Verlag, Inc.
12. Kubler-Ross, E.: On death and dying, New York, 1969, Macmillan Inc.
13. Livingston, P., and Zimet, C.: Death anxiety, authoritarianism, and choice of specialty in medical students, Journal of Nervous and Mental Disease **140**:222-230, 1965.
14. Pearlman, J., Stotsky, B., and Dominick, J.: Attitudes toward death among nursing home personnel, Journal of Genetic Psychology **114(1)**:63-75, 1969.
15. Schulz, R., and Aderman, D.: How medical staff copes with dying patients: a critical review, Omega **7(1)**:11-21, 1976.
16. Shady, G.: Death anxiety and care of the terminally ill: a review of the clinical literature, Canadian Psychological Review **17(2)**:137-142, 1976.
17. Shneidman, E.: Death: current perspectives, Palo Alto, 1976, Mayfield Publishing Co.
18. Simonton, O. C., and Simonton, S. S.: Belief systems and management of the emotional aspects of malignancy, Journal of transpersonal psychology **7**:1, 1975.
19. Waechter, E.: Death anxiety in children with fatal illness, Dissertation Abstracts **29**:2505, 1969.

16

The coronary-care unit: an appraisal of its psychologic hazards

THOMAS P. HACKETT, N. H. CASSEM, and HOWARD A. WISHNIE

The frequency of psychiatric difficulties in intensive-care units ranges from 30 to 70 per cent. Confinement in these units is described as an "ordeal,"[1] and the patient's expected psychologic response is presented as one of "catastrophic reaction."[2] Although the study from which this last term developed was conducted on postcardiotomy patients in the setting of the recovery room, there has been a growing tendency to apply it to all situations of intensive care. This is an unfortunate application because intensive-care settings differ remarkably as do the emotional responses of the patients they house. The question of whether patients in coronary-care units are subject to the "new madness of medical progress"[3] led to the work described below.

Although most investigators agree that organic factors play an important part in causing postcardiotomy delirium,[4-6] some maintain that the environment of intensive care is more to blame.[7,8] These authors cite sensory monotony and sleep deprivation as the principle causal factors. The equipment of intensive care, especially cardiac monitoring devices, is almost universally regarded as conducive to the patient's psychologic decline. Witnessing cardiac arrest and proximity to other critically ill patients have also been indicted for contributing to delirium, but no study has systematically divided the complex environment of intensive care into components suitable for study and comparison. Only by examining the patient's response to a series of variables found in all intensive-care units and comparing the findings with those in special units, such as recovery rooms, shall we be able to focus on the source of psychiatric trouble. The present study is the beginning of such an effort.

METHODS

Fifty patients, ranging in age from 37 to 74 (mean of 58), comprise our sample. All were admitted to the unit with the diagnosis of myocardial infarction. Thirty-five were males, and 15 females. Their average time in the coronary-care unit was four and eight-tenths days. Four died during the study. Patients were selected in a random fashion. The only criterion for inclusion was the ability to speak English. Thirty-seven were general-hospital patients in a four-bed intensive-care ward. Thirteen were private patients and had individual rooms on an intensive-care floor. The four-bed ward was a cramped, essentially windowless place, as cheerless and drab as a

Reprinted by permission from the New England Journal of Medicine, 279:1365-1370, December 19, 1968.

From the Department of Psychiatry, Massachusetts General Hospital (address reprint requests to Dr. Hackett at the Massachusetts General Hospital, Boston, Mass. 02114).

Work performed under a contract (PHS-43-67-1443) with the National Institutes of Health, Public Health Service, United States Department of Health, Education, and Welfare.

room in a tenement. Beds were separated by heavy, retractable, ceiling-to-floor curtains. There was no sound proofing. Sexes were mixed. The nursing station was adjacent to the unit, but not in visual contact. The only difference between the ward and private accommodations was privacy.

In the four-bed ward monitors were placed on a wall shelf above and behind the patient's bed. This made it difficult for the patient to observe his own oscilloscope, but easy to see his neighbor's. In the private rooms the monitor was on a bedside cart with the cathode screen usually visible. Constant intravenous therapy was carried out on all patients, and most had indwelling urethral catheters. Vital signs were taken hourly or more often, invariably awakening each patient.

The investigators introduced themselves to the patient within a day of his admission to the unit. We identified ourselves as part of a project interested in finding out what patients thought of intensive care. We indicated special interest in providing more comfort. Each patient was asked if he would help us and if he would mind our recording the interview on tape. Only one patient preferred not to be interviewed when she learned that the investigator was a psychiatrist. Interviews lasted from five minutes to an hour, depending on the patient's state of health and desire to participate. Questions were asked in the context of the patient's medical illness. Emotional issues were not pursued, and there was no psychologic probing. In general, the interview was designed to be as nonthreatening as circumstances could allow. It was closed at the first sign of distress. Each patient was seen between three and 10 times during his hospital stay. We assumed no direct role in the immediate care of the patient.

FINDINGS

Our data are broken down into 10 groups. The number of patients in each group is sometimes less than 50 because our data could not always be completed before the patient died or was otherwise lost to us.

The setting

Not one of the 48 patients questioned spontaneously complained about the atmosphere of the unit. Upon being asked specifically, eight agreed that the quarters were small or depressing or both. Six of the eight were lifelong claustrophobes. We could elicit no suggestions for improving the design of the unit, and most patients preferred to have no television or music.

The cardiac monitor

Twenty-six of the 50 patients questioned were reassured by the bedside presence of the monitor. Eighteen were neutral to its presence, and six disliked it. There was a trend indicating that women respond more positively than men to the monitor's presence. Thirty-nine did not object to the monitor's sound (three even found it comforting), and 11 considered it annoying.

Fourteen wanted to watch their own electrocardiographic tracings and made an effort to do so even though it meant twisting about uncomfortably to look over their shoulders. Three objected to seeing their oscilloscope patterns, and the remainder were neutral to it. Sixteen patients enjoyed watching the monitor of others; this group included five patients who did not want to observe their own. Men were far more interested than women in watching the oscilloscope.

There was no apparent correlation between the patient's knowledge of the monitor's purpose and his response to its sight, sound or presence.

The alarm accidentally sounded for 19 patients. The fact that only five of them admitted being frightened may be the result of previous explanations of the monitor's function and anticipation of the possibility of false alarm.

Transfer out of the unit

Responses were obtained from 45 patients. Thirty-three were reassured by being transferred from the unit. They interpreted the transfer as tangible evidence of improvement. Eight experienced a sense of loss with the transfer; each missed the attention that he received in the unit and the security of constant observation. Four were transiently frightened about the function of their hearts without a monitor.

Delirium

Five patients out of the 50 were delirious. Four were confused and disoriented in time and place, and in the fifth paranoid delusions developed as well (a response that was thought to be caused by atropine-like eye drops since it cleared within a day after the medication was discontinued). The predominant moods of the delirious patients are included in the next section. All five were anxious, of these, two were also hostile, and two others depressed.

Mood

Judgments of predominant mood for each of the 50 patients were made from comments in the hospital chart, nursing notes, observations by relatives, impressions of the investigator and subjective reports from the patient himself. At least two corroborating sources were required to confirm each investigator's observation. There was no disagreement between these sources.

Anxiety was judged to be present when the patient complained of being anxious or when he appeared nervous, sweaty, fidgety or restless or constantly asked for reassurance or sedation. Agitation, as we use the term, refers to patients who were notably hyperactive and whose motor restlessness evoked comment from all who cared for them. Depression was judged to be present either when the patient appeared despondent and was seen to cry or if he admitted to sadness or discouragement during our interview.

Forty of the 50 patients were judged anxious. Eight were agitated, and 11 expressed anger at fate or circumstances; hostility, however, was not directed against individuals. Twenty-nine admitted being de-

pressed or exhibited behavior consistent with depression. The depression was a reaction to coronary disease and judged to range from mild to moderate in intensity. In no case was the depressive reaction incapacitating; none of the patients required psychiatric treatment after discharge for the six-month period of our follow-up observation. Although the fact may be incidental, all four of the patients who died during our study were rated as depressed.

Sense of time

While in the coronary-care unit, 17 out of 38 questioned lost their temporal sense for the time of the day or the day of the week or the date in the month or any combination of these. The remaining 21 were fully oriented. Regardless of whether the patient retained his sense of time or lost it, only seven out of 36 questioned wanted a wall clock. Of the 33 asked, five wanted a wall calendar.

Twelve of the 38 patients had a complete amnesia for their time in the emergency ward as well as for most of their confinement in the coronary-care unit. A review of their charts disclosed that five contained notes to the effect that the patient was confused or disoriented, but the remaining seven contributed nothing to explain this memory lapse. Apparently, the doctors and nurses were unaware of any perceptual impairment during the period in question.

Dreaming

Thirty out of 40 patients questioned denied dreaming during their hospital stay. Of the 10 who dreamed seven had nightmares. Four of these patients were the survivors of cardiac arrest.

Witnessing cardiac arrest

Eleven of the 50 witnessed a fatal cardiac arrest. Seven of these denied fear either during or after the arrest. Only three admitted fear. These data were not collected on the eleventh patient. The initial response to watching the arrest was irritability and annoyance at the patient affected. This was rapidly followed by astonishment at the efficiency of the arrest team. All who witnessed the event described the activity with remarkable clarity. Sounds and imagination must have been involved because most accounts came through as if the bed curtain had not been drawn. For example, one patient "knew the doctor was massaging the heart." Another "knew they were opening the chest." In neither case was a thoracotomy performed, and the bed curtains were pulled shut in both.

One patient was reassured by the arrest drill because the victim was an elderly woman. He mused that if they did that much for her, they would go all out for him because he was so much younger. When asked if he worried more about himself after seeing the arrest he replied, "Oh, no, she was an old lady." Although empathy for the victim was expressed by all 11, none identified himself with the patient affected.

Survival of cardiac arrest

Nine of the 50 had cardiac arrest. Three died without recovering consciousness, and six survived—one, however, for only 13 days. Only two could remember anything about the event. A male patient vaguely recalled being thumped on the chest and hearing doctors' voices. The second, a woman, was unsure whether what she reported really happened or took place in a dream. "A funny experience . . . a hand down my throat squeezing my heart . . . I felt it was happening . . . but I don't know if it happened in a dream." Two patients had nightmares immediately after the arrest. A woman dreamed of smothering in a fire, and a man of being caught trying to smoke cigarettes. Two others had nightmares only after they returned home. One blamed sleeping medication for her bad dreams because they stopped when her bedtime barbiturate was discontinued. The other patient complained of "troubled dreams" that stopped once she returned to work. Traumatic neuroses with chronic anxiety and emotional invalidism have not developed in the three patients who are alive

at the six-month follow-up interval. Two have returned to work, whereas the third remains inactive because of physical disability. One of the two who died after leaving the hospital had signs of chronic anxiety and overdependency on his wife; the other man was emotionally stable until his death.

None of the six considered themselves unique as a result of having survived a period of heart stoppage. Two regarded their arrests as the equivalent of dying, but did not elaborate on this even when urged to do so by the investigator.

Denial

The defense mechanism of denial is defined as the conscious or unconscious repudiation of part or all of the total available meaning of an event to allay fear, anxiety or other unpleasant affects.[9] The term "major denial" is used to describe patients who stated unequivocally that they felt no fear at any time throughout their hospital stay; 20 of the 50 examined were in this group. The term "partial denial" is applied to the 26 patients who initially denied being frightened but who eventually admitted feeling at least some fear. "Minimal denial" is used to describe patients who complain of anxiety or who readily admit being frightened. In this group of four patients no consistent criteria for denial could be found. What little attempt they made to deny was transparent and ineffective.

The major denier usually had a lifelong pattern of reacting to emotional stress by simply repudiating it. The cliché was a common method of renouncing danger. Typical of the major denier's response was the following. We had asked a 52-year-old longshoreman why the prospect of another cardiac arrest did not bother him. "Why worry? If the marker's got your name on it, you've got to buy it." Another, disclaiming any concern about being attached to a cardiac monitor, said, "Some people would be scared [by the machine] but not me. I'm called the 'iron man.'" A third, when asked how he could have gone through four days in the unit, including witnessing a fatal cardiac arrest, without having a thought or a care for death answered, "My middle name is Lucky."

The partial denier often gave the same initial impression as his major counterpart. He might begin by disclaiming all fear, but its presence was revealed in subsequent statements. For example, one patient began saying, "I wasn't afraid because if I'm gonna go, there is nothing I can do about it. When my number's called, I'm gonna go—why panic?" This was followed by, "You've got to be alarmed a little, but why go all to pieces." A major denier would not have acknowledged the presence of alarm.

Denial is apt to be more evident when the alternative is to acknowledge fear. For example, 28 of 45 patients admitted they had thought of death during confinement in the unit; however, only 11 of 42 admitted experiencing fear during that time. Consequently, it appears that thoughts of dying do not necessarily produce an admission of fear in these patients.

Statistical analysis of our data demonstrated no significant relation between denial and the patient's mood. Anxiety, depression, hostility and agitation were equally dispersed among the deniers. Neither age nor sex correlated significantly with the patient's use of denial. However, there was a definite trend for deniers to respond positively to the cardiac monitor. None of the minimal deniers found monitoring reassuring.

Although the numbers are small, it is noteworthy that an inverse relation exists between denial and mortality. Not one major denier died during the study; two of the four deaths were in minimal deniers. The minimal denier, representing 8 per cent of the total sample, contributed 50 per cent of the mortality. Chi-square analysis shows this relation to be significant beyond the 5 per cent level.

DISCUSSION

Since some of our findings disagree with the concept of intensive care developed by others[1,2,5,7,10,11] we must question whether our unit and population differ from the others. They do in two respects, the first being that our work was done in a coronary-care unit whereas most of the other investigations were carried out in recovery rooms. Although the threat of sudden death is common to both settings, they differ in important ways. Recovery rooms usually contain more patients, are noisier and more brightly illuminated throughout the day and night, and have a hospital odor, more equipment and more rush and turmoil. The second point is that our cases were nonsurgical whereas samples used by previous investigators were largely postcardiotomy. The surgical patient is apt to be more obtunded and uncomfortable in the days after surgery than the patient with a myocardial infarction. Much of the varience between our data and those of others can be explained simply by these two differences. The reason for calling attention to what may seem obvious is the growing tendency to speak in terms of an "intensive-care syndrome"[10] as though intensive care, *sui generis,* induces a psychiatric condition. Our findings and those of others[12,13] indicate that this need not be the case.

In general, occupants of the coronary-care area are undercomplainers. There are three possible explanations: it is obvious to each patient that discomfort experienced in the unit is more than counterbalanced by the care and personal attention received; the patient is apt to be so preoccupied with his illness that surroundings are hardly noticed; and since the patient's welfare is almost entirely dependent upon the unit, to complain or criticize, even when asked to do so, is to risk good will. In follow-up studies done at intervals of three and six months after discharge, patients can recall service shortcomings, but seldom complain. Generally, the unit and its personnel are lavished with praise, most of which is deserved.

The fact that the majority of patients were either reassured by the monitor or indifferent to its presence is consistent with earlier work.[14] Unless these patients pretended this response or totally repressed fear, their reactions indicate that the machine has an immense potential for giving security—one that has largely been overlooked. If the monitor is introduced by the nurse as a "mechanical guardian angel,"[15] expressly designed to keep the heart functioning at maximum efficiency, the patient is apparently more inclined to accept the machine as such rather than to dwell upon its minatory significance. Even the potentially shattering experience of having an accidental alarm need not produce panic if the patient has been prepared for this event.

Although a few patients expressed curiosity about the machine, none asked specific questions even when they were invited to do so. They accepted what was told them with what seemed to be implicit faith. Consequently, the lifesaving properties of the monitor could be exploited in a manner most propitious to the patient's emotional well-being.

The 16 patients who claimed to enjoy watching the electrocardiographic tracings of their neighbors could give no reason for it. Perhaps the principal motive had to do with what they could read into the tracing. For instance, six of the 16 claimed their own tracings were more stable than those of their roommates, although there was no basis for this in fact.

Despite the high percentage of positive responses to the unit, most patients were glad to leave when the time came. Their reasons were all the same: transfer out signified tangible proof of their improvement. The eight out of 45 patients who felt a sense of loss upon leaving the unit mainly missed the instant attention given their needs by the nurses; the four who suffered weaning anxiety were all helped within hours by reassurance and sedation.

With the exception of a study by Parker and Hodge,[16] the occurrence of delirium in our population was lower than has been reported in previous work on critical care. The absence of postcardiotomy patients in our population and that of Parker and Hodge probably largely accounts for this. Another factor that may have had a bearing on the few cases of delirium among our patients was the house officer's tendency to undermedicate patients for pain, apprehensiveness and sleep. As a result, narcotics, sedatives and tranquilizers were not likely to enhance disorientation and confusion. Nonetheless, it is remarkable that so few major psychiatric complications arose in a setting that provided sleep deprivation, violent fluctuations in sensory input, ranging from monotony to sudden terror, and always the constant threat of death.

It is not surprising that many patients were anxious and depressed. Our surprise is directed more to the absence of serious panic reactions and major depressions. The defense of denial, so actively employed, may account for the mildness of the affective response. Whether or not the patients were pretending to be calm cannot be answered now. With the help of a polygraph and biochemical measures we hope to obtain a more objective method of assessing response to stress.

Disorientation in time occurred in less than half the sample. It was mild, occasioned no trouble to the patient and was easily corrected by nurses or relatives. The most unexpected finding was that time cues offered by wall clocks and calendars were not wanted by most patients. Since neither clocks nor calendars were present in the unit, patients may have minimized their importance to avoid seeming to complain.

The paucity of dreams, including nightmares, in our patients may be explained, in part, by the sparse amount of sedatives and sleeping medication given them. Druss and Kornfeld[11] report that eight of 10 survivors of cardiac arrest had violent nightmares. They also list persistent insomnia as occurring in nine out of 10 such patients. Our figures on nightmares support this finding, although two of the four patients who suffered from them after arrest blamed sleeping pills and idleness for their occurrence and reported abrupt cessation once these factors were corrected. Insomnia was not admitted to, although early wakefulness was present in one case.

The response of our patients to the witnessing of cardiac arrest offers a good example of how patients can grasp the most comforting meaning from an event while denying the more threatening. Even when the patient with arrest was the same age as the patient onlooker, some reason was always found to differentiate the onlooker's condition from that of the victim. If death occurred, the staff quickly reassured the survivor that the deceased's heart was much worse than his. No matter how obvious the excuse, patients seemed to accept it without question or reservation. The tendency was to extract from the situation only the elements that could bolster denial and thus restrain fear.

We question whether these responses represent the patient's true feelings. There is some evidence in our data that witnessing an arrest may cause the observer to ask for a private room in subsequent admissions for coronary care. More evidence through such unobtrusive measures, combined with biochemical and polygraphic studies, is required before we can draw conclusions from these data.

Like the patients described by Druss and Kornfeld,[11] those of our series who experienced cardiac arrest were unable to recall much of the event. The vague recollections of two are reported in the findings. Largely because of the total amnesia for the arrest, none of the six could assimilate it as part of the hospital experience. Even the two who spoke of having died and returned made little of it. We had the impression that with the passage of time, unless constantly reminded, they would forget that their heart had required assistance to regain its beat.

The use of denial as a defense against fear and anxiety has been dealt with at length in psychiatric literature. It is, perhaps, the most commonly used mental mechanism to cope with acute emotional stress. The reason for identifying three types of denial has to do with their management and perhaps their prognosis as well. It is important to

separate partial from major denial because patients with the former want reassurance but do not know how to ask for it directly; they also may be much more apprehensive than they appear and might benefit from sedation. Reassurance, encouragement and heavy sedation would also be the treatment of choice for the minimal denier. It is difficult to offer a method of approach for the major denier because we know less about him. The fact that none died during our study may indicate that the ability to deny to this extent has value for immediate survival, at least. Man has a faculty for defending himself against emotional stress in endlessly inventive ways, not the least of which is denial. We know very little about how he manages to deny obvious stress and less about whether this ability to deny can protect his cardiovascular system. The little we have learned ought to make us wary of drawing conclusions from impressions.

REFERENCES

1. Egerton, N., and Kay, J. H. Psychological disturbances associated with open-heart surgery. *Brit. J. Psychiat.* **110**:433-439, 1964.
2. Meyer, B. C., Blacher, R. S., and Brown, F. Clinical study of psychiatric and psychological aspects of mitral surgery. *Psychosom. Med.* **23**:194-218, 1961.
3. Nahum, L. H. Madness in recovery room from open-heart surgery or "They kept waking me up." *Connecticut Med.* **29**:771, 1965.
4. Blachly, P. H., and Starr, A. Post-cardiotomy delirium. *Am. J. Psychiat.* **121**:371-375, 1964.
5. Blachly, P. H., and Kloster, F. E. Relation of cardiac output to post-cardiotomy delirium. *J. Thoracic & Cardiovasc. Surg.* **52**:422-427, 1966.
6. Gilman, S. Cerebral disorders after open heart operations. *New Eng. J. Med.* **272**:489-498, 1965.
7. Kornfeld, D. S., Zimberg, S., and Malm, J. R. Psychiatric complications of open-heart surgery. *New Eng. J. Med.* **273**:287-292, 1965.
8. Abram, H. S. Adaptation to open heart surgery: psychiatric study of response to threat of death. *Am. J. Psychiat.* **122**:659-667, 1965.
9. Weisman, A. D., and Hackett, T. P. Predilection to death: death and dying as psychiatric problem. *Psychosom. Med.* **23**:232-256, 1961.
10. McKegney, F. P. Intensive care syndrome: definition, treatment and prevention of new "disease of medical progress." *Connecticut Med.* **30**:633-636, 1966.

11. Druss, R. G., and Kornfeld, D. S. Survivors of cardiac arrest: psychiatric study. *J.A.M.A.* **201**:291-292, 1967.

12. Sgroi, S., Holland, J., and Marwit, S. J. Psychological reactions to catastrophic illness: comparison of patients treated in intensive care unit and medical ward. Presented at twenty-fifth annual meeting. American Psychosomatic Society, March 29-31, 1968.

13. Pentecost, B. L., Mayne, N., and Lamb, P. Organization of coronary care unit in general hospital. *Brit. M. J.* **3**:298-301, 1967.

14. Browne, I. W., and Hackett, T. P. Emotional reactions to threat of impending death: study of patients on monitor cardiac pacemaker. *Irish J. M. Sc.* **6**(496):177-187, 1967.

15. Craffey, R. Cardiac pacemaker. *Quart. Rec. Massachusetts General Hospital Nurses Alumni A., Inc.* **10**(3):8-10, Fall, 1960.

16. Parker, D. L., and Hodge, J. R. Delirium in coronary care unit. *J.A.M.A.* **201**:702, 1967.

17

The hospital environment: its impact on the patient

DONALD S. KORNFELD

> It is not enough for us to do what we can do; the patient and his environment, and external conditions have to contribute to achieve the cure.
>
> *Hippocrates*

With the growth of modern hospital technology, there has been increasing concern by physicians for the emotional impact of the hospital environment on patients. In the past, the hospital environment has been studied primarily by social scientists[1-5] who have examined it as a social system. Few studies, however, have been done by physicians. This probably reflects two facts:

1. Members of the medical profession develop the necessary psychological defense mechanisms which allow them to work in this environment but in doing so, prevent themselves from appreciating its effect on others.

2. Physicians have not, until recently, appreciated that clinically significant reactions to the hospital environment can occur.

While space-age electronic gadgetry has dramatized the problem, the hospital has probably always been a frightening place for patients and their families. Certainly on one psychological level patients can appreciate hospitalization as a reassuring thing. We all know that "modern medicine" is now able to perform "miracles," but that big building with its special sights, sounds, and smells remains for most people a very frightening place. The hospital, however, is staffed by special people who have chosen to be there. It is merely the place where they work and they pass through its doors each morning with no more anxiety than business executives and secretaries entering an office building. Obviously, it is important that a medical staff be able to work without the emotional upheavals experienced by patients. They must, therefore, develop psychological defenses to allow themselves to deal objectively with the serious problems they must face each day. As a result, most of them do not appreciate the stress of hospitalization on the average patient.

A patient's maladaptation to the hospital environment can produce important clinical changes. The cardiovascular and endocrine responses associated with anxiety are well known. More recently we have begun to identify physiological changes which may accompany depression. It is reasonable to suspect that such psychophysiological responses can influence the course of illness. However, the environment can produce effects which are more obviously a threat to a patient's physical well-being. For example, the agitated psychotic patient

Reprinted in abridged form from Advances in Psychosomatic Medicine **8**:252-270, 1972.

in the open-heart recovery room with tachycardia and rising blood pressure is in danger of compromising his cardiac status. The patient who signs out of the hospital against medical advice because she misunderstood a remark made at bedside rounds runs all the risks of delayed diagnosis and treatment. Therefore, to consider the impact of the hospital environment on patients is not mere compassion, but a medical necessity.

What is the hospital environment? Bricks, machines, people. Each, in its own way, contributes to the atmosphere of the institution and its effect on the individual patient. Hospital architecture is a specialty which has concerned itself, until recently, primarily with creating efficient space in which medical people can work. There is little written regarding the impact on patients of hospital design. Architects are, therefore, forced to extrapolate from the body of knowledge available from home and office planning. However, the hospital patient is sick and helpless, and aspects of the physical environment which are relatively unimportant when one is well can become important when one is confined to a hospital bed. The healthy client can make adjustments in his environment. He can rearrange furniture; he can move about to avoid unpleasant noises, odors, or lights. The hospital patient must, for the most part, accept the environment as given.

THE HOSPITAL ENVIRONMENT—
AN OVERVIEW

Certainly, most people do regard hospitalization with considerable apprehension. We view the hospital as a more efficient place in which to study and treat our patients; however, for the patient, the act of hospitalization implies the presence of illness too serious to be treated in a doctor's office. This fact alone can be terrifying. It means the patient must abandon his role in society and face the reality of his own mortality. Man does not usually live with this anxiety in the forefront of his consciousness. It is hard to do otherwise in the hos-

pital where one is surrounded by serious illness and death 24 hours a day. Certainly, each patient deals with this situation in his own way but each one must come to grips with it. The question is, how does the hospital environment affect the individual patient in his struggle with this anxiety-provoking situation?

First, we must examine in more detail those aspects of the hospital situation which we see as "routine." Many of what we regard as standard procedures, to a patient, are new and very anxiety-provoking experiences. No diagnostic test is "routine" to the patient upon whom it is done. Such "standard" items as EKG machines, oxygen tents, and intravenous fluids may be new and terrifying experiences for some patients. What then of radioactive counters, cardiac catheters, arteriography and cobalt therapy machines? How much unnecessary anxiety is produced because we are unaware of these reactions? Patients often assume we are too busy to answer their "foolish questions." We must therefore, anticipate their anxiety and take the initiative, since simple explanations can usually provide adequate reassurance.

What are the effects of "routine" bedside rounds on a teaching service?[6,7] On the positive side, patients report they feel there is great benefit in having the talent of so many doctors applied to their problem. The potentially harmful effects of rounds are apparent. The presentation of the history and laboratory data along with a detailed discussion of the diagnostic and treatment possibilities may reveal information for which the patient has not been prepared. The use of euphemisms to avoid this is not very effective as patients become increasingly sophisticated. Similarly, the barrage of medical terms at the bedside can just as easily lend themselves to inaccurate assumptions. The "cancer" discussion between the attending and the intern could very well have been related to the last patient visited, but for the patient at whose bedside it occurs, this may not be so apparent. The physical exposure of patients without concern for their privacy does occasionally occur but should not require additional comment. Perhaps the most disturbing phenomenon at bedside rounds is the heated discussion regarding diagnostic and therapeutic possibilities. What a dilemma for the patient to see the physicians in apparent disagreement regarding her problem and how best to treat it. What a blow to see her doctor, a house officer, publicly chastised for some omission. We should be grateful for the mental mechanism of denial which allows most patients to deal with these situations. Certainly rounds can have a therapeutic function. The history presentation and discussion need not take place at the bedside. Most hospital wards have a room nearby where the group can assemble and discuss these matters. The patient can then be visited to have physical findings corroborated. At this time, he can be given an opportunity to ask questions and receive emotional support from the professional staff.

The entry into the hospital environment can also have very acute effects. The first psychiatric patient most interns have to treat is a little old lady who becomes disoriented at night and too often climbs out of bed and fractures a hip. She is probably suffering from an acute organic brain syndrome. Despite her chronically impaired cerebral functioning, she had been able to function adequately in her familiar home environment. In the hospital, often under the influence of sleeping medication, the darkness and unfamiliar surroundings produce a more acute disorganization of her mental faculties. The problem is often solved by canceling the sleeping medication and leaving a night light burning. A more severe form of this syndrome can exist with disorientation, confusion, agitation and, occasionally, paranoia, persisting day and night. Here the patient becomes disorganized by the strangeness of the environment and a senile psychosis occurs. While phenothiazines may give some symptomatic relief, the introduction of familiar people and objects can be helpful. Obviously, the treat-

ment of choice is to return the patient to the familiar environment of home where rapid improvement usually occurs.

Similar response can also be seen in patients who require eye-patching.[8] This is especially true in those who are also immobilized. They may react to the diminished sensory input with delusions, hallucinations, disorientation, and agitation. The treatment of choice is early patch removal and mobilization but in the meanwhile, the introduction of frequent meaningful auditory cues can help.

SPECIAL HOSPITAL AREAS

As medicine has become increasingly specialized, a need has arisen for separate hospital units in which highly trained staff and special equipment can be concentrated to allow for efficient care. Some of these units are unique environments and the observations which have been made on their psychiatric effects will be reviewed.

Isolation units

Our understanding of sensory deprivation effects has also provided some insight into the occasional acute psychiatric problems which occur in isolation rooms for patients with infectious disease or where reverse precautions are needed. Here the patients are in individual rooms visited only by gowned and masked staff and family. The need for the mask and gown undoubtedly reduces the number of visits. Those visits which do occur take on a strange quality as the masked figures go about their chores. Family members become less familiar and reassuring. This environment can therefore easily intensify whatever anxiety the patient may be experiencing regarding the nature and seriousness of his condition. For an occasional patient, this setting can trigger an acute psychotic reaction, often with paranoid trends. If transfer out of the unit is impossible, measures must be taken to relieve anxiety and increase meaningful stimulation. The patient's physician should attempt to explore possible misconceptions regarding the illness. The nurses should increase the frequency and length of their visits and these should be made to socialize and not just to perform tasks. The introduction of a television set and telephone can also be therapeutic. Phenothiazines can be used to provide symptomatic relief.

Holland et al.[9] have studied a group of acute leukemia patients treated in "germ-free units." These are plastic bubblelike enclosures or plastic-lined rooms in which patients are literally separated from all direct contact with anyone. They are touched only through plastic gloves at the end of plastic arms built into the walls or by individuals dressed in "space suits" wearing gloves. The average patient stayed 28 days.

Twenty percent of patients eligible for treatment in these units declined such treatment or were rejected as unsuitable. Twelve patients were studied. Eleven reported that they could have stayed longer if necessary. No acute psychiatric problems related to the environment were reported. All stated that the personality of the nurses contributed to their ability to tolerate the totally dependent situation. The most significant complaint by patients was their inability to touch or be touched directly by another human being. As one patient put it, "About a week ago, it started to get on my nerves in the bubble and not being able to feel other people and hoping I could come out soon. I felt like I couldn't stand it anymore. I just had to feel other people. I wanted to feel somebody; touch another human being. If I could have done this, I could have stuck it out longer in the bubble."

Dr. Holland observes that physical contact is an important way of providing emotional support and comfort to someone who is ill. The pat on the shoulder, the squeeze of the hand, are often so automatic that we are unaware of how often it occurs between the patient and his visitors, both staff and family. Physicians apparently cannot underestimate the continuing importance of "the laying on of hands" in the practice of medicine.

Intensive care units

The intensive care unit (ICU) in its various forms has come under special scrutiny. McKegney[10] has referred to an "intensive care syndrome" and called it a new disease of medical progress. These are indeed psychiatric problems which appear to be a reaction to the unique environment of the ICU itself and these phenomena will be reviewed. However, intensive care is applied in a variety of medical and surgical settings and the nature and extent of the psychiatric problems can vary. Sgroi et al.,[11] for example, report no meaningful difference in the incidence of psychiatric symptoms in a group of patients in a general medical ICU when compared with comparably ill patients treated in the ward. Above all, one must realize that in any setting in which there are very sick patients, a variety of psychiatric problems can emerge. It would be unfortunate if the concept of the ICU syndrome were overemphasized and other possible causes of psychiatric difficulties in that setting were overlooked. This is especially true of the acute organic brain syndrome (delirium) which can be the product of a variety of metabolic, cardiovascular, neurologic, or pharmacologic factors. These possibilities must be ruled out before one can assume that the patient's delirium is a reaction to the environment alone.

Open-heart recovery room

The concept of an ICU syndrome developed out of reports of a high incidence (38-70%) of delirium following open-heart surgery.[12-14] The delirium developed in the open-heart recovery room (OHRR) after a lucid postoperative interval. While a variety of preoperative and operative factors appeared to contribute to the delirium, some felt that the environment of these rooms played a major contributory role.[12-14] The typical OHRR was a large open area with 5-7 beds, separated by a movable curtain. The patients were attached to EKG cables, intravenous tubing, and a bladder catheter. Although movement was possible, most patients remained relatively immobile as a result of pain and the implied limitation of motion produced by the cables. An electronic monitor with an oscilloscope was placed next to the bedside and flashed constantly. The patient was placed in a plastic oxygen tent which produced a constant background humming and hissing noise. Nurses and house officers arrived at frequent intervals to perform their chores. The room's overhead light was constantly on. There was always the possibility of an emergency with the associated activity. Thus, for the 4-6 days that most patients were there, they were subjected to an experience which combined elements of a sensory monotony experiment with sleep deprivation. This was similar to the experience of patients with polio placed in tank respirators. Having possibly had their cerebral function partially compromised by the cardiac bypass it was not surprising that these cardiac surgery patients had a high incidence of delirium. The typical patient would appear lucid for the first 3-4 days. He would then experience an illusion, for example, sound arising from an air-conditioning vent might begin to sound like someone calling him. This might then progress to auditory and visual hallucinations and frank paranoid delusions. Disorientation to time, place, and person could occur. In a typical case, the delirium would clear within 24-48 hours after the patient was transferred to a standard hospital environment where he would have a sound sleep.

On the basis of these findings, it was suggested that certain modifications in the design of these rooms and the nursing procedures associated with them might reduce the incidence of delirium.[14] The authors suggested: (1) Nursing procedures should be modified to allow the maximum number of uninterrupted sleep periods; the usual day-awake, night-asleep cycle should be maintained wherever possible. (2) Patients should be placed in individual cubicles. There they would not be awakened or made more anxious by activity occurring around other patients. (3) Monitoring equipment

should be maintained, when possible, outside the patient's room. Bedside monitors could be turned on whenever needed. This would reduce the anxiety in those patients who are aware of the significance of these signaling devices and the danger implicit with any change in their pattern. (4) Patients should be allowed increased mobility by removing as many wires and cables as possible. Telemetry equipment would achieve increased mobility and allows for the use of remote monitors. (5) The constant noise of oxygen and cooling tents should be modified or removed wherever possible. (6) Each room should be equipped with a large clock and calendar. (7) An outside window should be visible to the patient to allow for orientation.

Lazarus and Hagens[15] found that modifications in the OHRR and its routines which were designed to lessen anxiety, sensory monotony, and sleep deprivation did produce a lower incidence of delirium after open-heart surgery. Heller et al.[16] also reported a reduction in the incidence of delirium in recent years. Diminished time required on the heart-lung machine may have contributed to this decline; however, modifications in the environment of the OHRR which allow for more sleep and reduce anxiety may also have played a role.

Operating room

The operating room had been considered one area where a patient's psychological responses could be temporarily ignored. Recent reports have suggested that this may be a false assumption. The work of Cheek[17] and Levinson[18] indicates that patients may perceive remarks made while they were apparently anesthetized. They have demonstrated through the recall under hypnosis that patients can recall statements made during surgery by the operating team. A remark which suggests that the patient may have been in danger seems to be most readily recalled. This type of recall is most common in patients being operated upon with regional or spinal anesthesia where the accompanying sedation still allows some awareness of what is being said. However, it can apparently also occur with patients under general anesthesia. The problem is complicated by the use of muscle relaxants which can obscure a patient's true level of awareness. Unexplained postoperative anxiety or depression have been attributed to the effects of remarks made during surgery and been successfully treated with hypnosis and ventilation therapy.[17]

Recovery room

Until very recently little attention has been paid to the psychological responses of patients in the surgical recovery room. However, a paper by Winkelstein et al.[19] questions the assumption that patients in the recovery room are too obtunded to be aware of what goes on about them or to communicate their concern regarding their recent surgery. They interviewed a series of patients in recovery room and demonstrated that very shortly after emerging from surgery they were able to relate quite directly with an interviewer. They were also able to recall 24 hours later much of the content of these interviews. Therefore, what many have felt to be a pharmacologically induced obtundity may very well be the use of the mental mechanism of denial to blot out the unpleasantness of surgery and the frightening sights and sounds which surround the patient in the recovery room itself. This is not to suggest that denial may not be the most effective mental mechanism to be used by an individual in such circumstances. But it should be noted that such patients are not as oblivious as may first appear to what is happening to them. This knowledge should be applied to the management of the recovery room experience for patients.

What are the frightening aspects of the recovery room? Typically, a recovery room is a large, open area in which a group of patients lie about at various levels of consciousness; an area in which one patient may be lying for 3 hours waiting for spinal anesthesia to wear off, while across the room a patient who has suddenly begun to bleed is being frantically worked upon by a group of physicians and nurses. In the same room, a patient emerging from anesthesia is screaming loudly for pain relief while another patient, awaiting transfer to her floor, lies quietly, staring off into space apparently oblivious to what goes on about her. In one corner, a patient appears to doze as two surgeons discuss the pathology found at frozen section. In another corner of the room, a child who has just had a tonsillectomy lies terrified watching this group of sick adults. The picture I have just painted is perhaps not typical of all recovery rooms but demonstrates the psychological problems which do exist there: unnecessarily exposing patients to frightening experiences by allowing them to observe all that goes on about them; inadequate analgesia for patients left with only postoperative orders to be administered upon return to their hospital floor, unnecessarily exposing patients to frightening remarks by staff who believe they are oblivious to these comments. There is especially the problem of the impact of this generally horrifying scene upon the mind of a child.

What can be done to reduce the anxiety-provoking aspects of this room? One basic change can be made in the structure of the room itself. It is possible to construct a room with a central nursing station and individual cubicles for patients. In this way, patients are not totally exposed to the sights and sounds of other patients about them. While it is true that with limited nursing staff one must provide easy access to all patients, there is still no reason why partitions cannot be built so that the patient, lying flat on his back, is not exposed to the problems on either side of him. Curtains can also be provided on an overhead track which can be used to provide complete privacy when indicated. Hopefully, someone will remember to close them at those times. There is a special danger that with increasing reliance upon electronic monitoring equipment, the recovery room could too quickly become a place in which patients attached to machines are watched from afar by nurses and medical staff. This would be most unfortunate. Patients coming out of anesthesia are in particular need of human contact for reassurance that all is well.

It is strongly recommended, whenever possible, to have a separate recovery room for children. The surgical experience is difficult enough for them without their being exposed to the recovery room of a general hospital. Some of the suggestions made for the adult recovery room could be applied here. A special preoperative preparation room could be of great value. Here a child could be adequately premedicated and perhaps have a final reassuring visit from a physician. If possible, the route by which children enter the operating suite should not take them past the recovery room. The recovery room could be constructed as suggested for adults so that patients are separated in cubicles and thus not completely exposed to whatever disturbing scene may occur in their vicinity. Children awaiting transfer back to the hospital proper could also be separated from those still recovering from anesthesia. The special pediatric recovery room also provides a group of nurses specially trained to deal with the specific problems of children, both psychological and physiological. These nurses develop an expertise in dealing with children which can be remarkably effective.

Despite all efforts to diminish the anxiety-provoking features of the recovery room, there are certain limits to what can be done. I would, therefore, recommend that patients be removed from the recovery room to their hospital quarters as quickly as possible. It was striking, for example, that even in a special pediatric recovery room frightened children would stop crying when placed on the stretcher returning them to their hospital bed. Returning to the hospital proper removes the patient from the stresses of the recovery room scene and also indicates to him that all is well. A delayed departure for some administrative reason, e.g., waiting for a nursing shift to take place, may be interpreted as a sign that some surgical problem still exists.

SUMMARY

I am sure that there are few surprises for the average physician in what he has just read. Most of the observations have been made by psychiatrists, i.e., physicians not involved in the primary care of these patients. They were able to identify the effects of the environment because they were not initially a part of it. Their recommendations are often obvious to the physicians involved once these observations are brought to their attention. The modifications in the environment can often be readily incorporated into a hospital routine with gratifying results. Therefore, what is needed is for all physicians to increase their awareness of the potential environmental hazards which they encounter each day. What is essential is that we enhance our ability to empathize with patients, i.e., to recognize the meaning of the hospital situation for them, without our overidentifying with the patients themselves. In this way, using good common clinical sense, we can do a great deal to make the environment at the bedside, which is the most important of all, truly therapeutic.

REFERENCES

1. Brown, E. L. The use of the physical and social environment of the general hospital for therapeutic purposes. I. Newer dimensions of patient care, New York: Russell Sage Foundation, 1961.
2. Coser, R. L. Life in the ward. E. Lansing: Michigan State University Press, 1962.
3. Field, M. Patients are people. New York: Columbia University Press, 1967.
4. Friedson, E. (Ed.) The hospital in modern society. New York: Free Press, 1963.
5. Dichter, E. The hospital–patient relationship. *Modern Hospital* **83** (1954).
6. Kaufman, M. R., Franzblau, A. M., & Kairys, D. The emotional impact of ward rounds. *Journal of Mt. Sinai Hospital* **23**: 782-803 (1956).
7. Romano, J. Patient attitudes and behaviour in ward round teaching. *Journal of the American Medical Association* **117**:664-667 (1941).
8. Linn, L., Kahn, R., Coles, P., Cohen, J., Marshall, D., & Weinstein, E. A. Patterns of behavior disturbance following cataract extraction. *American Journal of Psychiatry* **110**:281-289 (1953).
9. Holland, J., Harris, S., Plumb, M., Tuttolomondo, A., & Yates, J. Psychological aspects of

physical barrier isolation. Observation of acute leukemia patients in germ-free units. *Proceedings of the International Congress of Hematology* (1970).

10. McKegney, F. P. The intensive care syndrome. *Connecticut Medicine* **30:**633-636 (1966).

11. Sgroi, S., Holland, J., & Marwit, S. Psychological reactions to catastrophic illness. A comparison of patients treated in an intensive care unit and a medical ward (abstract). *Psychosomatic Medicine* **30:**551-552 (1968).

12. Egerton, N., & Kay, J. H. Psychological disturbances associated with open heart surgery. *British Journal of Psychiatry* **110:**433-439 (1964).

13. Blachly, P. H., & Starr, A. Post-cardiotomy delirium. *American Journal of Psychiatry* **121:**371-375 (1964).

14. Kornfield, D. S., Zimberg, S., & Malm, J. R. Psychiatric complications of open-heart surgery. *New England Journal of Medicine* **273:**287-282 (1965).

15. Lazarus, H. R., & Hagens, J. H. Prevention of psychosis following open-heart surgery. *American Journal of Psychiatry* **124:**1190-1195 (1968).

16. Heller, S., Frank, K. A., Malm, J. R. et al. Psychiatric complications of open-heart surgery. A re-examination. *New England Journal of Medicine* **283:**1015-1019 (1970).

17. Cheek, D. S. Unconscious perception of meaningful sounds during surgical anesthesia as revealed under hypnosis. *American Journal of Clinical Hypnosis* **1:**101 (1959).

18. Levinson, B. W. States of awareness during general anesthesia. *British Journal of Anaesthesia* **37:**544 (1965).

19. Winkelstein, C., Blacher, R., & Meyer, B. Psychiatric observations on surgical patients in recovery room. *New York State Journal of Medicine* **65:**865-870 (1965).

PART V

Personal encounters with life-threatening illness

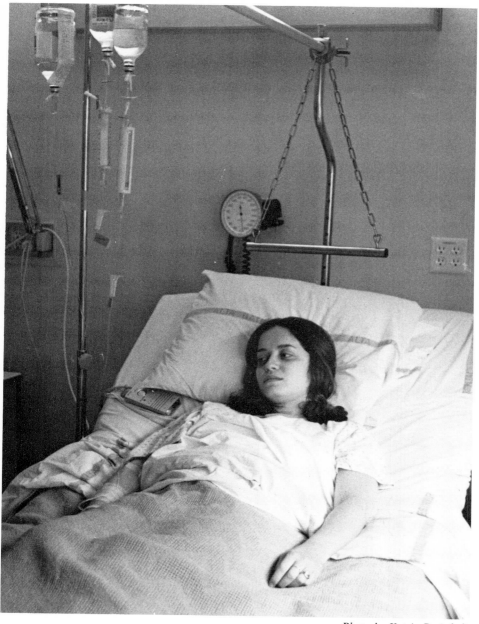

Photo by Katrin P. Achelis

18

Anatomy of an illness (as perceived by the patient)

NORMAN COUSINS

Ever since the publication of Adam Smith's much-talked-about *Powers of the Mind* some months ago, people have written to ask whether his account of my recovery from a supposedly incurable illness was accurately reported. In particular, readers have been eager to verify Mr. Smith's statement that I ''laughed'' my way out of a crippling disease that doctors believed to be irreversible.

I have not written until now about my illness, which occurred in 1964, largely because I was fearful of creating false hopes in other persons similarly afflicted. Moreover, I knew that a single case has small standing in the annals of medical research. I had thought that my own episode might have anecdotal value—nothing more. However, since my case has surfaced in the public press, I feel justified in providing a fuller picture than was contained in Mr. Smith's account.

In August, 1964, I flew home from a trip abroad with a slight fever. The malaise, which took the form of a general feeling of achiness, rapidly deepened. Within a week it became difficult to move my neck, arms, hands, fingers and legs. I was hospitalized when my sedimentation rate hit 80 mm per hour. The sedimentation rate continued to rise until it reached 115.

Reprinted by permission from the New England Journal of Medicine 295:1458-1463, December 23, 1976.

There were other tests, some of which seemed to me to be more an assertion of the clinical capability of the hospital than of concern for the well-being of the patient. I was astounded when four technicians from four different departments took four separate and substantial blood samples on the same day. That the hospital didn't take the trouble to co-ordinate the tests, using one blood specimen, seemed to me inexplicable and irresponsible. When the technicians came the second day to fill their containers with blood for processing in separate laboratories, I turned them away and had a sign posted on my door saying that I would give just one specimen every three days and that I expected the different departments to draw from it for their individual needs.

I had a fast-growing conviction that a hospital was no place for a person who was seriously ill. The surprising lack of respect for basic sanitation, the rapidity with which staphylococci and other pathogenic organisms can run through an entire hospital, the extensive and sometimes promiscuous use of x-ray equipment, the seemingly indiscriminate administration of tranquilizers and powerful painkillers, more for the convenience of hospital staff in managing patients than for therapeutic needs, and the regularity with which hospital routine takes precedence over the rest requirements of the patient (slumber, when it comes for an ill person, is an uncommon blessing and is not to be wantonly interrupted)—all these and other practices seemed to me to be critical shortcomings of the modern hospital.

Perhaps the hospital's most serious failure was in the area of nutrition. It was not just that the meals were poorly balanced; what seemed inexcusable to me was the profusion of processed foods, some of which contained preservatives or harmful dyes. White bread, with its chemical softeners and bleached flour, was offered with every meal. Vegetables were often overcooked and thus deprived of much of their nutritional value. No wonder the 1969 White House Conference on Food, Nutrition, and Health[2] made the melancholy observation that the great failure of medical schools is that they pay so little attention to the science of nutrition.

My doctor did not quarrel with my reservations about hospital procedures. I was fortunate to have as a physician a man who was able to put himself in the position of the patient. Dr. William Hitzig supported me in the measures I took to fend off the randon sanguinary assaults of the hospital laboratory attendants.

We had been close friends for more than 20 years, and he knew of my own deep interest in medical matters. We had often discussed articles in the medical press, including the *New England Journal of Medicine* and *Lancet*. He felt comfortable about being candid with me about my case. He reviewed the reports of the various specialists he had called in as consultants. He said there was no agreement on a precise diagnosis. There was, however, a general consensus that I was suffering from a serious collagen illness. I had considerable difficulty in moving my limbs and even in turning over in bed. Nodules appeared on my body, gravel-like substances under the skin, indicating the systemic nature of the disease. At the low point of my illness, my jaws were almost locked.

Dr. Hitzig called in experts from Dr. Howard Rusk's rehabilitation clinic in New York. They confirmed the general opinion, adding the more particularized diagnosis of ankylosing spondylitis.

I asked Dr. Hitzig about my chances for full recovery. He leveled with me, admitting that one of the specialists had told him I had one chance in 500. The specialist had also stated that he had not personally witnessed a recovery from this comprehensive condition.

All this gave me a great deal to think about. Up to that time, I had been more or less disposed to let the doctors worry about my condition. But now I felt a compulsion to get into the act. It seemed clear to me that if I was to be that "one case in 500" I had better be something more than a passive observer.

I asked Dr. Hitzig about the possible cause of my condition. He said that it could have come from any one of a number of causes. It could have come, for example, from heavy-metal poisoning, or it could have been manifested by the aftereffects of a streptococcal infection.

I thought as hard as I could about the sequence of events immediately preceding the illness. I had gone to the Soviet Union in July, 1964, as chairman of an American delegation to consider the problems of cultural exchange. The conference had been held in Leningrad, after which we went to Moscow for supplementary meetings. Our hotel was in a residential area. My room was on the second floor. Each night a procession of diesel trucks plied back and forth to a nearby housing project in the process of round-the-clock construction. It was summer, and our windows were wide open. I slept uneasily each night and felt somewhat nauseated on arising. On our last day in Moscow, at the airport, I caught the exhaust spew of a large jet at point-blank range as it swung around on the tarmac.

As I thought back on that Moscow experience, I wondered whether the exposure to the hydrocarbons from the diesel exhaust at the hotel and at the airport had anything to do with the underlying cause of the illness. If so, that might account for the speculations of the doctors concerning heavy-metal poisoning. The trouble with this theory, however, was that my wife, who had been with me on the trip, had no ill effects from the same exposure. How likely was it that only one of us would have reacted adversely?

There were two possible reasons, it seemed to me, for the different responses. One had to do with individual allergy. The second was that I was probably in a condition of adrenal exhaustion and I was less apt to tolerate a toxic experience than someone whose immunologic system was fully functional.

Was adrenal exhaustion a factor in my own illness?

Again, I thought carefully. The meetings in Leningrad and Moscow had not been casual. Paper work had kept me up late nights. I had ceremonial responsibilities. Our last evening in Moscow had been, at least for me, an exercise in almost total frustration. A reception had been arranged by the chairman of the Soviet delegation at his *dacha,* located 50 to 65 km outside the city. I had been asked if I could arrive an hour early so that I might tell the Soviet delegates something about the individual Americans who were coming to dinner. The Russians were eager to make the Americans feel at home, and they had thought such information would help them with the social amenities.

I was told that a car and driver from the government automobile pool in Moscow would pick me up at the hotel at 3:30 p.m. This would allow ample time for me to drive to the *dacha* by 5:00 p.m., when all our Russian conference colleagues would be gathered for the social briefing. The rest of the American delegation would arrive at the *dacha* at 6:00.

At 6:00, however, I found myself in open country on the wrong side of Moscow. There had been a misunderstanding in the transmission of directions to the driver, the result being that we were some 130 km off course.

We didn't arrive at the *dacha* until 9:00 p.m. My host's wife looked desolate. The soup had been heated and re-heated. The veal was dried out. I felt pretty wrung out

myself. It was a long flight back to the States the next day. The plane was overcrowded. By the time we arrived in New York, cleared through the packed customs counters, and got rolling back to Connecticut, I could feel an uneasiness deep in my bones. A week later I was hospitalized.

As I thought back on my experience abroad, I knew that I was probably on the right track in my search for a cause of the illness. I found myself increasingly convinced, as I said a moment ago, that the reason I was hit hard by the diesel and jet pollutants, whereas my wife was not, was that I had had a case of adrenal exhaustion, lowering my resistance.

Assuming this hypothesis was true, I had to get my adrenal glands functioning properly again and to restore what Walter Cannon, in his famous book *The Wisdom of the Body,*[3] called homeostasis.

I knew that the full functioning of my endocrine system—in particular, the adrenal glands—was essential for combating severe arthritis or, for that matter, any other illness. A study I had read in the medical press reported that pregnant women frequently have remissions of arthritic or other rheumatic symptoms. The reason is that the endocrine system is fully activated during pregnancy.

How was I to get my adrenal glands and my endocrine system, in general, working well again—both physically and emotionally?

I remembered having read, 10 years or so earlier, Hans Selye's classic book, *The Stress of Life.*[4] With great clarity, Selye showed that adrenal exhaustion could be caused by emotional tension, such as frustration or suppressed rage. He detailed the negative effects of the negative emotions on body chemistry. He wrote, for example, about the increase of hydrochloric acid in the stomach. He also traced changes in corticoids and anticorticoids under conditions of emotional stress.

The inevitable question arose in my mind: What about the positive emotions? If negative emotions produce negative chemical changes in the body, wouldn't the positive emotions produce positive chemical changes? Is it possible that love, hope, faith, laughter, confidence and the will to live have therapeutic value? Do chemical changes occur only on the downside?

Obviously, putting the positive emotions to work is nothing so simple as turning on a garden hose. But even a reasonable degree of control over my emotions might have a salutary physiologic effect. Just replacing anxiety with a fair degree of confidence would be helpful.

A plan began to form in my mind for systematic pursuit of the salutary emotions, and I knew that I would want to discuss it with my doctor. Two preconditions, however, seemed obvious for the experiment. The first concerned my medication. If that medication were toxic to any degree, it was doubtful whether the plan would work. The second precondition concerned the hospital. I knew I would have to find a place somewhat more conducive to a positive outlook on life.

Let's consider these preconditions separately.

First, the medication. The emphasis had been on painkilling drugs—aspirin, phenylbutazone (Butazolidin), codeine, colchicine, sleeping pills. The aspirin and phenylbutazone were anti-inflammatory and thus were therapeutically justifiable. But I wasn't sure they weren't also toxic. With Dr. Hitzig's support, we took allergy tests and discovered that I was hypersensitive to virtually all the medication I was receiving. The hospital had been giving me maximum dosages: 26 aspirin tablets a day; and 3 phenylbutazone tablets four times a day. No wonder I had hives all over my body and felt as though my skin was being chewed up by millions of red ants.

It was unreasonable to expect positive chemical changes to take place so long as my body was being saturated with, and toxified by, painkilling medications. I had one of my research assistants at the *Saturday Review* look up the pertinent references in the medical journals and found that drugs like phenylbutazone and even aspirin levy a heavy tax on the adrenal glands. I also learned that phenylbutazone is one of the most powerful drugs being manufactured. It can produce bloody stools, the result of its antagonism to fibrinogen. It can cause intolerable itching and sleeplessness. It can depress bone marrow.

The hazards of phenylbutazone are explicit. Aspirin enjoys a far more auspicious reputation, at least with the general public. The prevailing impression of aspirin is that it is not only the most harmless drug available but also one of the most effective. When I looked into research in the medical journals, however, I found that aspirin is quite powerful in its own right and that it warrants considerable care in its use. The fact that it can be bought in unlimited quantities without prescription or doctor's guidance seemed indefensible. Even in small amounts, it can cause internal bleeding. Articles in the medical press reported that the chemical composition of aspirin, like that of phenylbutazone, impairs platelet function. Did the relation between platelets and collagen mean that both drugs do more harm than good for some sufferers from arthritis?*

It was a mind-boggling train of thought. Could it be, I asked myself, that aspirin, so universally accepted for so many years, was actually harmful in the treatment of collagen illnesses?[5]†

The history of medicine is replete with instances involving drugs and modes of treatment that were in use for many years before it was recognized that they did more harm than good. For centuries, for example, people believed that drawing blood from patients was essential for rapid recov-

---

*I realize, of course, that the implications here are not entirely negative in view of the fact that the same properties of aspirin that prolong bleeding also prevent clotting. Aspirin is therefore useful to some patients with cardiac disease and those for whom clotting is a danger.

†The scientific verification that aspirin can be harmful in the treatment of collagen disease came in 1971 and is discussed later in this article.

ery from virtually every illness. Then, midway through the nineteenth century, it was discovered that bleeding serves only to weaken the patient. King Charles II's death is believed to have been caused in large part from administered bleedings. George Washington's death was also hastened by the severe loss of blood resulting from this treatment.

Living in the second half of the twentieth century, I realized, confers no automatic protection against unwise or even dangerous drugs and methods. Each age has had to undergo its own special nostrums. Fortunately, the human body is a remarkably durable instrument and has been able to withstand all sorts of prescribed assaults over the centuries, from freezing to animal dung.

Suppose I stopped taking aspirin and phenylbutazone? What about the pain? The bones in my spine and practically every joint in my body felt as though I had been run over by a truck.

I knew that pain could be affected by attitudes. Most people become panicky about almost any pain. On all sides they have been so bombarded by advertisements about pain that they take this or that analgesic at the slightest sign of an ache. They are largely illiterate about pain and so are seldom able to deal with it rationally. Pain is part of the body's magic. It is the way the body transmits a sign to the brain that something is wrong. Leprous patients pray for the sensation of pain. What makes leprosy such a terrible disease is that the victim usually feels no pain when his extermities are being injured. He loses his fingers or toes because he receives no warning signal that he is being injured.

I could stand pain so long as I knew that progress was being made in meeting the basic need. That need, I felt, was to restore the body's capacity to halt the continuing breakdown of connective tissue.

There was also the problem of the severe inflammation. If we dispensed with the aspirin, how would we combat the inflammation? I recalled having read in the medical journals about the usefulness of ascorbic acid in combating a wide number of illnesses—all the way from bronchitis to some types of heart disease. Couldn't it also combat inflammation? Did vitamin C act directly, or did it serve as a starter for the body's endocrine system—in particular, the adrenal glands? Was it possible, I asked myself, that ascorbic acid had a vital role to play in "feeding" the adrenal glands?

I had read in the medical press that vitamin C helps to oxygenate the blood.[6] If inadequate or impaired oxygenation was a factor in collagen breakdown, couldn't this circumstance be another argument for ascorbic acid? Also, according to some medical reports, people suffering from collagen diseases are deficient in vitamin C.[5] Did this lack mean that the body uses up large amounts of vitamin C in the process of combating collagen breakdown?

I wanted to discuss some of these ruminations with Dr. Hitzig. He listened carefully as I told him of my speculations concerning the cause of the illness, as well as my layman's ideas for a course of action that might give me a chance to reduce the odds against my recovery.

Dr. Hitzig said it was clear to him that there was nothing undersized about my will to live. He said that what was most important was that I continue to believe in everything I had said. He shared my sense of excitement about the possibilities of my recovery and liked the idea of a partnership.

Even before we had completed arrangements for moving out of the hospital, we began the part of the program calling for the full exercise of the affirmative emotions as a factor in enhancing body chemistry. It was easy enough to hope and love and have faith, but what about laughter? Nothing is less funny than being flat on your back with all the bones in your spine and joints hurting. A systematic program was indicated. A good place to begin, I thought, was with amusing movies. Allen Funt, producer of the spoofing television program "Candid Camera," sent films of some of his "CC" classics, along with a motion-picture projector. The nurse was instructed in its use.

It worked. I made the joyous discovery that 10 minutes of genuine belly laughter had an anesthetic effect and would give me at least two hours of pain-free sleep. When the painkilling effect of the laughter wore off, we would switch on the motion-picture projector again, and, not infrequently, it would lead to another pain-free sleep interval. Sometimes, the nurse read to me out of a trove of humor books. Especially useful were E.B. and Katherine White's *Subtreasury of American Humor*[7] and Max Eastman's *The Enjoyment of Laughter*.[8]

How scientific was it to believe that laughter—as well as the positive emotions in general—was affecting my body chemistry for the better? If laughter did in fact have a salutary effect on the body's chemistry, it seemed at least theoretically likely that it would enhance the system's ability to fight the inflammation. So we took sedimentation-rate readings just before as well as several hours after the laughter episodes. Each time, there was a drop of at least five points. The drop by itself was not substantial, but it held and was cumulative.

I was greatly elated by the discovery that there is a physiologic basis for the ancient theory that laughter is good medicine.

There was, however, one negative side effect of the laughter from the standpoint of the hospital. I was disturbing other patients. But that objection didn't last very long, for the arrangements were now complete for me to move my act to a hotel room.

One of the incidental advantages of the hotel room, I was delighted to find, was that it cost only about one-third as much as the hospital. The other benefits were incalculable. I would not be awakened for a bed bath or for meals or for medication or for a change in the bed sheets or for tests or for examinations by hospital interns. The sense of serenity was delicious and would, I felt certain, contribute to a general improvement.

What about ascorbic acid and its place in the general program for recovery? In discussing my speculations about vitamin C with Dr. Hitzig, I found him completely open-minded on the subject, although he told me of serious questions that had been raised by scientific studies. He also cautioned me that heavy doses of ascorbic acid carried some risk of renal damage. The main problem right then, however, was not my kidneys: it seemed to me that, on balance, the risk was worth taking. I asked Dr. Hitzig about previously recorded experience with massive doses of vitamin C. He ascertained that at the hospital there had been cases in which patients had received up to 3 g by intramuscular injection.

As I thought about the injection procedure, some questions came to mind. Introducing the ascorbic acid directly into the bloodstream might make more efficient use of the vitamin, but I wondered about the body's ability to utilize a sudden massive infusion. I knew that one of the great advantages of vitamin C is that the body takes only the amount necessary for its purposes and excretes the rest. Again, there came to mind Cannon's phrase—the wisdom of the body.[3]

Was there a coefficient of time in the utilization of ascorbic acid? The more I thought about it, the more likely it seemed to me that the body would excrete a large quantity of the vitamin because it couldn't metabolize it that fast. I wondered whether a better procedure than injection would be to administer the ascorbic acid through slow intravenous drip over a period of three or four hours. In this way we could go far beyond the 3 g. My hope was to start at 10 g and then increase the dose daily until we reached 25 g.

Dr. Hitzig's eyes widened when I mentioned 25 g. This amount was far beyond any recorded dose. He said he had to caution me about the possible effect not just on the kidneys but on the veins in the arms. Moreover, he said he knew of no data to support the assumption that the body could handle 25 g over a four-hour period, other than by excreting it rapidly through the urine.

As before, however, it seemed to me we

were playing for bigger stakes: losing some veins was not of major importance alongside the need to combat whatever was eating at my connective tissue.

To know whether we were on the right tract, we took a sedimentation test before the first intravenous administration of 10 g of ascorbic acid. Four hours later, we took another sedimentation test. There was a drop of nine full points.

Seldom had I known such elation. The ascorbic acid was working. So was laughter. The combination was cutting heavily into whatever poison was attacking the connective tissue. The fever was receding, and the pulse was no longer racing.

We stepped up the dosage. On the second day we went up to 12.5 g of ascorbic acid, on the third day, 15 g and so on until the end of the week, when we reached 25 g. Meanwhile, the laughter routine was in full force. I was completely off drugs and sleeping pills. Sleep—blessed, natural sleep without pain—was becoming increasingly prolonged.

At the end of the eighth day I was able to move my thumbs without pain. By this time, the sedimenation rate was somewhere in the 80's and dropping fast. I couldn't be sure, but it seemed to me that the gravel-like nodules on my neck and the backs of my hands were beginning to shrink. There was no doubt in my mind that I was going to make it back all the way.

Two weeks later, my wife took me to Puerto Rico for some sustained sunshine. On the first day, friends helped support me in the breaking surf. Within a few days I was standing up by myself. At first the soles of my feet were so sensitive that I felt as though I were standing on my eyeballs. But walking in the sand was the best possible therapy, and within a week I was able to jog—at least for a minute or two.

The connective tissue in my spine and joints was regenerating. I could function, and the feeling was indescribably beautiful.

I must not make it appear that all my infirmities disappeared overnight. For many months I couldn't get my arms up far enough to reach for a book on a high shelf. My fingers weren't agile enough to do what I wanted them to do on the organ keyboard. My neck had a limited turning radius. My knees were somewhat wobbly, and, off and on, I had to wear a metal brace.

But I was back at my job at *Saturday Review* full time again, and this was miracle enough for me.

Is the recovery a total one? Year by year the mobility has improved. During the past year I have become fully pain free, except for my knees, for the first time since I left the hospital. I no longer feel a sharp twinge in my wrists or shoulders when I hit a tennis ball or golf ball, as I did for such a long time. I can ride a horse flat out and hold a camera with a steady hand. And I have recaptured my ambition to play the Toccata and Fugue in D Minor, though I find the going slower and tougher than I had hoped. My neck has a full turning radius again, despite the statement of specialists as recently as 1971 that the condition was degenerative and that I would have to adjust to a quarter turn.

It was seven years after the onset of the illness before I had scientific confirmation about the dangers of using aspirin in the treatment of collagen diseases, which embrace the various forms of arthritis. In its May 8, 1971 issue, *Lancet* published a study by Drs. M. A. Sahud and R. J. Cohen[5] showing that aspirin could be antagonistic to the retention of vitamin C in the body. The authors said that patients with rheumatoid arthritis should take vitamin C supplements since it has often been noted that they have low levels of the vitamin in their blood. It was no surprise, then, that I had been able to absorb such massive amounts of ascorbic acid without kidney or other complications.

What conclusions do I draw from the entire experience?

The first is that the will to live is not a theoretical abstraction, but a physiologic reality with therapeutic characteristics. The second is that I was incredibly fortunate to have as my doctor a man who knew that his biggest job was to encourage to the fullest the patient's will to live and to mobilize all the natural resources of body and mind to combat disease. Dr. Hitzig was willing to set aside the large and often hazardous armamentarium of powerful drugs available to the modern physician when he became convinced that his patient might have something better to offer. He was also wise enough to know that the art of healing is still a frontier profession. And, though I can't be sure of this point, I have a hunch he believed that my own total involvement was a major factor in any recovery.

People have asked what I thought when I was told by the specialists that my disease was progressive and incurable.

The answer is simple. Since I didn't accept the verdict, I wasn't trapped in the cycle of fear, depression and panic that frequently accompanies a supposedly incurable illness. I must not make it seem, however, that I was unmindful of the seriousness of the problem or that I was in a festive mood throughout. Being unable to move my body was all the evidence I needed that the specialists were dealing with real concerns. But deep down I knew I had a good chance and relished the idea of bucking the odds.

Adam Smith, in *Powers of the Mind*,[1] says he discussed my recovery with some of his doctor friends, asking them to explain why the combination of laughter and ascorbic acid worked so well. The answer he got was that neither laughter nor ascorbic acid had anything to do with it and that I probably would have recovered if nothing had been done.

Maybe so, but that was not the opinion of the specialists at the time.

Two or three doctors, reflecting on the Adam Smith account, have commented that I was probably the beneficiary of a mammoth venture in self-administered placebos.

Such a hypothesis bothers me not at all. Respectable names in the history of medicine like Paracelsus, Holmes and Osler have suggested that the history of medication is far more the history of the placebo effect than of intrinsically valuable and relevant drugs. Physicians in the past who favored such modalities as bleeding (in a single year, 1827, France imported 33 million leeches after its domestic supplies had been depleted); purging through emetics; physical contact with unicorn horns, bezoar stones, mandrakes or powdered mummies—the physicians prescribing such treatments no doubt regarded them at the time as specifics with empirical sanction. But today's medical science recognizes that whatever efficacy these treatments may have had—and the records indicate that the results were often surprisingly in line with expectations—was probably related to the power of the placebo.

I have wondered, in fact, about the relative absence of attention given the placebo in contemporary medicine. The literature on the subject is remarkably sparse considering the primacy of the placebo in the history of medicine. The late Henry K. Beecher[9] and Arthur K. Shapiro[10] are among the small number of contemporary medical researchers and observers who have done any noteworthy thinking and writing about this phenomenon. In connection with my own experience. I was fascinated by a report citing Dr. Thomas C. Chalmers,[11] of the Mount Sinai Medical Center in New York, which compared two groups that were being used to test the theory that ascorbic acid is a cold preventive. "The group on placebo," says Dr. Chalmers, "who thought they were on ascorbic acid had fewer colds than the group on ascorbic acid who thought they were on placebo."

I was absolutely convinced, at the time I was deep in my illness, that intravenous doses of ascorbic acid could be beneficial—and they were. It is quite possible that this treatment—like everything else I did—was a demonstration of the placebo effect. If so, it would be just as important to probe into the nature of this psychosomatic phenomenon as to find out if ascorbic acid is useful in combating a high sedimentation rate.

At this point, of course, we are opening a

very wide door, perhaps even a Pandora's box. The vaunted "miracle cures" that abound in the literature of all the great religions, or the speculations of Charcot and Freud about conversion hysteria, or the Lourdes phenomena—all say something about the ability of the patient, properly motivated or stimulated, to participate actively in extraordinary reversals of disease and disability. It is all too easy, of course, to raise these possibilities and speculations to a monopoly status—in which case the entire edifice of modern medicine would be reduced to little more than the hut of an African witch doctor. But we can at least reflect on William Halse Rivers's statement, as quoted by Shapiro, that "the salient feature of the medicine of today is that these psychical factors are no longer allowed to play their part unwittingly, but are themselves becoming the subject of study, so that the present age is serving the growth of a rational system of psychotherapeutics."[10]

What we are talking about essentially, I suppose, is the chemistry of the will to live. In Bucharest in 1972, I visited the clinic of Ana Aslan, described to me as one of Rumania's leading endocrinologists. She spoke of her belief that there is a direct connection between a robust will to live and the chemical balances in the brain. She is convinced that creativity—one aspect of the will to live—produces the vital brain impulses that stimulate the pituitary glands, triggering effects on the pineal glands and the whole of the endocrine system. Is it possible that placebos have a key role in this process? Shouldn't this entire area be worth serious and sustained attention?

If I had to guess, I would say that the principal contribution made by my doctor to the taming, and possibly the conquest, of my illness was that he encouraged me to believe I was a respected partner with him in the total undertaking. He fully engaged my subjective energies. He may not have been able to define or diagnose the process through which self-confidence (wild hunches securely believed) was somehow

picked up by the body's immunologic mechanisms and translated into anti-morbid effects. But he was acting, I believe, in the best tradition of medicine in recognizing that he had to reach out in my case beyond the usual verifiable modalities. In so doing, he was faithful to the first dictum in his medical education; *primum non nocere*. He knew that what I wanted to do might not help, but it probably would do little harm. Certainly, the threatened harm being risked was less, if anything, than the heroic medication so routinely administered in extreme cases of this kind.

Something else I have learned. I have learned never to underestimate the capacity of the human mind and body to regenerate—even when the prospects seem most wretched. The life-force may be the least understood force on earth. William James[12] said that human beings tend to live too far within self-imposed limits. It is possible that those limits will recede when we respect more fully the natural drive of the human mind and body toward perfectibility and regeneration. Protecting and cherishing that natural drive may well represent the finest exercise of human freedom.

REFERENCES

1. Smith A: Powers of the Mind. New York, Random House, 1975, pp 11-14.
2. White House Conference on Food, Nutrition and Health: Final report. Washington, DC, Government Printing Office, 1969.
3. Cannon WB: The Wisdom of the Body. New York, WW Norton and Company, 1963.
4. Selye H: The Stress of Life. New York, McGraw-Hill, 1956.
5. Sahud MA, Cohen RJ: Effect of aspirin ingestion on ascorbic-acid levels in rheumatoid arthritis. Lancet 1:937-938, 1971.
6. Hamburger E: A two-stage study of plasma ascorbic acid and its relation to wound healing. Milit Med 127:723-725, 1962.
6a. Kinderlehrer J: Vitamin C: The best thing that ever happened to antibiotics. Prevention 26:71-75, 1974.
6b. Klenner FR: Observations on the dose and administration of ascorbic acid when employed beyond the range of a vitamin in human pathology. J Appl Nutr 23:61-87, 1971.
7. White EB, White KS: A Subtreasury of American Humor. New York, Capricorn Books, 1962.

8. Eastman M: The Enjoyment of Laughter. Johnson Reprint of 1937 edition, 1971.

9. Beecher HK: The powerful placebo. JAMA 159: 1602-1606, 1955.

10. Shapiro AK: Factors contributing to the placebo effect: their implications for psychotherapy. Am J Psychother 18: Suppl 1:73-88, 1964.

11. Blake K: Vitamin C: the case looks stronger, but . . . *Pastimes* [Air-shuttle edition] (Eastern Airlines) March, 1976.

12. James W: Psychology. New York, World Publishing Company, 1948.

19

Cancer is not a four-letter word

LEONARD SHLAIN

I would like to share with you a very personal encounter I had with cancer at age 37. The title of my talk, which was suggested by my wife, alludes to the fact that, although we devote many hours of formal teaching to the scientific aspects of disease, very little is said about what is the impact in personal terms of a serious diagnosis. I am somewhat embarrassed to be up here because I know that what I dealt with is not unique or all that unusual. What is different is my perspective. As a surgeon I must often be the bearer of terrible news as well as serve on occasion as Charon, the boatman, to convey patients across the river Styx to the other side. During my training I spent two years as a Research Fellow of the American Cancer Society where it was my task to administer chemotherapy to dying patients. Since having to undergo the personal transformation that was associated with my first finding out that I had a malignant non-Hodgkins lymphoma and undergoing surgery followed by 5 months of radiation, I have changed the way I perceive many things.

Since all of you are in one way or another involved with this problem I hope that sharing these perceptions with you will somehow be helpful. I have no charts or graphs, as it is a very personal story, so please bear with me.

Let me first comment on the phenomenon of why there is so much popular interest in this subject. Why now? It seems hardly a week goes by that I don't receive some brochure about another seminar on this subject. Since the only uniformly 100 percent fatal condition that I know of is life, death has always been with us. Why all this fascination? I believe we as a society are grieving. We are grieving the loss of our most cherished beliefs. I think that in the 1960s and 1970s, what with the student riots, Vietnam, and Watergate, there was not a single aspect of our society that in the past we had taken for granted that was not held up to the harsh light of examination and then found wanting. You name it. The military, our government, our religious beliefs, the FBI, and our educational system all were found flawed. This included also the wonders of medicine. Many of us became cynical; almost all of us grieved in some way for the loss of our innocence. It is out of this collective grief that I believe this whole study of thanatology was born.

Let me give you a little background of where I was in my life when this happened. Carl Jung pointed out that Western mythology and literature mainly concerned itself with the struggles of the first half of a man's life. Over and over the theme is repeated whether it be Perseus, Jason, Moses, or Oedipus.

The young man given an impossible task against all odds succeeds and becomes king. There is little in the culture to prepare you for what to do once you become king, that is, what to do with the second half of your life. Any one who has persisted in attaining a difficult goal, whatever it be, will not feel uncomfortable with this comparison. At age 37 I had begun to address myself to what should be my concerns in the second half of my life. I had a good marriage, three bright young children, and a thriving practice. It was here that everything changed.

The medical details are long and complicated and I won't go into much of it. To simplify the story, I noticed a small lump at the angle of my jaw while shaving one morning. It was with more curiosity than dread. What could happen to me? I was full of myself and invincible. Doctors as a general rule, after going through that terrible phase in medical school known as morbid medicans, when we think we have all the symptoms of the diseases we are studying, develop a unique ability to think of themselves as impervious to the sea of misery that we navigate through each day.

My denial systems were activated and I ignored it. Time went by. I remember being asked on my orals, "What is the differential diagnosis of a lateral mass in the neck?" At the time I spit the answer back like a computer. Now, I was dumb. When it slowly enlarged I showed it to physician friends in a casual way. They said not to worry. Maybe they didn't and I didn't hear them, but this brings me to an important point.

I would like to call your attention to what I call the blind spot phenomenon. If a close friend seeks your advice or you seek your medical advice from friends, beware; your friend does not want to see you ill. He loves you and because of that love will tend, not always, but often to underdiagnose, undertreat, or minimize. He may also overcompensate and overtreat. Beware if a close doctor friend stops you in the hall and after some chitchat offhandedly mentions what sounds like a minor medical problem. He wants your reassurance that all is well, and because you want him to be well you might unwittingly give him that unwarranted reassurance. I strongly recommend that, if you find yourself on either end of this interchange, make it official. Do it with an appointment in someone's office so that it is official. Hallway consultations can be traps whether you be the seeker or the seekee. It is important, if you are involved either as a

patient or treating physician, to sometimes, not always, doublecheck your findings with a third party who is disinterested and has no emotional involvement.

Finally one night at a dinner party a psychiatrist's wife with no medical training said that the emperor has no clothes. She said, "What is that thing under your jaw?"

Still believing all was well, I saw a surgeon who scheduled a biopsy. When I awakened from anesthesia I had a sense of foreboding. Nothing was said, but my alarm system began going off. The slides could not be read; they were not sure; they would have to send them off to a lymph node specialist. It was the weekend and my concern began to mount. On Monday I was told we would not have an answer until Tuesday. In the midst of all this I received a phone call on Monday that my 7-year-old son was hit by a car while riding his bicycle and knocked unconscious; he was being rushed to the hospital by ambulance. If you want to know what will immediately take your mind off anything, it is the sight of your child with a broken leg and brain concussion lying on a stretcher. At the time my wife and I thought it was an incredible coincidence; now I am not so sure. I believe that the anxiety my wife and I were experiencing was transmitted to our children even though we had discussed nothing of the possibilities.

The next afternoon while I was operating, the circulating nurse came and informed me that my personal physician had called and asked that I call him as soon as I was finished. That could only be the results, and I remember cursing the perversity of the common bile duct stone I was trying to extract from the patient's biliary duct. The operation was long, and when I finally called him I asked him what the results were. He said he wanted to discuss it with me and my wife personally, not on the phone, which was understandable. However, I knew what that meant. I said, "You mean it's cancer." He said he would discuss it with me when I met him at the children's ward where my wife was.

I remember hanging up the phone, and it

was as if someone had thrown a hand grenade into my brain. I was totally alone. I felt like I was cut off from everything. I have often maintained that someone should be present when news like this is given, but at that moment I was glad I was alone because there was nothing anyone could say. The reality was such a shock that I needed a few moments by myself just to comprehend it. I got in my car and am totally amnesiac about how I got from one hospital to the next. I remember pulling over to the side of the road, burying my head in my hands, and crying, trying to pull myself together. I did not want my wife or anyone to see me like this. After this experience, I try never to let a patient or relative drive anywhere by himself when news of this kind is given. It is a wonder that I did not kill someone in an accident.

When I got to the hospital and saw my wife, I knew she knew. My doctor, who was at that point dealing with two very scared human beings, again told me what I found impossible to hear: cancer. I submit to you that, in the entire dictionary, in any language, you will not find a single word that carries with it such emotional impact as cancer. Lawrence LeShan once defined the elements of a nightmare. He said there are three:

1. Someone or something is doing something terrible to you.
2. You have no idea how long it will last.
3. You have no control over it.

That definition fits nicely for cancer. At that moment in my life I was consumed by fear. Later, in a more reflective moment, I had a chance to analyze what exactly it was that I feared. Certainly fear of death itself was one, even though rationally I have always believed that death is an endless sleep or beginning or something else. In either case, rationally there should be little to fear. No one ever said that fear was rational. It was the thought of suffering, of dying slowly, and in the end dying, not as I was in life, but rather as a shriveled ghost of myself. My vanity loathed the idea that my children, my wife, my friends would see me thus. I feared I would be the object of pity

and that people would be afraid of me and withdraw.

I remembered in the movie "The Black Orpheus" that there was a character representing death. He wore the costume of a skeleton. At the height of the carnival, the revelers were always being reminded of their own mortality by his presence. I would now be wearing that costume. I feared my fear would be contagious and people would treat me differently. I feared for my wife and children. They were my responsibility, and because of circumstances beyond my control—you know the rest. I feared I would be damaged in some way that I would not be able to work again in surgery, the thing I love so much. I even feared that I would flunk dying. I have been so geared to doing well on examinations that I feared I would screw up this final examination, that somehow I would not have the courage when things went badly. Yet I now know that dying is just an extension of living, and I have observed that people die in the same style that they lived. The whiny complaining person dies saying, "Why me?" The flamboyant die flamboyantly; the quiet mousy person who never said "boo" during his life usually dies in the corner of a nursing home; and the person who has handled most of life's vicissitudes well usually handles dying well. Last, my greatest fear was the loss of control over my own destiny. I would have to hand it over to faceless x-ray technicians and people I did not know.

Mixed into all this fear was the overwhelming grief of the knowledge that I might not have a chance to see how it all turned out. No one has ever come back from the other side to tell us what it's like. So we spend a lot of our energy speculating about this. But the one thing I knew for sure was that, regardless of what would happen after death, I sure as hell wouldn't be *here*. To be absent from all the important milestones in my wife's and children's lives was a sad thing to contemplate. Also I have to mention the great sadness I felt for my body, which I knew would have to undergo considerable damage before this was over. My age of innocence was over. My wife's life and my life were unalterably changed, regardless of the outcome.

Franz Kafka's short story "Metamorphosis" made a deep impression on me when I read it in college. There have been many interpretations given about what it meant, but now let me give you mine. It is the story of a young man who one morning wakes up to discover he has been converted into a beetle. There he is lying on his back, unable to turn over in bed; his legs are flaying, and he is unable to speak. His family finally comes to see why he has overslept, and their initial reaction is to recoil in horror. Then they are unable to find words for the catastrophe that has befallen them. The next phase is that they accept his condition and become very solicitous. They clean his shell, feed him, and protect him from the outside world. Because sympathy is such a difficult emotion to sustain over a long period of time, they slowly withdraw, and the end of the story is that he dies from dehydration because they neglected to care for him. To me this was an allegory of how the world treats someone with cancer.

My doctors recommended that I should enter the hospital immediately for the staging tests, culminating in the staging surgery. You see, we knew the verdict and the verdict was cancer, but we didn't know the sentence. These tests would determine how extensive the process was, which in turn would predict the prognosis. I must tell you that in this whole experience, which spanned an entire year, nothing, I repeat nothing, was as terrible as the anxiety associated with the staging. The *not knowing* was almost unbearable. As a result of this experience, I try to never make patients wait for appointments regarding biopsies or results when this kind of information hangs in the balance. If I tell a woman she needs a breast biopsy, I try to schedule it the next day. The psychic expenditure of energy spent worrying is enormous, and the sooner the results are known, the sooner the patient can either break out the champagne or screw his courage to the sticking place and get on with it.

As soon as I was rehospitalized, the news spread quickly. I was immediately confronted by two major problems: what to tell my children, ages 5, 7, and 8, and what to tell my parents, ages 73 and 75. It took me a long time to resolve what to tell my children, and I will discuss that later. As for my parents, I held off as long as possible. How could I do that to them? I was the youngest, their doctor, the apple of their eye, and I had to call them long distance and tell them that I might precede them out of this world. When I called, my mother immediately said, "Something terrible has happened." She thought we were hiding something from them about their grandson. But she knew. Tell me psychic phenomena do not exist.

The reactions from the people I love, the people I work with, and the people who know me were very interesting. Generally there were three reactions. The first reaction was no reaction. Some people could simply not deal with it. I don't judge them harshly. They simply could not come to see me. One doctor I know quite well saw me walking down the hall in slippers and a bathrobe and quickly averted his eyes. Later he told me that he didn't drop by because he didn't want to disturb me. This was quite common. Actually I needed reassurance that people would not abandon me, so for me this was the opposite of what I wanted.

The second reaction from some people was an almost hysterical attempt to reassure me that everything was going to be alright. I found this highly offensive: I surely didn't know everything was going to be alright, how in the hell did they? What they said was, "It's okay. I knew someone once who had this and he's fine and everything is going to be alright." What I heard was, "Oh my God, you're going to die." While in the hospital I received as gifts three pairs of pajamas and one bathrobe. I was to be the best dressed dying man in the hospital. The gifts all came from people who assured me that everything was going to be alright.

The third reaction, the one I appreciated

the most, was when a friend I didn't know that well came in, looked at me, started to cry, and said, "I don't know what to say." I replied, "it's okay because there is nothing to say." The emotions involved are greater than mere paltry words. One good friend just came and sat. He listened to my ravings and said little, but he was a very calming influence. His silence said more than all the reassurances. I found a kinship with anyone else who had confronted death, knowing that I belonged now to a peculiar order and that only by having experienced it would someone else understand it.

I knew that, if any of the staging tests were positive and they showed tumor in more than the two places I already knew about, then school was out. All the tests were frightening, but the gallium scan was uniquely diabolic. A radioactive dye was injected into my bloodstream, from whence the tumor would pick it up. A scanning device slowly swung back and forth over me, beginning with my head and going down to my toes. As each swing was made, the read-out appeared on a screen that I was able to watch. Slowly, I watched the general outline of my entire body begin to make itself evident. I knew that if any "hot spots" lit up in my chest or abdomen it would be bad news indeed. I now understand how the victim felt in Poe's story "The Pit and the Pendulum." The bone marrow biopsy was the single most painful experience I ever had in my life. If you do these, make sure you use plenty of sedation.

Next came the surgery. Surgeons make lousy patients, and the major issue was loss of control. To fight this I made an incredible nuisance of myself. I adjusted my I.V.s, ordered my own x-ray films, and even took my own stitches out. (After all, I wouldn't hurt me, would I?) Let me give you my theory of the horizontal and vertical positions. I believe that, when two people are vertical, the kind of exchange they have, no matter what it is, is somewhat decided by the fact that they are both standing facing each other. However, if one person be-

comes horizontal and the other remains vertical, a whole different kind of interchange takes place. Anyone who has had to lie in bed while someone standing over him talks to him will know immediately what I'm talking about. I believe it is important to sit down and talk to the person on the same eye level.

Let me elaborate on this part a little. Many times house staff members and nurses catch a lot of hostility from patients and it's unwarranted. I think what's going on is that, when you take people who have a strong sense of themselves and put them in a hospital bed with a life-threatening illness, they find themselves in a relationship with their doctor much like a child and his parents. During serious illness patients must give up control over their lives. After all, as a surgeon I come around each morning and write something call orders—what could be more authoritative than that? I decide when they can eat, when they can go to the bathroom, and when they can get out of bed. Most people react to this kind of helplessness and authority just like they did as a child, with a great deal of ambivalence. They put their faith in the attending physician, hoping that he will make them well, but they also harbor a great feeling of anger for being put in their dependent position in the first place. Their anger has to manifest itself somehow and it usually is misdirected at nurses, interns, and residents. So the next time you are dealing with an angry patient, consider from whence it is coming.

Aside from a record-breaking ileus, I survived the surgery and finally left the hospital. The nurses were so happy to get rid of me that *they* gave *me* the box of candy, instead of the other way around. Here I must digress. I can no longer leave out the most important person in this story, my wife Carole. Someone said that cancer makes a weak marriage weaker and a strong marriage stronger. Certainly the latter has been true for us. Most doctor's wives suffer from a syndrome in which, because their husband is receiving so many rewards in the form of satisfaction, strokes, prestige, and money, the wife feels thwarted in her ability to emerge as a person on her own. What this experience did was let my wife show what she is made of: courage, steadfastness, and iron will. I knew I loved her; now I found out how much I needed her. The treatment had weakened me, and she was someone who gave me her strength. She moved her bed into my hospital room and never budged. We cried together, oh how we cried together. To the rest of the world it was all stiff upper lip and a lot of jokes, but between us it was fathomless emotion. I will never let any husband or wife try to play "I've got a secret." This is too powerful and beautiful an experience, as painful as it is, to try and protect the other person, and God knows many of my patients try and do this. "Don't tell her, she'll never be able to handle this," etc. When people know they are writing the last chapter of their story, they usually can summon a great deal of courage to make it a good one.

After the surgery was over, I began the radiation treatment. This consisted of radiating every lymph node area of my body with 4,400 rads. As a medical student, intern, and resident, I don't think I've been to a radiation department but once and that was just to pick up some x-ray films. Radiation therapy departments are hidden in the bowels of the hospital fortified by lead walls, and most practicing doctors know little, if anything, about what goes on there. I chose to have my treatments at Stanford, which meant an hour's drive each way each day. To sit in the waiting room of the Stanford Radiation Department awaiting my turn is an experience difficult to describe: to see in the faces of young children and old men the same haunted look, while just outside birds are singing and the shopping center nearby is filled with people who are making plans.

It just so happened that the start of my treatment coincided with Stanford's Radiation Department's remodeling drive. This meant that my first introduction to an actual cobalt machine was in a room where the tiles had been removed. There was just this strange machine surrounded by exposed wires, conduits, and bare concrete. Fellini could not have created a more frightening tableau.

After the technician positioned me on the table with the admonition not to move (as if I'd move), everyone quickly exited and a heavy lead door clanged shut, leaving me alone with my machine. Since this illness creates a devasting feeling of being an island unto yourself, being cut off in this room only serves to drive home how alone you are. So that I would know when the machine was turned on, a red light would suddenly go on accompanied by a spine-jarring discordant buzzing noise.

Since this went on for 5 months, it was interesting for me to watch my feelings toward this machine change. After a while, I came to develop a certain affection for it. I considered it my daily journey to a center of a star. How ironic that I had to drive an hour each day to find this machine that emitted the stuff of the universe. After all, this kind of radiation fills the interstellar spaces and is inimitable in life. Yet I was depending on it to cure me. It is interesting that the main forms of treatment for cancer—surgery, radiation and chemotherapy—are all previews of coming attractions. In case you didn't know what dying was like, these forms of treatment are all introductory courses. It is ironic that the side effects are exactly the symptoms of the disease in its last stages.

In addition to losing the indefinable thing called one's sense of well-being, I had a new problem with which to contend. This was depression. It was once said that there is nothing as depressing as depression. How true. It is a vicious cycle that feeds on itself. It made the time I spent with my children poignant, and poignancy is a joyless emotion. My wife was a great source of strength. She planned activities to keep me busy, and this is an important point. Vacations are bummers. Vacations have large blocks of time to turn inward and to begin to descend into that black pit. I do not recommend them. At a time like this, it is not wise to leave your support system; by that I mean friends, relatives, and family. It is probably more important to keep busy with work, projects, or whatever. Although I felt lousy every day and knew I would throw up exactly 3 hours after each abdominal treatment, I still went to work almost every day. If you have a friend or associate who is going through a depression for any reason, I recommend that you try to monitor his work. This is where friends and colleagues can help. It is easy to make mistakes when you are busy fighting demons.

It took 5 months for Stanford to finish the radiation. During this time there was a daily ritual I went through each morning while shaving. I carefully inspected my face. What a strange, sad, pathetic thing it was to watch the slow but steady disintegration of health. I felt like Rip Van Winkle in reverse. With each passing day the radiation was internally aging all of my organs, so that I was a 37-year-old man whose body was aging 20 years in 5 months. I must admit that my fears about what might happen were greater than the reality.

Interestingly enough, it was only afterward that I started to come apart. This is common. The main need for support may not be during the crisis. People can call on great reserves to handle crises. At the time of the diagnosis everyone wants to help. Usually this is not the time it is needed. I was in shock, and after that passed I was summoning up the courage to go through what lay before me. The trouble actually began after it was all over. Although I thought that at last the depression would lift, I found that it still took very little to trigger it: the sight of old people in an elevator, meeting the teenage child of a colleague, staring out an airplane window. Any of these incidents could cause the ground in my head to suddenly lose its firmness and become an inky swamp. As a surgeon, one of the most common questions I'm asked is, "How long will it take the scar to heal?" I answer that question by saying it takes approximately 2½ years for an incision to finally become what it is going to be. I guess

that is approximately right for psychic scars as well. It is reassuring, I think, to know that it is okay to still be depressed a year later. It is important to know that there will come a morning when the first thing that swims into your consciousness on opening your eyes will not be this terrible word and that life will return to a modicum of normalcy.

After the radiation was over, I received conflicting advice regarding my need for chemotherapy. Some said I should take another 6 months just to be sure. Stanford said no. I didn't know who to believe. Obviously if I made the wrong decision it could cost me my life either way, so I began to read and doctor shop. I flew around the country consulting all the wise men, and that was an awful experience. As a physician, I understood their language and knew what they were talking about, and I still came away confused. God help the ordinary patient who falls into this maze. Many of the chemotherapists thought I should have 6 more months of treatment. Henry Kaplan, the grand old man of Stanford, said definitely not. That was an awful time. Finally one night I had a dream. In the dream, I was on a witness stand and all the chemotherapists were telling me to take their medicine. Henry Kaplan was sitting way in the back and was speaking softly, saying "Don't do it." In the dream I could only hear Kaplan's voice. When I awoke, I turned to my wife and said, "It's settled; I won't take it." After months in the library pouring over arcane articles and statistics, here I was, the scientist, making one of the most important decisions in my life on the basis of a dream.

This whole experience has produced a strange schizophrenia in the way I have to live my life. Now, if I were to ask each of you what you would do if you knew you only had a year left to live, I think each one of you would be able to come up with an answer. This question has been the theme of countless novels, articles, and even a television series. But for me that was not the question. I did not know if I was cured or in remission, which makes it a little more sticky. Should I live my life as if I'm going to die? In that case I would go around the world with my family. But suppose I'm alright; then I will have neglected those aspects of living that need tending. Supposing I live my life as if everything is going to be fine. In that case, if it isn't and I find a lump while showering tomorrow, I will have done the wrong thing. So my mind travels on two tracks. The main one is that I'm alright, but the other one is always there cautioning me to be prudent, spend time with my family, take many vacations and try to live a quality life, and God knows that's hard enough to do.

You may be curious to know how this has changed me as a physician. It has been very helpful. I believe I can be much more supportive and empathetic with both patients and families in this situation. When appropriate, I share freely the information that I also was once the recipient of the news that I am giving them. I think it is quite reassuring to them to see that the word "cancer" is not synonymous with death. There is a doctor here in town who has survived 20 years with the same diagnosis as mine. I am always glad to see him.

Now I must tell you that all and all I had excellent medical care, both from doctors and nurses but one of the hardest things for me to deal with was the lack of tact on the part of many staff members. Being sick is undignified enough just as it is, but being treated as an object is degrading. I remember one of my first radiation treatments at Stanford. I was lying on the table, my anxiety a mile high, and the technician was adjusting these little lead blocks that would protect my spinal cord, vocal cords, and few other important structures from receiving too much radiation. A young resident came into the room. Totally ignoring me, he began a conversation with the technician that went something like this (remember now, I'm horizontal and they are vertical):

"Hey Joe, the VA just sent two old goners with brain tumors over, and I'm wondering can we fit them in today."

"Gee, I'm busy and we're swamped today."

"I know that, but I have to let them know at the VA and I really want to get them started today."

Back and forth this conversation went, while I was lying there in a modified crucifixion position. Finally I could restrain myself no longer. I do not remember my exact words, but they were explicit.

Another doctor would turn to my wife and ask playfully, "Well, has he been behaving himself?" I suppose now, after 4 years, it seems like an innocent remark, but at the time my dignity was very important to me and I bristled at anyone who tried to treat me like a child.

After my illness I began to read everything about cancer, including its psychologic effects. I was contacted by many well-meaning people that we in organized medicine refer to as the fringe. Being a believer that all truth is not circumscribed by the scientific tradition, I explored some of these paths. I spent a weekend with Dr. Carl Simonton; I'm sure many of you are familiar with his techniques. This is in keeping with the times. There is a turning away from the traditional forms of treating cancer. It seems that, as the technologic advances become more specialized and remote, there is a swing to the holistic forms of treatment. I would like to comment on this.

First let me tell you about a study that was done at the M. D. Anderson Cancer Hospital in 1952. A psychologist did a personality profile on all admitted patients. He did not know their diagnosis or prognosis. With only a psychologic profile he was able to develop an 80 percent predictability regarding prognosis. I am sure that this is no surprise, since we know the will to live is an important part of getting well. Since this is the 1970s and we are all told in the many forms of the human growth potential movement that we are all responsible for creating our own experiences, I have to address the question "How did this happen to me?" and more important, "Did I do this to myself and, if so, why?'' Obviously, there is a continuum of responsibility that begins at one end, for instance, with this room being randomly struck by a falling 747, in which case we would have had little to do with creating our collective demise. The other end of the spectrum is the person who jumps off the Golden Gate Bridge and takes his own life. In between are all the rest. Some things are out of my control but some are not.

I wanted to marshall all the energy I had into conquering that part that I had control over. The idea of Simonton, and most of the others, is that you must stop playing victim and make yourself well. His techniques deal with meditation, but there are many alternatives including diet, medication, flying to the Philippines, and going to Mexico City. Certainly his contributions are the most valuable in my opinion. I can say that this part is a helpful thing. The patient feels like he is retaining some control over his life. The problem with this approach is that, if you accept that you could make yourself well, you must have made yourself sick in the first place, and he has you examine this. All is well so far—he is able to report on some startling successes with some patients, and for a certain group of people I think this is very helpful.

However, one thing bothers me, and I have used his techniques with several patients: Suppose that you use his techniques and they don't work, as in most cases they will not. Then the person not only is dying but also is feeling guilty about it because he has been told that he has the power to make himself well. I have seen this and it is a two-edged sword. It is fine while it works but quite cruel when it fails, because it robs the patient of valuable time that he needs to come to terms with his dying.

This brings me to the subject of the will to live. When I finished my residency, one of my mentors told me, ''Lenny, if you have your choice between being a lucky surgeon and a good one, choose to be a lucky one.'' At first I did not understand what he meant;

now I do. There is more to this healing art than just science. There are some doctors, not always the smartest or the most technically proficient, who consistently get patients well when others fail. I have noted again and again in the literature that one man may achieve results that no one else can duplicate. He is usually suspected of fudging, but there is something else going on. It is something that can never be statistically measured and that has to do with two separate entities. One of them is the physician. There are doctors and there are Physicians, with a capital P. If a patient feels that you really care and want them to get well, they will respond. The great physicians I have met are, first and above all, loving human beings.

This phenomenon also applies to types of patients as well. Let us suppose that there are two women who on the same day in Sioux City, Iowa, are told that they have breast cancer. One meekly lies down and allows whatever needs to be done, and then says, ''Poor me.'' This is the classic victim. Suppose the other says, ''I'm not going to let this do me in,'' and then gets on a plane and flies to see whatever big name doctor is currently being featured in Ladies Home Journal.

You will never be able to compare a series of those two patients who have identical diseases because the second one that I have described, due to force of will and some hidden ability of the physician, is going to live longer and in general do better. That is why I am so suspicious whenever I read the scientific literature or hear popular accounts of dramatic cures. The feisty patient generally does better than the placid one in the long run.

The one issue that is slowly becoming resolved is what to tell my children. They saw me when I was very ill and even accompanied me to Stanford for my radiation treatments on occasion. If we sat them down and explained all the implications to them at their young age and if it turned out that I was alright, then we would have needlessly frightened them. On the other hand, I wanted to be open. I have had talks with my two oldest children and explained to them what happened. I cannot bring myself yet to do it with my little one.

My children's reactions to my illness varied with each child. My youngest daughter, who was 4, seemed unaffected by it, but she was the best prognosticator of how I was doing. During my treatment she said to me, "Did you know I see colors around people?" I replied, "Oh really, what color is your brother?" She squinted her eyes, looked across the room and said, "He's green."

"And what color is your sister?"

"She's yellow."

"How about Mommy?"

"She's orange."

Finally, I looked at her and asked what color I was. She looked at me a long time and then said, "I see you as black." That really scared me.

Several months later, after the treatments were over, I tried again. She looked at me, gave me a sly smile, and said, "I see you as magenta." I started feeling much better from that day on.

My oldest daughter has told my little one recently that "Daddy almost died but he's okay now." She was very sympathetic and caring when I was sick. My son was furious. Here he was in the hospital with a cast on—the most important event in his 7-year-old life—and his father upstaged him. At one point he demanded to know why everyone was concerned about me since it was clear that he was the one with the broken leg. My son and I are very close, and I am convinced he and I were resonating like two tines of a tuning fork. We both were admitted to the hospital the same time. One night, a month later, while I was receiving the radiation treatment, my son was getting ready for bed and was putting his pajamas on. My wife and I simultaneously saw an egg-sized mass in his axilla. My wife consulted our pediatrician who immediately advised her to see a pediatric oncologist. It turned out to be mononucleosis, but that's just too much of a coincidence.

Finally, this experience has caused me to reexamine that age-old question, "What's it all about?" It is an interesting exercise for anyone to consider the universe without them in it. This was especially pregnant for me; as those who know me well will tell you, humility is not one of my long suits. I had to ask myself the question of what the effect of my departure would be. When I thought about that I realized that the galaxies would continue in their outward journey. Not one planet would budge from its orbit. Medicine in San Francisco would go on; no one who needed an operation would go without one. Of course my friends would miss me and they would be sad for a while, but no vacations would be canceled or cocktail party invitations go unanswered for long. The greatest impact would be on my wife and children, but she would not be history's first widow, and my children would grow up into adulthood and stand or fall on the foundations that had already been laid. So what meaning did my life have? I was forced to conclude that the major meaning of my life was in my family relationships, not in work or material things.

At first I thought, "My God, I've got to tell this story. I've got to write it all down and tell everybody." But then I realized it has all been said before and I had no blinding insights for the world. Pangloss was right after all. So I finally came to terms with my companion, the man in the skeleton costume. At first, when my fear was great, I had tried to run from him, but it was like trying to escape my shadow. In the beginning not a day passed in which I didn't at sometime or another think about him. In the beginning it was "Oh my God, what are you doing here?" Now it is just, "Ain't that a shame."

Before this happened, I was like the Soviet Politburo. I had a 5-year plan, a 10-year plan, even a 20-year plan. That is no more. What I realized was that I could only die in the future, but I was alive right now and I would always be alive in the here and now. I savor many things more appreciatively now, although I must confess that I have begun backsliding and once again am making long-range plans.

It has been interesting for me, your standard-issue scientist, to stand back and watch the slow transformation of that scientist into a mystic. When I was younger I was an existentialist agnostic. Life was a kick, but it had to be basically random and absurd. Anyone growing up in World War II would have to conclude what I thought. Now, I am not sure. Camus once said, "Science has many truths but no truth." I find this experience one of delving into what were ancient universal truths before science decreed them all nonsense because they could not be subjected to a random double-blind study. In fact, I must admit that, in terms of personal growth, this has been a very enlightening period in my life. Robert Frost once said in a poem, "You only get to see the light from your star when it gets dark."

20

A therapist encounters the possibility of an early death

HOWARD KOGAN

Beginnings and endings are a part of everyone's life. In the therapist's life, since so many other lives are intimately opened to his view, it is an intensified experience. Birth and death emerge in fantasy, in dreams, in recollections; in direct and symbolic forms, on all levels of consciousness and in the near and remote unconscious. There is throughout a pervasiveness and a depth in feeling and meaning to things that are ending and to things that are beginning anew. For most of us the only end that is not also a beginning anew is death. That is a part of its terror and the part that is hardest to comprehend.

My encounter began on a Saturday morning in January 1972 when I visited a physician because of a minor scalp infection. In the course of his examination he commented that my thyroid gland seemed "rather full." The next few weeks I watched the invisible "rather full" stage quickly become a visible lump. A lump in the throat. What pregnant symbolism. A life's accumulation of sadness unexpressed now turning to devour the self? Or perhaps something I just can't swallow and can't vomit out? Lump finally translated only one way to me; cancer. It wasn't likely, but it was a real possibility.

I had felt for years that I would die in my mid-fifties as my father had and as his father had before him. Both died of cancer. Since

Reprinted from Voices, pp. 82-86, Summer, 1973.

I was now only 31, the fantasy brought with it a sense of omnipotence for the present and for that and many other reasons I cherished it. The fantasy, however, had only the power of a wish or a fear which could be great but was not equal to the power of this growing lump in my neck.

Patients had often told me of the terror the night can hold. The day with its work and demands and the forced interaction with others supports an outer directedness that can be comforting. The night is a confrontation with the self. I would lay down to sleep and feel suddenly and intensely awake. I would read until I seemed almost fully asleep, or watch T.V., or pour a few nightcaps; nothing really helped. Regardless of what I would do, there was in each night an hour or two, or more of sadness and fear, of thinking and ruminating, of bitching or crying.

I felt I wanted to keep my worse fears and fantasies to myself but I did not. I would wake Libby in the middle of the night and tell her, and when they had become too much for her I had only my analyst left who could listen to me and not ask me to stop. I was admitted to the hospital on a Sunday evening in March and was scheduled to be operated on the following Tuesday morning. The "nothing to be concerned about" of January had become an "it ought to come out." I had told my patients I was having minor surgery and planned to return in three weeks. I was still scared about the possibility of cancer, but I was more confident now that it was only a remote possibility. At least I wanted very much to believe that and I did and I didn't.

Fifteen years before at sixteen I had said goodbye to my own father after a tense, bickering drive to the hospital. He died a few days later. This came back to me in the flurry of my last minute preparations to leave for the hospital. Douglas is five and I told him I loved him and I kissed him and I kept on wanting to do it again so that would last him if it had to. Susan at two didn't quite comprehend what was happening. The melancholy feeling left me as I drove to the hospital. This was to be a learning experience; that was the mind-set.

I was in the hospital scarcely two hours before there was a nurse sitting at bedside telling me of her boyfriend and their problems. I had risen like a phoenix from the patient role and was a therapist again. She in crisp whites and me in a hospital gown; not a bad session. The next morning I learned that I was to have a student nurse assigned to me to go through the pre-op, the operation and the post-operative period. I was going to be her term paper and I was delighted. When I wasn't having tests I spent my time telling Janet, the student nurse, of my fantasies of the operation. In an exhibitionistic, manic tour de force I produced one fantasy after another, each replete with psychodynamic explanations and references to my childhood experiences. Mostly it was a diversion and a denial and a manic defense, but I was enjoying being the ham and entertaining Janet.

I awoke Tuesday about five in the morning feeling relaxed and optimistic. I was fascinated by the trip to OR and the wait in the crowded hallway. We were all lined up side by side, flat on our backs, being pushed and pulled about by orderlies. Though we easily could have, none of the patients seemed to want to look at or to talk to the person on the stretcher along side. The look of the OR (like a huge dormitory shower room) and the smell (very medicinal) and the sound (noisy with a rock radio station in the background) filled me with questions. It soon became apparent even to me that I was intensely interested in anything except my own surgery. When I went under I still had enough questions to last another few hours.

As I was coming out of the anesthesia I heard Janet's voice very close to me and I asked her if it was cancer. She said "yes," and I took a long slide back into the dark. The dark was broken first by one doctor then another calling my name loudly and saying things I don't remember. *The heat of their breath on my face is the clearest memory.* The word cancer had registered and it was louder than the other words.

Libby was there sometime later, but I only smiled at her in the brief moments of wakefulness. We didn't talk. I did test my voice and found it still sounded like me. The possible loss of my voice due to nerve damage during surgery had been a major concern. How could I do therapy without a voice or with a hushed, loudly whispered voice? People like my voice and I was happy to still have it.

I felt better, more alert after my visitors left and I began to think about cancer. I felt I needed to work it through for myself before I could talk to Lib. My first reaction was strangely positive. If I had cancer, then I would never do anything I didn't want to do again. I had a weapon with which to intimidate my rather severe super-ego. No more demands, no more being middle-class, no more work, no more conformity; using my cancer as a shield against my conscience, I would enter nirvana. I wasn't sure whether it was my trump card in the battle of the chamber pot or if the possibility of death made me embrace life more and reminded me I had only one life and I needed to be for me *now*. Maybe they're both true.

I was still uncomfortable physically and the pain and stiffness in my neck kept pulling me away from my thoughts. I had a shot of Demerol and fell asleep. It's hard to put the next two days in any kind of order. Slowly I was feeling better and in less pain. I talked to the nurses, my doctors and visitors, but I was mechanical and used a few pat lines over and over with whoever showed their faces at bedside. I was a little angry with Janet because she saw me joking before and I wasn't now. I wished I wasn't her term paper and that she would stop trying to draw me out or cheer me up.

I felt incredibly guilty. Sue was only two and Doug five and Libby only 28. What right did I have to do this to them. We had moved into a new house only six months before and I didn't even have enough insurance to cover the mortgage. Reel after reel I went through a dozen fantasies about my death and how they would react to it. It hurt so much that I still can't bring myself to write them all down.

Though Lib is Jewish now, she was raised a Christian and I worried and grew angry thinking that she would be closer to her family than mine after I died and that Douglas might not even think of himself as a Jew. Surprisingly, Judaism seemed very important, not for me but for Doug; it was as though the religion would become his new father. He would have as his new father all of the great rabbis and story-tellers.

Somehow it was in connection with this thought that I hit bottom. I realized Susan and Douglas probably wouldn't remember me. Susan couldn't, I was sure. Douglas might remember a little. A favorite question of mine in the beginning of therapy is to ask for a patient's earliest memory. I searched my memory going from patient to patient to see how many people recalled things from age five or younger. A good number had, in fact I had at least a few memories that were clear and went back to age three or four. The one patient who lost a father when she was four had no memory of him. I alternated from being depressed to angry about my not being remembered.

I thought about the places my name had appeared; in a local newspaper, on case records in social agencies, in a high school and two college commencement bulletins.

There were other places but none seemed to be a source of immortality. It seemed that that was attainable only through my children. It was something that only they could confer on me. At the time it seemed completely voluntary.

At some point I reminded myself that I wasn't dead now and that I would have at least some time at home with the children. The doctors were saying I'd have lots of time, but I wasn't listening to them yet. My plan for the time remaining was to be super-father. I would go home and sell the new house, move the family into an apartment that could be maintained after I died, and spend the time remaining being the kind of father I wanted to be. The children had to feel loved by me and not deserted by my death, and I still wanted to be remembered. I thought about how many hours a father spends with his son and and daughter in a year and added up the years till both would have reached 21. Putting in twelve hours a day, seven days a week, I would be a typical father if I lived another year and a half. This solution was short lived as I realized that what was needed was an hour or two of fathering everyday not an intensive marathon of fathering. The essence of fathering seemed now to be presence. I decided to write a book for the children about my life, my father and mother, stories about an uncle who died in a concentration camp and about another who came to the United States alone as a child and who became wealthy and used his money to rescue other relatives from the Nazis. Year by year I would tell more and speak more maturely. I would include needed information, advice, and my favorite books, music and foods. I hoped that they would come to the book the way religious people can go to the bible for comfort and guidance and strength.

The possibility of Lib remarrying occurred to me and it seemed like a good idea for her but I grew increasingly sullen and resentful as I thought of my children having a new father. I stopped thinking about it. If I wasn't going to die now, when, I wondered, would be the best time. When Doug is eight he'll be pretty much on his way, but Sue will be very involved with me oedipally and it is very hard for a girl to lose her father at that time. When Sue is eight, Douglas will be eleven and though it is not the worst time to die there are so many father and son kind of things to do at that age he'd feel terrible without me. I carried that on for quite a while but never really found a good time to die.

It was very late in the evening on Thursday night when I tried again to really relate to someone. By now it had become apparent to the trio of physicians treating me that the mature, optimistic, strong person they had known had been replaced by a very depressed and withdrawn one. They must have conspired because they all came in that day mouthing almost the same words and vieing with each other to see who could "snap him out of it." The first in that day was the one I knew best. He asked me how I was feeling and without really waiting for an answer said that I was doing fine. He repeated that one way or another about ten times before he left. He is a sweet guy and I would have liked to respond but I was still much too heavily involved in my own inner world. The surgeon stated things directly: "I'm telling you the truth, I don't believe in telling people who have cancer the truth; so if I'm telling you about cancer, it means you don't have it." I didn't even try to think that one through. I did stir me enough, however, to think that medical doctors don't seem to know enough about people in the psychological sense. It was my first "professional" thought since surgery.

I wasn't any more open to the final doctor's approach except that his showing up so late at night surprised me. He took me into an examination room behind the nurses station and we talked. He got the same mechanical agreement as the others had, but he knew it wasn't real and persisted. Finally I felt ready to talk realistically about having cancer and I asked a few questions and got what seemed like straight answers. At one point I guess I was coming across in such a distrustful way that he showed me

my charts and the pathology lab report. I concluded he was probably telling me the truth and that the time had come for me to begin to relate to that. I had had cancer but it had been successfully removed and I could now expect an almost normal life span. It seemed so certain: he absolutely knew I didn't have cancer now but he wanted to do more tests even though he knew the results would be negative. That piece of medical double-talk almost pushed me back into my own "bell jar" but Manny read real and I was able finally to begin to take the hope he was offering.

I returned to work just thirteen days after the surgery, feeling that I wanted to be myself again, the sooner the better. Subsequent testing proved negative and as the days passed and my scar slowly settled into a thin raised line concealed by the crease of my neck, I found myself wondering if this experience would make any difference at all in my life. In certain ways, however, it already had. I had been seeing two terminally ill patients for the prior year. One, an angry manipulative woman, would flagellate me with her dying and create a survivor's guilt strong enough to make confrontations with her sadistic behavior almost impossible. It was in the midst of a difficult session with her when I realized she was no longer able to justify her behavior to me by using her illness. In fact, I was feeling more firm and urgent about trying to resolve some of her problems *now* because she would be dead in a few years. A second patient and I had gently danced around the periphery of her impending death. I felt willing to talk about her dying, yet I had usually found some hint from her that she needed not to talk about it and I would go along with that. Now we had a long talk about dying and she welcomed it. I considered telling her about my brush with cancer, but did not. At first I felt I might only worry her and inhibit her fully expressing her own feelings, but later I began to feel it had more to do with the fact that I had survived my brush with cancer while she would die from hers. So we talked together and cursed and mourned all the things that wouldn't get done and finally returned to thinking about life and treating it in a properly precious way.

Death had lost some of its mystique; it seemed now to be more a part of life, more normal less otherworldly, less alien. I feel committed to the idea that any meaningful change in personality takes a long time. Years of work for most. But I ask myself more and more these days if each patient and I are moving as fast as we can. It's not pleasant to keep remembering such things but at least it helps me stay in touch with my own mortality and hence with the value of every day.

While I was writing this paper on a hot July morning four months after my surgery, the secretary of the Training Institute called to inform me of a faculty member's death. About five weeks before we had spent an hour together and I had decided to use him as my control analyst in the fall. He apparently got sick about a week after our talk and died quickly of a malignant brain tumor. We had made an appointment for September the fifth, shook hands and exchanged wishes for a good summer. Appointments made in the future cannot ward off an impending disease though in an illusory way it seems to ward off the dis-ease. One of us is having a good summer and one

of us is dead. Did he wish harder for me than I for him? So much for plans and schedules and the routine that denies death.

The day after saying goodbye to Irwin at the chapel, it was the day of his funeral, my family and another couple took the ferry out to Fire Island; we spent the hottest day of the summer walking through the Sunken Forest, swimming, body surfing and playing ball. Susan had to be carried throughout most of the trek in the Forest but she was singing part of the time and teasing Lib by kissing me and shouting out that she was ''smooching'' with daddy. I almost liked carrying her. Doug spent about five minutes resenting his having to walk while Susie was carried but then he was able to get involved in being a scout and tour guide. Running ahead of us, he would come back full of grave warnings about the steepness of the trail or the poison ivy that seemed to be everywhere.

On the way back on the ferry the kids fell asleep and Libby and I exchanged glances, smiles and a few words about how nice the day had been and what we would have for supper. Most of the words were lost in the oscillating drone of the engines. We decided to have a pizza with green peppers. It was the right choice.

21

Observations by a doctor who's been a CCU patient

JAMES A. ABBOTT

On July 20, 1973 I had a myocardial infarction. Following this I was hospitalized for 22 days days in a large Detroit hospital which is part of the Wayne State University Medical School complex. I was in the coronary care unit during the first six days and during the remaining period I was in the intermediate care unit.

During my hospital stay and during the time that has followed, I have had a chance to reflect on my experiences. I would like to discuss these observations, particularly as they apply to the psychology of the patient in the coronary care unit.

Let us start with the circumstances that surround the patient's admission to the hospital. A person can approach a serious operation with a certain degree of emotional preparation. He can gear himself up to it. In other sudden and severe medical conditions there are usually prodromal symptoms that enable the person to become accustomed to the idea of being sick. But a heart attack is a sudden, unplanned and unexpected event. One moment the person is pursuing his daily activities and an hour later he is being wheeled into the coronary care unit. When he arrives at the unit and has been "hooked up" to the monitor, he is told that he must be more or less completely passive.

We have, therefore, a situation in which a person, who is often a vigorous and active person, is suddenly and unexpectedly thrust into a strange world in which his life is in some danger and in which, to enhance his chances for survival, he must be as passive as possible.

In our culture, most self-sufficient adults look upon passivity as a weakness, a reminder of childhood. In addition, perhaps without realizing it fully, some people regard a passive role as a dangerous one, exposing the person to rejection and to an inability to cope with the aggressions of others. Particularly if the patient has a strong unconscious wish to be passive in the first place, will he find the stress of the passive position in the coronary care unit a difficult one to deal with.

From the reading that I have done, I do not think that this factor has been given sufficient attention or even recognition. Most articles stress the anxiety arising from the fear of dying. This is, of course, a factor. But it seems to me that a person is going to be confronted more relentlessly by his feelings about being passive (because of the necessary routine of the coronary care unit) than by his fear of dying.

It goes without saying that the benefits of the coronary care unit are so unequivocal that, except for psychosis, any disturbance of the patient's emotional state is distinctly of secondary importance. Nevertheless, I here offer a few thoughts on alleviating the strain of this particular emotional stress.

1. It would be beneficial to mention to

Reprinted from Michigan Medicine, p. 104, February, 1976.

191

the patient at the beginning that the demands of his passive situation are *temporary* and that in a few days he will start to resume gradually more normal activities.

2. It seems to me that allowing a patient to have as many choices in as many areas as possible would help to neutralize, to some extent, his feelings about having nothing to say about his activities. An example that comes to mind is choosing the menu for the day from two or more choices for each item.

3. I feel that having a clock and calendar in view helps to give the patient a feeling of being "on top" of things, of participating in events.

4. My personal opinion is that being able to turn one's head and look at the monitor helps in the same way, although I can imagine some patients being made uneasy by all the gadgetry.

5. It hardly needs mentioning that, having impressed on the patient the importance of being passive, it would place an intolerable burden on him if his efforts to cooperate by being passive were met with impatience or annoyance.

6. When the time comes to "unhook" the patient from the monitor and move him to the intermediate care unit, this can cause, without any pun being intended, a separation anxiety. I think that this situation can best be handled by adequate preparation for the move, by reassurance and perhaps by a little more attention by the nurses of the intermediate care unit than is physically warranted for the first half day or so.

One thing that impressed me a great deal was the autonomy of the nurses on the coronary care and intermediate care units. The new attitudes and responsibilities of nurses were undreamt of during my internship of nearly 30 years ago. They are absolutely essential for the proper running of the coronary care unit and the intermediate care unit and they represent real progress.

In summary, the coronary care unit is a relatively recent innovation in cardiology and it represents a most valuable weapon against the ravages of cardiovascular disease. In order to utilize it to its utmost potential, it is important to recognize and study the various psychological implications inherent in its use.

22

Private experience and public expectation on the cancer ward

LEA BAIDER

ABSTRACT—A sociologist relates her experiences with staff and patients on a cancer ward. Within a short time the staff perceived her as a threat to their system of efficiency-oriented norms and regulation, a system which she, in turn, came to regard as an institutionalized defense against that-which-could-not-be-confronted. In becoming acquainted with the patients themselves, the phenomenon of pain was brought to the fore. The patient's existence sometimes was dominated by pain, and yet there were significant differences from one cancer patient to another in how they interpreted and related to pain. These variations included positive valuation of pain as a symbol of life. Ethnic differences in the interpretation of pain, especially between people from Latin and Anglo-Saxon background, were observed. In general, pain behavior in terminal patients was strongly colored by the individual's feelings concerning impending death. The observer also shares some of her personal feelings of the rhythms of hospital life and their impact upon the individual.

My initiation rites upon entering the hospital and the cancer ward as a sociological observer were both instructive and puzzling. The staff quickly noted my disorientation and naivete. They smiled among themselves with the mature and experienced air of those who knew what was to be expected. My back was patted comfortingly. Yet this solicitation felt to be absurd and Kafkaesque. In a place where the beds are filled with men and women suffering and perhaps awaiting death, why should the staff comfort and console *me*?

At our first encounter, the head nurse

Reprinted from Omega **6**:373-381, 1976. This article is based upon a section of the author's dissertation study, *Family Structure of the Process of Dying: A Study of Cancer Patients and Their Family Interactions.* Waltham, Mass: Brandeis University, 1973.

conveyed the message that "This is a hospital; here sentimentality is disruptive and interferes with work. There is no reason to ask patients anything. They listen to what we tell them about themselves. We, not they, know how they feel and what is wrong with them." Her words served both as prologue and epilogue. During the next five months, the professional staff provided me with both direct and indirect advice about "not getting involved" with the patients' personal lives, and even less with their families. The staff had a rationale for this advice: the hospital is a place to provide specific medical services, and *not* a place to solve the patient's emotional and personal problems. Bothering with the latter would interfere with the effectiveness of the hospital's work.

The slogans for efficiency struck me as a

pretext to block out that which could not be confronted. The alternative was clear and was not permitted further consideration. Either one professed a type of institutionalized belief system, accepting its norms and regulations, or one must be outside the system and, in some sense, an enemy.

The staff knew that I had given my home telephone number to the patients. This provoked the first formal reprimand. Other "misconducts" included my occasional visits to the patient's homes, and informal chats with those patients who did not have their names on my strict "list." These actions were considered as disruptive, and as important enough to provoke necessary disciplinary measures. The smiles stopped, ditto the friendly advice. The questions about my role, my visits, and my function became ever more inquisitional. The silences and pseudo-denial of my presence became more intense. Later, anger and irritation cropped up overtly.

Looking back on all this, I can detect on the part of the staff a rhythm in three movements, an undulating pattern whose curves reflected all the ambiguity and doubt my presence awoke. At the beginning of the cycle, the situation was somewhat unusual for all of us, but smooth, because no one clearly understood my function, and because the staff was sure that the patients sought only "medical attention" and not "chats with visitors." Later came the questions, the disagreements, and the acrimony. Finally, the norms, oriented toward preserving the already established and regulated situation, took on the force of totalitarian power. Yet it was not I, Lea, whom they rejected, but rather that which I represented. Unintentionally, I had become a threat to the staff who could not understand my function nor what I might have to offer to the patients.

It was true that I doubted the institutionalized "efficiency religion." This "atheism" led me to search for new questions and answers. But also—perhaps in the same way as the patient—it led me to an encounter with a solitude that cannot be shared, and for which adequate answers are seldom found, namely, pain and death.

THE PATIENT IN THE HOSPITAL
Pain

My experience with the patients brought out a recurrent theme: the *pain*. Bodily pain could become a dominant part in the patient's existence at a certain point in the progress of his or her disease.

Bakan formulated a theory of pain and disease from a phenomenological point of view, using the concept of *distality* to understand the pain as an externalized object to which the patient relates. He defined distality as the psychological distance between an event or an object and the person, or, how far away from the person something appears to be. Although there are substantial correlations between the physical and the psychological distance from the body to an external object, the distances are not necessarily the same.

Following Bakan's ideas, it is worth observing how the patient looks upon pain as a strange presence in his body, a phenomenon which produces unpleasant sensations, which intrudes between his life and his body. The symptoms of pain which the patient feels do not always seem to be related to his sickness. When the pain recedes and the patient says he feels much better, he may then start to believe that the sickness, the danger of his impending death, might also have disappeared. The pain becomes not only the link between the self and the body, but it also develops into, and takes over, a central part in the illness.

But the type of response manifested by a person in pain depends also upon specific social situations, e.g., whether the person is at home or in the hospital, alone, or with his friends. Discomfort, pain, and illness often are clearly related to the psychological state of the patient. This relationship can be exemplified by quotations from three patients with whom I became familiar.

Mr. O. made increasing requests for medication. He would ask any one at any time to bring medication: "I just prefer to sleep all day . . . day and night. . . . I can't stand the pain. . . . I don't want to suffer . . . I could see day and night my pain . . . and nobody does anything about it. . . . The nurse gives me just one dose per day . . . one during all day. . . . Why can't I have three, or four, often. . . . I feel the pain . . . I could touch it. . . . Yes. . . . They don't believe me. . . . Nobody sees my pain."

Mrs. S. was described by the nurses and physicians as a "very good" patient. She never complained about anything, never asked about anything. I never heard her moan. Mrs. S. wanted to present herself as very strong, and capable of enduring her own suffering: "You know, sometimes I find myself biting my blankets . . . not to scream . . . not to ask for help . . . because really . . . I don't need help . . . and I don't want that anybody will see me weak and in despair. . . . I don't suffer . . . and if something hurts me it is my problem. . . . I want that they will see me strong and peaceful . . . like I always was. . . . Because this is how one should be. . . ."

Mrs. A. was a sixty-two year-old Puerto Rican who constantly refused to take any medicine, even when in great pain. Her rationale was similar to other Puerto Rican patients I met. Doctors don't know as much as they think they do about the person's body. Each body has a soul, and if the doctor cannot see the soul, then he cannot see the body. "I know, I know that my family does not want that I suffer . . . but suffering is part of life . . . and without it you are not a man. No medicine can help with any pain . . . or, sometimes it could help putting all your body asleep . . . like a baby . . . and then it takes away my pain . . . but it also takes away all that I feel and see. If I could feel the pain I also can feel my body . . . and then I know that I am still alive."

As a warning signal, pain acquires a symptomatic significance for most of the patients. It may be welcomed, as we saw with Mrs. A., for whom pain is an indication of life. In some cases the absence of pain would signify total or partial death. Pain then becomes a symbol of life.

If "pain expectancy" can be defined as the anticipation of pain in association with a specific physical, social, or cultural situation, then "pain acceptance" is the willingness to tolerate this sensation. Both at-

titudes will lead to a tendency to inhibit or to amplify the reflex reactions by emotional and behavioral responses.

The close relationship between pain on the one hand and life and death on the other is also apparent in the fact that in certain situations pain, whose primary function is to provoke apprehension, also fulfills the function of an anxiety-reducing device. Thus, for instance, many patients have expressed satisfaction with the fact that they feel pain in the injured parts of the body because it gave them the assurance that the injured leg or arm was not dead.

I noticed with surprise how differently patients would react toward pain. Coming as I do from a Latin country where priority is given to emotional behavior, the rational Anglo-Saxon temperament seemed to me divorced from any concrete reality: most of my Anglo-Saxon patients tried to be rational, controlling their behavior very carefully. They felt that their effort should be directed toward alleviating their condition, and evaluated according to their effectiveness. Screaming, crying, and childish complaining belong to the category of things that do not help and therefore should be avoided. The patients' avoidance and control of any emotional manifestations of pain and discomfort could be seen as part of their own philosophy about the uselessness and aimlessness of these behaviors, supported also by the strong disapproval of the hospital personnel.

This tendency to conform to an ideal mode of behavior, does not mean, however, that many of them would not have liked to behave differently. Covertly or overtly, many of the patients wanted to be more expressive, more free and less controllable in the expression of their own feelings and emotions.

Pain behavior in terminal patients can be strongly colored by the individual's feelings concerning his impending death. Expression of pain often is a substitute for the expression of feelings of helplessness, dependency, hopelessness, fear of separation, and of being abandoned. But the

Puerto Rican patients I knew did not have to use their pain to establish communication, or as a search for help and understanding. For them, pain became shameful, something that bothers the rest of the family, and for which many times they blamed and cursed God for having brought it upon them. One of the reasons offered for this strong denial of pain complaints is the fear of being taken to a hospital, and being unable to die in one's own home.

These patients attitude toward hospitals, doctors, and medicine is distrustful. When you enter a hospital, nobody knows if you will be able to leave alive. The patient prefers to rely more on his own home treatment, especially when feeling that he is in his final stage and that only God can decide his fate.

Time, space, and solitude

On the other hand, many of the patients I came to know had already been in the hospital for several months. Their lives and time perspectives changed slowly, imperceptibly, without any conscious decision or effort. In the hospital they had learned the codes and norms regulating the patients' rights and demands. Very soon they knew with whom and when they could be submissive, dependent, or aggressive. After being long enough in the hospital they learned to hide most physical manifestations of sadness and despair, so that only proper physical complaints are presented to the observers (doctors, nurses). The patient will then be very careful as to how he behaves himself. He will test all the possibilities for gratification and attention, and avoid the potential threat of acting against specific regulations. He starts developing new ways of interaction, new modes of dealing with himself and the external world. All his private experiences, sometimes painful, sad and desperate, become part of a new identity that the patient himself is creating.

When the patient is taken to the hospital, he becomes essentially alone. In a new environmental setting he is in a dependent, submissive role, alone to perceive how his body, his reaction to treatment, his pain, become part of a new self-image. He does not know what to expect, from whom, or when. The interaction between his family and himself will be essentially in terms of "behaving as normally as possible." He keeps to himself most of the experiences that he is undergoing, all the fears of possible separation, the feeling of being deserted by his family, the anger and frustration that arises from it, and the slowly coming to terms with his life, himself, but with the constant hope that maybe a new "miracle" in terms of treatment will take him away from all this. Time and space become united. The patient's body, mind, room, become his one and only place, where time moves back and forth between the hope of seeing a familiar face and his slow withdrawal into a world of dreams and recollection. Some patients become wholly involved within the bounds of evocation —they use all their energy in order to remember past experiences and fix them in their mind. They cannot share it with anybody and their secret will remain their own, sometimes as a dream, without knowing if it really took place.

During my months of work in the hospital, I heard neither cries, nor screams, nor any external manifestation of emotion. In the final period of the disease, everyone was usually very quiet, the family members smiled timidly and still tried to look as if nothing was happening or was going to happen.

Usually the patient dies alone, without family knowing about it until the hospital informs them. The body is removed immediately from the room and goes from the hospital directly to the funeral home. Nothing then is left besides nebulous memories.

And memories can themselves be forgotten.

"I want to share this experience with you"—this was the recollection of a young man, one day after his wife, one of my patients, died. Mrs. C. was twenty-three years old, and he was twenty-nine.

. . . Then the door closed and a nurse with her head down and very silent announced that she had died. A doctor came to the room; he looked at me without knowing what to say. Immediately another nurse, possibly the head of the floor, called me to fill out some papers, and another doctor asked me about the autopsy. I was there with technical forms the whole afternoon. (Silence.) Later, I remember thinking about the cars, who would sit in what cars.

I wanted to remember, to remember her face wrinkled with pain, shrunken from not eating. I wanted to recall her expression. To see her completely, absolutely completely . . . and talk to her . . . talk openly and freely as never before we did . . . It all lasted only an instant, an instant which my memory has already begun slowly to forget . . . I wanted to cry, to cry from pain, from loneliness, from being deserted and abandoned, as when I was a child. . . . But I couldn't I couldn't . . . I began to feel all around me my impotence and my frustration . . . And my image, my stupid image, molded by the outside . . . It was years since I cried . . . Someone taught me how to behave . . . how to be a man . . . And now, I forgot, I have forgotten how to cry. . . .

He didn't continue. He started crying, crying like a child, like a man, realizing the suffering of his own pain.

LONELINESS IN THE NIGHT—MY OWN EXPERIENCES

I experienced dinner time on the cancer ward as an intermediary time process between the flow of visitors, the noise of farewells, the clarity of the afternoon, which seemed to move very swiftly, and the slow encounter with the solitude of the night. Night, at the Hospital, began with dinner. It was like a boundary line separating dual facets of life and death. The image of the dinner-hour produced in me an effect quite the reverse of what might be expected to stimulate the appetite.

The food itself, hygienic, nutritious, protected by nylon wrappings from any exterior contact, was grouped on the trays according to the different diets of the patients, in accord with the vastly impersonal handling of objects, people, situations which defined the 5th Floor. I also used to think

that both the patients and the food they had to eat were denied the chances of pleasure that smells and taste can produce. The noise of dishes, of teeth chewing, of liquids gurgling down throats, would make me shudder. I never understood very well just why —but I think it was because somehow all that noise was like an ironic comment on a great lie.

I would walk down the halls, empty of voices, and could glimpse through the open doors of private rooms a solemn, automatic kind of eating, a habit which allowed the double activity of watching a television screen and of chewing.

Dinner time was no more pleasurable than any other time; it was simply another dimension which marked the sequence between a before and an after—but an "after" which was awaited anxiously, as confirming the probability of our existence within the future.

The nurse would distribute the trays, her arms, her body, moving in consistent, repetitive patterns, each a part of a chain of reflexes acquired by time and trained actions.

I once asked to accompany a nurse on her routine of distributing the trays during dinner-time—special permission was necessary, since my request, seen as disruptive to the nurse's duties and the effectiveness of her work, was granted for one time only. After following the nurse into several patients' rooms, we entered a room with four beds, but with only two patients in it. The nurse, with repetitive, almost mechanical efficaciousness, placed a tray on a table by one of the empty beds. After she had served food to the two patients, and just before she was about to leave the room, I asked her about the third tray; she glanced casually at me, and said, "Oh, here we don't need one," and, withdrawing the tray, went on with her job.

Slowly I began to build a kind of rhythm, an internal rhythm of times, of preambles, of spaces, between an anxiety which grows with solitude and with the silence of the night or remain temporarily suspended during the chores of the day. The rhythm of waiting, from one event to another, the need to integrate into the hospital routine, with its times of frenzied activity, of fears, and of solitude, began to be a part of my own needs and rhythm.

During the morning hours, the rooms were filled with the sounds of cleaning, with the movement of groups of interns and nurses which corresponded to the movement of the doctors, with unforeseen and occasional visitors who accompanied the patients at lunch. Then the afternoon would arrive, and with it, the uncertainty as to which relatives might come, the anxiety to see them again, even if it meant forcing conversations and avoiding silences.

Later, after the noise of the visitors (with their gifts of unopened magazines, flowers, candy, all put aside and forgotten where they were left), after the smiles, the farewell phrases, after the doors finally closed behind them, after all that, there began, for me, the true waiting period.

The approach of night would bring me face to face with the unasked questions of the patients, with their silent stares which transcended any vision of time and memory, with their monologues—raised fantasies which could not, at least at that time, open into dialogue.

Ever since I began to work in the Hospital, the night time (not just those hours of it I would spend in the Hospital—*all* the night) began to acquire the meaning of capturing and controlling one hour after the other, until one could perceive that one had reached, alive, the doors of a new day, a day which fully belonged to one by right of conquest, by *feeling* oneself within it.

And then and there my questioning began: what to do in the face of death? I attempted to live myself, to see how I would react, faced by my own inevitable death, or by the imminent death of the person I most dearly loved. I have no answer. And I do not believe any final answer may be found, or even exist. None, when all is said and done, can be supplied *a priori,* even by a deep knowledge of philosophy or by deeply felt faith. The awareness of the feeling of death cannot be apprehended through the teachings of others as impartial observers. The experience is unique, unrepeatable, profoundly individual. Still, I am convinced of the relevance of the values which a culture imposes and imparts through its socializing process. These basic values are the ones which will determine our attitudes, within that culture, towards life and death. And I have found in myself that certain values of my own culture helped me when confronted with the shock of the process of dying, of a patient's death.

I tried to become involved with the patients insofar as I was able to overcome my involvement with my own self, with my awareness of my own fears, desperation, and sorrow. In other words, I tried not to place a barrier between them and myself, not to restrict myself to certain theoretical techniques whereby my feelings would be very far removed.

One of the things I found (and in this I differed widely from the professional staff) was that the way most of the staff, as well as the patients' families, would attempt to flee from death, to cloak their feelings, by raising defensive systems (each within his or her role) so ingrained socially, that they were convinced that of course they were dealing with the riddle of death. During all those months in the Hospital, I came to understand that what was taught about how to deal with the process of death and dying was in face an efficient system of defenses in order to control and avoid the experience of death. The chance of talking about the issue was denied; but so, also, was the chance to remain silent, whenever that silence implied assuming and confronting the endless sorrow of loss and separation.

My work in this Hospital is finished; it is here and now that my true travail begins.

PART VI

Survival: social and psychologic support

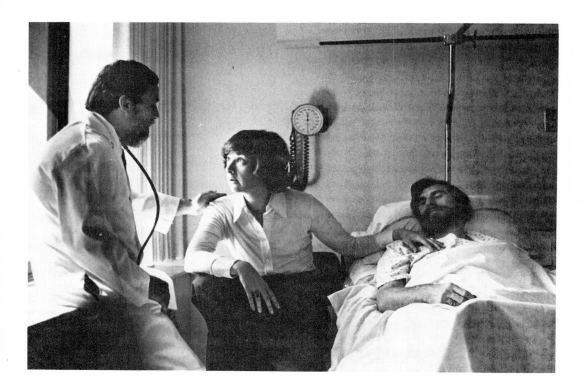

23

Psychological management of the myocardial infarction patient

THOMAS P. HACKETT and NED H. CASSEM

The acute coronary experience is divided into three parts. In the first, the pre-hospital phase, attention is devoted to the widespread phenomenon of patient delay. Evidence is given to indicate that the source of delay is entirely psychological and centers around the inability to decide whether or not to seek help. The second part, or hospital phase, describes the response of the patient to the various aspects of the coronary care unit, including monitoring, false alarms, witnessing and sustaining a cardiac arrest. The third phase, the post-hospital convalescence, centers on the principal psychological problem of this period, depression. Its causes, manifestations, and methods of management are discussed.

The psychological management of the patient with an acute MI can be divided into three sections, each with its specific problem: 1) the pre-hospital phase, in which the main issue is delay; 2) the hospital phase, in which anxiety about the present and future predominates; and 3) the post-hospital or convalescent phase, which centers around the management of depression. Although the response to any acute illness can be similarly divided, there are factors which separate myocardial infarction from most of the others. The two most important are its prevalence—it is nearing epidemic proportions in the USA—and its lethality. Coronary heart disease is America's number one killer. There is an average of 1,000 coronary deaths a day in this country. Nearly half of our total death rate is due to coronary disease and well over half of those who die

before their 65th birthday succumb to this disorder.

PRE-HOSPITAL PHASE

In the last five years a number of studies have been published on the extent of delay in coronary heart disease.[1,2,3] All of their findings agree that the average man or woman struck down with severe chest pain will delay four or five hours before seeking medical help. Since it is estimated that well over 60 percent of coronary deaths occur between one half to one hour after the onset on chest pain, it is apparent that delay of this sort occurs at the very time when the patient is in most danger of dying. Many of these deaths would be preventable if the patient were treated properly at the time the symptom developed. It is estimated that a good 50 percent of these deaths could be avoided by prompt, proper treatment.

The most common response that seems to occur in an individual experiencing sudden intense chest pain which lasts more

Reprinted from Journal of Human Stress, pp. 25-38, September 1975.

201

than five minutes is not to call a doctor but to reach for an antacid. Eighty to ninety percent of patients queried attribute their distress to acute indigestion. Even though the symptoms may be unlike any attack of indigestion the person has ever experienced, he still prefers to think it stems from the stomach rather than the heart. The reason, of course, is that the stomach is a safer organ to have afflicted than the heart. If the thought of having a heart attack crosses the person's mind, it is usually countered by the rationalization, "It couldn't happen to me." We have examined patients who responded to chest pain by doing vigorous push-ups or running up a flight of stairs —reasoning that they could not be experiencing heart attack, since the exertion had not caused them to drop dead. Others drink tea or coffee or alcohol, in a vain attempt to diminish or extinguish the pain. In this respect it is important to point out that the pain in all of the studies cited is of sufficient magnitude to curtail the individual's activity. In other words, the coronaries we are discussing do not fall into the category of the "silent coronary."

The following is a typical case of delay. A 47-year-old man was visiting a city for a business meeting. After a heavy meal he retired to a hotel room and began to experience severe pericardial pains. Immediately, he took two aspirin followed by sodium bicarbonate. The pain did not abate; he began to pace the room rapidly and then did some sitting-up exercises in an attempt to "bring up the gas." When this was unsuccessful he took a sleeping pill and consumed four ounces of bourbon—his customary nightcap. Upon his lying down, the pain spread into his left arm and caused him to think he was having an attack of bursitis, a condition he had had in the past. Even though his bursitic pains always had been confined to the shoulder and left arm— totally unlike the chest pain he was experiencing—he was able to take comfort from this diagnosis and went into a light sleep. About an hour later he was awakened by an increase in the severity of his chest pain.

By this time he felt "as though a truck had run over my chest." Until then the thought that he was having a heart attack had not crossed his mind—even though he had a family history of coronary disease, including a father who had angina pectoris. Rather than call the hotel physician he phoned his wife and described his situation to her, hoping to gain some reassurance. Instead, she instantly thought of a heart attack and insisted that he call the hotel physician. Knowing that he had a tendency to procrastinate, she made the call for him. The next thing he knew, a doctor was knocking at his door. After a cursory examination the physician sent him to the hospital where a diagnosis of anterior myocardial infarction was confirmed. The time lapsed between the onset of chest pain and his arrival at the hospital was four and one-half hours.

Often we have heard it said that delay in coronary heart disease is confined chiefly to the uneducated or to the lower socioeconomic classes. In our study and in others the phenomena of delay cuts across all of the usual socioeconomic variables. Age, sex, level of education, socioeconomic status and even history of a previous heart attack do not appear to reduce the tendency to delay. The delay times of the physicians we have interviewed, including three cardiologists, have not been distinguished by the swiftness of their response.

While there has been a tendency for delay times to be less when the severity of the pain mounts, the relationship between these two factors is by no means direct. Certainly, it has been our experience that the presence of severe pain in no way insures a speedy response. Originally we had thought that a symptom such as shortness of breath might be an added inducement for the patient to respond quickly, but this finding has not been reported.

Many of our colleagues have expressed the opinion that delay is explained by traffic or by the necessity to arrange for transportation in getting to the hospital or in finding a doctor for examination. More recent work points out that three-fourths of the time taken up by delay is used to make the decision to consult the doctor.[2,3] In fact, approximately 10 percent of the total delay time was accounted for by traffic or transportation. It would seem then that the principal cause for delay is psychological. The decision making process gets jammed by the patient's inability to admit that he is mortally sick.

How can one reduce delay? Since the patient's chance of dying is lessened by one-third once he reaches a hospital, it is obvious that this is a major goal. There are a few clues for developing a strategy to cut down delay. One is that a patient's response to obtain help quickens when he recognizes that the heart is the source of his difficulty. However, of all the factors that work in favor of getting an individual to respond promptly, the one that is most effective is the advice of another party. If the patient is struck by chest pain at work and is told to visit the hospital by his foreman, he does so immediately. Similarly, the individual, clutched by pain in the midst of a busy sidewalk and spotted by a policeman, is much more apt to find himself in the emergency ward than he would if he had the same pain at home. Curiously, the least effective source of advice is the spouse. One could almost say that the more impersonal authority invested in the advisor the more swiftly the patient is to seek aid, and the time lag follows a linear decrement as a function of diminishing authority. A case in point has to do with the wife of one of our patients who stated that she had pleaded with her husband for three hours while he lay on the sofa racked with chest pain during his second MI. He kept insisting that it was indigestion from some goulash she had failed to prepare properly while she continued to goad him with the knowledge it was another coronary. We could not help but wonder why she did not take the initiative and simply call the police or their family doctor.

There are a few suggestions we can make in the hope of reducing delay time. The first is to anticipate with the patient that his initial tendency will be to explain chest pain by some means other than its coming from the heart. This will probably be true even when the patient has had a previous MI. As a consequence we give the following formula to patients:

When you find yourself reaching for an antacid and talking about indigestion with pain in the chest on either side that has lasted for longer than two-and-a-half minutes, rather than head for the medicine shelf, call your physician.

We also make it a point to inform the spouses of coronary patients or those in a high-risk category that they should take the initiative and make the necessary arrangements for an examination immediately when their spouse complains of chest pain lasting longer than two to three minutes.

Of equal importance in dealing with the immediate reaction to chest pain is to give the patient a background of factual information on coronary artery disease. We know that society often unfairly assigns the role of a cardiac cripple to those who have been stricken with this condition, even when there is no basis for doing so. It is important to point out that many leaders in the community have led successful and fulfilling lives after sustaining an MI and that individuals with uncomplicated MIs often return to the same level of work and physical activity which they enjoyed before. The simple information that most people who recover from heart attacks can work and lead normal lives often comes as a surprise to patients. Certainly the fact that the quality of life need not be markedly reduced is heartening information to survivors.

HOSPITALIZATION

The hospital phase begins when the patient arrives at the emergency ward or receiving area. In the majority of medical installations in this country a person with chest pain is ushered into an examining room immediately, thereby circumventing tedious and dangerous delays such as the gathering of insurance information. The fact that his symptom is taken seriously instantly, and that he is attached to a monitor, examined by a doctor and tended by a nurse is far more assuring than distressing to the majority of patients. Most express a feeling of great relief when they finally reach a medical center and find themselves cared for.

There are two potential sources of stress for patients immediately after entrance into the hospital. The first is being left alone and the second is having the last rites administered. It is a simple matter to assign a nurse or attendant to stay at the patient's side and in this way avert the first source of fear. If no one else is around it is well to leave a relative in the same room with the patient. Early in our work with coronary patients we made a special study of the effect of administering the sacrament of the sick to patients.[4] Our findings pointed to the obvious fact that patients can accept a great deal of adversity as long as the individual administering it is kind and tactful. The majority of Catholics who had the sacrament of the sick felt comforted by it but all agreed their response was almost entirely dependent upon the manner of the priest administering it. When the priest presented the ritual as a routine, stating that everybody with a possible heart attack received it and went about his task in a calm and relaxed way, he was apt to provide far more hope and comfort than distress. Women seem to respond more positively than men, and private patients more positively than ward patients. As would be expected, those to whom religion was important in premorbid life were the most appreciative responders.

When patients complained of being given last rites, invariably it was the manner of the priest that bore the brunt of their criticism. An example of this may be observed in the recollections of a 72-year-old boiler-room worker admitted with his first MI:

"The priest comes in and tells me, 'I come in a rush . . . They just called me up and told me they got you in here and to come and anoint you.'

" 'What do you mean,' I says, 'Anoint me? Anoint me for what?'

"He replies, 'For death, of course, 'cause we can't be too careful. Anybody with a heart attack can shuffle out in no time.'

"I laughed, he was so nervous. We joked about it for a few minutes and then went through with the formalities and I bid him goodbye."

Both the patient and his wife, who had been present, agreed that the priest's presentation could have been improved as it caused unnecessary anxiety which was not leavened by humor until later.

Although the majority of patients have amnesia for part or all of their emergency ward experience, some are able to recall emphatically what they were told by their admitting physician. Our research reveals two traits that were appreciated most in their doctors: compassion and forthrightness. One patient remembered a physician saying to him, "You've had a heart attack but it is not a large one. However, all heart attacks are serious and you will need our attention." He appreciated the double message—that it was not massive but was serious enough to warrant admission. It is worth mentioning that of the hundreds of patients we have examined, not one has complained of being told too much in the emergency ward. A possible rule of thumb for those physicians who are unsure of what to disclose could be, "It is safer to err on the side of openness rather than being close-mouthed." Needless to say, one should not run down a list of possible eventualities or emphasize all the conceivable complications. Confidence and enlightened optimism are the keynotes for this early phase of admission. Patients who are desperately in need of medical help are apt to respond positively to the smallest intimation of competence on the part of their physician, so the latter need not work very hard to embellish this impression.

Sources of stress

Once admitted to the hospital the patient is more than likely sent to the coronary care unit (CCU), where there are three main sources of psychological stress: the first is being continuously monitored; the second is witnessing a cardiac arrest in another patient; and the third is undergoing and surviving cardiac arrest.

Continuous monitoring

The experience of being monitored is central to occupying a bed in the CCU. In our first encounter with patients in the CCU, in 1958, we regarded the electrodyne monitor pacemaker as a formidable instrument. We believed it was bound to inspire a considerable amount of apprehension in the patients attached to it. The results of a preliminary study did anything but confirm our suspicions.[5] Far more patients were reassured by it. Even those who underwent painful external pacing regarded the machine with a mixture of awe and gratitude.

One of the principal reasons for their overall positive reponse had to do with the way in which they were introduced to the monitor. A nurse described the instrument as a "mechanical guardian angel." She went on to say, "As long as you're attached to it you couldn't die if you wanted to." This proved to be a remarkably effective stratagem in a population that was predominantly Irish Catholic. This humbling experience taught us three valuable lessons. The first is that when one identifies with a seriously ill patient and attributes to him emotions which one imagines one would feel in his predicament, there is bound to be a wide margin of error by virtue of the fact that the investigator is not seriously ill and as a consequence does not think like a sick man. The second lesson pertains to the value of explanations and how they can deflate much fearful fantasy. The third is the usefulness of the defense of denial in individuals faced with severe stress. A sick patient is apt to fix on the benefit he derives from an instrument and to negate its more threatening aspect, particularly if it causes no pain. He also will eagerly absorb explanations of its function, and his natural tendency will be to deny the connotation

that constant monitoring means his life may be in danger.

The psychological defence of denial is defined as the repudiation of part or all of the total available meaning of an event in order to reduce painful affects such as anxiety.[6] A simple example of denial occurs in everyday life when we board an airplane. We are far more concerned with the sleek design and the confident expressions of the pilot and copilot than we are with the possibility of midair collisions, hijackings, and faulty circuiting which might necessitate an emergency landing. Once aloft, we are less aware of defying gravity than we are of the scenery spreading beneath and of the prospect of a forthcoming cocktail or supper. We deny the sources of possible peril, a human virtue that is just as apt to be found in the CCU as aboard a luxury airliner.

Along with introducing the machine in the manner described, nurses routinely take the precaution of removing an electrode to demonstrate how this can set off a false alarm. In this way she is able to reduce the amount of "startle response" when the alarm sounds. She goes on to demonstrate how body movements can cause artifacts and static on the monitor screen. Pointing out the patterns caused by artifacts is particularly important in the case of blue-collar patients. We found that they are less apt to know about the machinery of intensive care than are their white-collar counterparts.[7] It is our belief that the more the patient understands the purpose and function of the mechanical devices in the unit the less fear these will produce.

In well over 700 patients whom we have followed through the CCU we rarely have found one who objected to being monitored. If criticism was voiced, usually it was directed toward the physical irritation caused by the electrode paste. Occasionally the "beeping" of the monitor was bothersome, but this occurred far less often than we would have supposed. The noise elicited more comment from staff and visitors than from patients. In fact, visitors impressed us as being more intimidated and frightened by the equipment than were patients. In viewing the response of patients to the instrumentation of intensive care such as pacemakers, respirators and monitoring systems, we have noted how infrequently one hears the fear of a mechanical failure. Whether this would be true in a less mechanically oriented culture is unknown; Americans seem able to put their trust in motors.

Witnessing cardiac arrest

To avoid the major stress of a patient's observing cardiac arrest in another person, there has been a trend in the design of newer coronary units which supplant the open ward with a series of cubicles that insure visual isolation. Of those patients in our series who witnessed a fatal cardiac arrest, about 20 percent readily admitted being frightened by the sight. The others claimed not to have been.[8] The initial response to watching the arrest was anger and annoyance at the afflicted patient. This seemed a particularly uncharitable response until we examined it. As we all know from personal experience, one of the best ways to reduce anxiety or fear is through anger. If a child, intimidated by a bully, can convert fear into anger, there is a consequent reduction in his anxiety. The same mechanism applies to the coronary care patient. What begins as fear for the arresting patient is quickly transformed into a more palatable and endurable anger.

In conjunction with anger a number of other responses quickly occur which may explain why only 20 percent of our patients were frightened by watching an arrest. The next response most commonly elicited was of being impressed by the speed at which the arrest team responded and by the amount of time they spent in revitalizing the patient. "They came in like gangbusters." "They just popped in out of the walls." "They worked on her for hours." These were typical comments. We also noted that, although the majority of onlookers empathized with the arresting victim, none identified with the person experiencing arrest or imagined himself/herself to be in the same position. This held true even when both the victim and the observers shared the same age, sex and social background. In general, unaided, the patient was able to find some difference to separate the arresting person's condition from his own. When death occurred, the staff quickly assured the survivor that the heart of the deceased had been much worse than his own. Even when the excuses given were quite obviously overdrawn, the survivor was apt to accept them without question or reservation. The response of those who witnessed an arrest offers a good example of how patients can grasp the most comforting meaning of an otherwise terrifying event while denying or overlooking the threatening aspects.

It would be unfair to imply that viewing an arrest is not a source of great stress. There have been reports by others, notably Bruhn,[9] that there is an increase in anxiety as well as in systolic blood pressure in patients who recently have been present at an arrest. Some of our nurses report that more requests for tranquilizers and pain medication occur in the wake of an arrest. Another reason to believe that watching an arrest takes an emotional toll has to do with room selection. We ask all patients whether they would prefer to be in a single room or a four bed ward should they require another hospitalization in the future. All of those occupying a four bed ward at the time of our question choose the same setting for readmission except those who have witnessed an arrest; these prefer a single room. They have no idea of the reason for our question except that it pertains to administrative needs. This unobtrusive measure tells its own story.

Survival of cardiac arrest

We have interviewed and followed a sizable number of people who have gone through cardiac arrest. The majority had difficulty remembering anything about the event. Some vaguely recalled being thumped on the chest and hearing voices, but the majority remembered nothing at all.

The most complete account we have was given by a young teacher. He was brought into the emergency ward by his fiancée after having been stricken by severe chest pain. While being examined in the emergency ward he arrested. After his resuscitation he recounted a vivid dream in which he found himself on a conveyor belt heading toward the checkout counter of a supermarket. He was trussed up like a package of meat. As he got closer to the cashier, he said to himself, and then aloud, "Oh no. Oh no, they don't. They're not going to check me out!" he awoke with a start after the second jolt of cardioversion. Looking around and finding himself encircled by men in white, he exclaimed, "Christ, what a batch of clerks in this butcher shop." Everybody laughed and then his doctor explained what had happened. If he had not been told what had occurred, this man probably would have had no clear recollection of the event or of its significance. It may have been remembered only as a bad dream whose basis in fact he may have doubted. This is by far the most common type of impression victims have of their arrest.

One of the first reports in the psychiatric literature of the aftermath of recovery from a cardiac arrest described the result in terms reminiscent of a traumatic neurosis.[10] The survivors had recurrent nightmares, existed in a state of chronic anxiety and depression and often felt unable to return to a normal way of life. They looked upon themselves as being different from their fellow men. It was as though they had died and then had been raised from the dead. With the passage of time more experience has been gained in the use of defibrillating techniques, and cardioversion has become more a standard part of the operating procedure in the CCU. Now patients are told what has happened to them after an arrest has occurred; also, they are told that being defibrillated does not necessarily influence their chance for recovery or alter their prognosis. When the aforementioned pioneer study was carried out, these techniques were not known, nor was there any established procedure outlin-

ing what to tell a survivor about the event. Subsequently, as more information became available and a routine of information dispersal developed, there have been far less emotional sequelae following recovery from an arrest.

In our series we have scarcely any traumatic neuroses or mental incapacity directly linked to a saved arrest. Dobson and his coworkers in Great Britain, who followed a series of arrest survivors for some years, report a uniformly good response.[11] In their opinion the best policy is to tell the patient what has happened, and to deal with it in a matter-of-fact way. The aim is to avoid making the patient feel singled out by fate as someone who has died and come back to life. We emphasize the fact that the purpose of the CCU is to provide exactly this type of service. There is nothing unique about sustaining a cardiac arrest and surviving. In this decade survivors number in the millions; many of them bear illustrious titles and have positions of signal importance in this country.

One of our patients felt that he enjoyed a unique status as the result of surviving an arrest. He was a man who wanted to be an astronaut and, in fact, had been enrolled in a program that eventually might have put him into space, but he was unable to complete his training. A brief time after returning to civilian life he suffered an unexpected myocardial infarction and arrested shortly after being admitted to the CCU. His resuscitation was uncomplicated and his recovery was complete. When told of what had happened he felt that his experience had been just as good as going to the moon. He described it as a true 20th-century journey, in which he had been to the other side and returned with the personal knowledge that insofar as he was concerned, there was no hereafter.

Aside from the three major sources of stress as described previously, what can be said concerning the ordinary variety of anxiety that is found in the coronary unit? We have observed elsewhere that anxiety is difficult to identify in the CCU because patients either simply do not experience it or, deliberately or unconsciously, they deny it.[12] If anxiety is present, it often takes the patient time to get around to expressing it in terms of specific fears. As a consequence, physicians who make their rounds hastily are not apt to be able to judge adequately their patient's mental condition. Often times the busy physician would do well to inquire of the nurse about the feeling tone of his patient. We believe that mild to moderate anxiety is more common than the outward appearance of patients in the unit might suggest. Since it is unreasonable to expect the busy practitioner to spend a sufficient amount of time with each patient to unearth covert anxiety, we believe it is advisable to regard every patient as anxious and to treat him accordingly, even though supporting evidence might be lacking. A minor tranquilizer (diazepam 5 mg. 4 i.d. or chlordiazepoxide 10 mg. 4 i.d.) is ordered for all patients with the stipulation that it can be deleted or decreased at the patient's bidding. Rather than place the medication on a p.r.n. basis we order it around the clock because CCU patients, in our experience, are apt to suffer in silence rather than trouble the nurse for more attention, as in requesting p.r.n. medication. We found the benzodiazepine group of tranquilizers to be the most effective in that they have a smaller number of side effects than do barbiturates and do not interfere with warfarin compounds.[13] In using them one must be alert to the possibility of their paradoxical effect of producing rage or lowered threshold for anger, although it rarely is encountered in our experience. It is useful to remember that bedtime sedation often can be provided by doubling or tripling the sedative dose of the benzodiazepines. Flurazepam HCl, because it has minimal interference with REM sleep, has been widely used in ICU settings and is considered a good hypnotic with a minimum of side effects.

Although most patients prefer to be sedated, there is a small percentage who dislike the feeling of being drugged. These should be given the privilege of having no tranquilizers if this is their desire. We believe it is necessary to emphasize the importance of mental rest and to assure patients that tranquilizers are CCU standard medications. Although their number seems to be decreasing, there are some men who equate the need for sedation with weakness and the lack of manliness. This kind of thinking must be corrected.

Depression is apt to be felt as the danger of the acute stage wanes. It occurs toward the end of the patient's stay in the CCU or shortly after being transferred to the convalescent ward. The depression is reactive in nature and generally centers around a fear for the future. In the hospital it is apt to be so mild that it escapes the doctor's attention. The standard signs are a saddened face, disinterest, listlessness, slowness of speech or, much less frequently, weeping. It is good practice to ask the patient about his state of mind, particularly about discouragement or depression because these are easier affects to hide than anxiety, and they are feelings which many individuals, particularly men, often feel ashamed to express. Depression focuses on concerns about reduced earning power, restrictions of activity, sexual incompetence, invalidism, premature old age and recurrence of illness.

The main issue in any depression is loss. The loss may be quite real, as in the death of a spouse or the bankruptcy of a business. It also may be symbolic, as in imagined loss of youth with the advent of gray hair. In either, the loss produces feelings of loneliness, inadequacy and sadness—all of which come under the heading of mourning. In order to cope with these feelings individuals develop a variety of defenses. Some quickly attempt to replace the loss (the rebound marriage is an example of this). Others attempt to deny it by suppression ("I simply won't think of it") or through minimization ("It really isn't too bad—after all, others have lived through the same type of thing"). None of these coping tactics is bad so long as it allows some mourning to be expressed. Long experience and research have demonstrated that grieving is a necessary and natural reaction to loss. To stifle or thwart appropriate sorrow is to block a natural function, the equivalent of censoring joy. The patient who has sustained an MI recently should be encouraged to express whatever sentiments of sorrow, frustration, anger or depression he harbours. It is altogether normal for him to have these feelings, and the sooner they emerge the more quickly something can be done about them.

POST-HOSPITAL CONVALESCENCE

As has been noted earlier, depression is one of the main psychiatric complications of convalescence. The latter is defined as the time between discharge from the hospital and the point of maximum yield in rehabilitation, in terms of job, family role and personal happiness. It has been said that the depression following MI causes unwarranted invalidism which, in turn, accounts for a tremendous loss of man hours. Certainly, as any rehabilitation counselor or family physician can attest, prodigious amounts of misery are suffered during coronary convalescence, much of which can be avoided.

Although not every person with coronary artery disease is a candidate for a post-MI depression, we favor a program of prevention which assumes that depression can occur in anyone who has sustained an MI. It is inaugurated in the CCU on or about the third day. The physician or a nurse-clinician trained in cardiology sits down with the patient to go over the facts of his/her illness. The nature of the infarction is explained, as is the process of repair. We have found that while white-collar patients are accurately informed about the damage to heart muscle and its repair through scar formation, the same cannot be said for their blue-collar counterparts. The latter understand infarction in terms of a damaged and weakened heart, but they are altogether unaware of the process of mending. As a consequence, some blue-collar patients picture their heart as permanently punctured. They conceptualize the infarct as a hole punched out of the heart that remains an eternal source of leakage. Providing information to remedy this conception can do more to insure peace of mind than any type of medication.

Since the largest part of the depression suffered by the post-coronary patient usually revolves about the fear of being unable to resume work and lead an active life, one can remedy this by providing both from the national scene and from the local community, examples of individuals who have sustained an MI and returned to an active and productive life. We have found that the majority of our patients are dogged by outmoded stereotypes which equate heart disease of any degree with permanent invalidism. Union practices and corporate policy bylaws often encourage this archaic mythology. The information that eight runners who completed a recent Boston marathon previously had sustained an MI is heartening news for a man in the CCU who is mourning what he regarded as the loss of his active life.

Aside from educating the patient through correcting misinformation and clarifying what he can expect in terms of his specific myocardial lesion, the next best treatment for depression is a program of physical conditioning. Some hospitals start patients with uncomplicated MIs on such a program by the third CCU day. By using carefully graduated passive then active exercises, function is slowly restored. The reports of all of these programs to date indicate that anxiety and depression are less troublesome when the patient is actively engaged in physical conditioning[14,15] which gives the patient a sense of participating in his recovery rather than being a passive recipient.

It is important to note that as in-hospital time is reduced in the treatment of MI, more privileges are allowed patients during their hospital stay. For example, businessmen who become restive and irritable when denied access to a phone are now sometimes provided with this and dictating equipment as well, assuming their cardiac status is stable or improving. Enforced passivity for some may be an exquisite form of stress.

We have used the term homecoming depression to describe the reaction of patients returning home after discharge from the hospital. The majority of patients are unprepared for the extent of the depressive reaction that occurs.[16] While hospitalized they eagerly look forward to being allowed home and welcome the actuality, as it means that the heart has been restored to a point where it can function on its own. Soon after arriving home and walking about, many patients experience a sense of sudden physical weakness. One reason for this is physiological; they are out of condition. In the hospital they were confined to a small area. Even though they could pace the halls they were in no way prepared for the amount of activity available to them upon coming home. Unfortunately, weakness often signifies to the patient that his heart is not as sound as he supposed. It sometimes serves to confirm a hidden fear that invalidism will be his lot. An example is that of a 39-year-old teacher who did very well following his MI—until he returned home. In his words, "I felt great in the hospital. No matter what anyone told me, I pictured myself breaking records in getting back to work. The first week home I could hardly walk the length of the house without being exhausted. I felt like a cooked goose, as if I were done for. It took me another two weeks until I started feeling better." This is a prototypical statement, one that would apply to the majority of patients in early convalescence at home. The sense of weakness often is the trigger that springs an underlying depression into the open.

At the point of hospital discharge, let us tally the number of restraints binding the convalescent cardiac patient:

- The omnipresent threat of recurrence and possible sudden death;
- depression due to inactivity and job uncertainty;
- deprivation or limitation of food, alcohol, excitement and sex; (One young man commented, concerning these restrictions: "No smokes, no booze, low salt, low fat, low energy, low sex or no sex—I feel like a cardiological capon!")
- depression due to possible disruption in interpersonal relationships. (Role changes in marriage are common following an MI—e.g., the wife must return to work to support the family, and she becomes the breadwinner. In this setting sexual problems are common. Premature ejaculation and potency disturbances have been found to be as high as 40 percent by some authors.[17])

What can be done about the homecoming depression? The favored method of approaching the problem is prevention, as has been mentioned. Anticipating with the patient that it will be normal if he feels depressed upon arriving home, and that a sense of weakness might dampen his spirits, is a good beginning. The doctor legitimizes the depression by predicting it. Realizing that others undergo the same sense of sadness makes the patient feel less unique and alone. The family should be informed as well.

We encourage the patient to take tranquilizers if they are needed. We emphasize the importance of sound sleep in the first three months and encourage the use of benzodiazepines as hypnotics. If early morning awakening is the problem he should be given a longer acting hypnotic such as chloralhydrate. Aside from using minor tranquilizers and selected hypnotics we do not rely on drugs to treat the post-MI depression. The tricyclic antidepressants are contraindicated, because their use is associated with disturbances of rate and rhythm. Along with the phenothiazines, they have been implicated by some investigators in sudden death. Similarly, the MAO inhibitors are unsafe to use in coronary convalescence because, in combination with tyramine bearing foodstuffs, they can induce hypertensive crisis.

Just as we did in the hospital we encourage patients who have returned home to become involved in programs of physical conditioning. This is perhaps the most important aspect of convalescence, in terms of its ability to control depression by raising self-esteem, a sense of independency and confidence in one's ability. Physical conditioning must be carried out through convalescence until it has become a way of life with the patient.

Many patients complain of having no structure to their days of convalescence. The doctor tells them to increase their activity slowly but does not specify where or how. Conditioning programs provide this guidance. In addition some patients, especially those with compulsive traits, must have a schedule or hourly activities set out for them. This can be done by a skillful nurse or physical therapist. It is surprising how much post-myocardial infarction patients need in the way of direction, especially those in the blue-collar category.

One of the bulwarks of our program is education. After taking a careful history which reveals how the patient regards his condition, and particularly his views about returning to a more active life, we specifically mention some common misconceptions. For example, we state that some people believe that recurrence of infarction is most apt to occur during orgasm. After laying this myth to rest, we ask whether or not the patient has any personal beliefs that might complicate his recovery. The most common myths are:

• Even mild exercise is dangerous.
• Sexual intercourse should never be attempted, because following a myocardial infarction one is "over the hill."
• Repeated infarctions or sudden death is more likely to occur at sexual orgasm.
• Driving must be avoided.
• The arms must not be suddenly raised above the head, especially the left arm.
• The patient is apt to die at the same age as a parent who had had heart disease.
• Recurrence is apt to take place around the anniversary of the first infarction.
• The heart is more vulnerable to repeat infarctions and sudden death while the patient sleeps.

Any educational efforts should include the patient's spouse and children. They must be taught not to make the father or husband a cardiac cripple or treat him as though he were an infant. Since the best way to determine how a family works together is to watch them in a group meeting, after the patient is discharged we feel it is a good policy for the physician or nurse clinician to visit the home and meet with the entire family. In the group setting it has been valuable to anticipate various responses. For example, one can predict that a wife will become angry at her husband when he tends to overeat and will tend to discipline him as she would a child. The patient may expect to be waited upon, particularly when objects need to be moved, and he may become resentful toward his children when they do not leap to help him. He must be told to express his desires in a pleasant and acceptable way. When it comes time for him to return to work, one can anticipate that he will feel anxious and apprehensive until he is able to perform to his satisfaction without developing cardiac distress. Similarly, the patient can be told that he/she will feel anxious when new types of activity are attempted or the range of accustomed activities is extended. In general, the tendency of the family is toward overprotection while the tendency of the patient is toward irritability. Highlighting these trends sometimes serves to reduce their impact.

We have found that conducting a telephone follow-up, at weekly intervals for the first three months following discharge, serves an important function. A nurse clinician makes the call and then talks to both the patient and to his/her spouse. The purpose of the call is to check on their progress and to find out if they have questions, or problems with which they need help. This service has been greatly appreciated by our patient population.

There have been studies over the past few years on the usefulness of discussion groups or "heart clubs" in coping with the problems of convalescence. Eight or ten patients get together on a weekly basis under the guidance of a nurse clinician and discuss their experience in managing diet, change in habits, medication, moods, etc. Often, these provide valuable forums for the exchange of information and for learning from the experience of others, with the nurse serving as a source of answers. The overall value of these groups has not been tested as yet in a scientific manner, but it is the impression of most of us who have worked with them that potentially they have great merit.[18,19,20]

The outlook for the individual who has survived an acute myocardial infarction is increasingly brighter. This is especially so since the advent of coronary artery bypass graft surgery. However, in spite of technological advances, there remains a miasma of myth and misinformation which works against the coronary survivor. It is our obligation as physicians to push back this ignorance and to give our patients the best and the most recent therapies available. We must let them know that they can live long lives that can be extended even more by proper care.

REFERENCES

1. Hackett, T. P., and N. H. Cassem. "Factors Contributing to Delay in Responding to the Signs and Symptoms of Acute Myocardial Infarction," *Am. J. Cardiol.,* Vol. 24, 1969, pp. 651-658.
2. Simon, A. B. et al. "Components of Delay in the Pre-hospital Setting of Acute Myocardial Infarction," *Am. J. Cardiol.,* Vol. 30, 1972, pp. 475-482.
3. Moss, A. J. et al. "Delay In Hospitalization During the Acute Coronary Period," *Am. J. Cardiol.,* Vol. 24, 1969, p. 659.
4. Cassem, N. H., H. A. Wishnie and T. P. Hackett. "How Coronary Patients Respond to Last Rites," *Postgrad. Med.,* Vol. 45, 1969, pp. 147-152.
5. Browne, I. W., and T. P. Hackett. "Emotional Reactions to the Threat of Impending Death: A Study of Patients on the Monitor Cardiac Pacemaker." *Jr. J. Med. Sci.,* Vol. 496, 1967, pp. 177-187.
6. Weisman, A. D., and T. P. Hackett. "Predilection to Death: Death and Dying as a Psychiatric Problem," *Psychsom. Med.,* Vol. 23, 1961, pp. 232-256.
7. Hackett, T. P., and N. H. Cassem. "Blue-Collar and White-Collar Responses to Having a Heart Attack," Psychosomatic Society National Meeting, Boston, 1972.
8. Hecket, T. P., N. H. Cassem and H. A. Wishnie. "The Coronary Care Unit: An Appraisal of Its Psychological Hazards," *N. Engl. J. Med.,* Vol. 279, 1968, pp. 1365-1370.
9. Bruhn, J. G. et al. "Patients' Reactions to Death in a Coronary Care Unit," *J. Psychosom. Res.* Vol. 14, 1970, pp. 65-70.
10. Druss, R. G., and D. S. Kornfeld. "Survivors of Cardiac Arrest: Psychiatric Study," *J.A.M.A.,* Vol. 201, 1967, pp. 291-296.
11. Dobson, M., et al. "Attitudes in Long-Term Adjustment of Patients Surviving Cardiac Arrest." *Br. Med. J.,* Vol. 3, 1971, pp. 207-212.
12. Cassem, N. H., and T. P. Hackett. "Psychiatric Consultation in a Coronary Care Unit." *Ann. Intern. Med.,* Vol. 75, 1971, pp. 9-14.
13. Hackett, T. P., and N. H. Cassem. "Reduction of Anxiety in the CCU: A Double-Blind Comparison of Chlordiazepoxide and Amobarbital," *Curr. Ther. Res.,* Vol. 14, 1972, pp. 649-656.
14. Sanne, H. "Exercise Tolerance and Physical Training of Non-selected Patients after Myocardial Infaction," *Acta Med. Scand [Suppl.],* No. 551, 1973.
15. Heinzelman, F. "Social and Psychological Factors that Influence the Effectiveness of Exercise Programs," *Exercise Testing and Exercise Training in Coronary Heart Disease.* John Naughton and Herman K. Hellerstein, eds., pp. 275-287, Academic Press, New York, 1973.
16. Wishnie, H. A., T. P. Hackett, and N. H. Cassem. "Psychological Hazards of Convalescence Following MI," *J.A.M.A.,* Vol. 215, 1970, pp. 1292-1296.
17. Hellerstein, H. K., and E. H. Freidman. "Sexual Activity and the Postcoronary Patient," *Arch. Intern. Med.,* Vol. 125, 1970, p. 987.
18. Rahe, R. H., et al. "Group Therapy in the Outpatient Management of Post-myocardial Infarction Patients," *Psychiatry Med.,* Vol. 4, 1973, pp. 77-88.
19. Bilodeau, C. B., and T. P. Hackett. "Issues Raised in a Group Setting by Patients Recovering from Myocardial Infarction," *Am. J. Psychiatry.* Vol. 128, 1971, pp. 73-78.
20. Adsett, C. A., and J. G. Bruhn. "Short-term Group Psychotherapy in Post-MI Patients and their Wives," *Can. Med. Assoc. J.,* Vol. 99, 1968, pp. 577-584.

24

Rehabilitating the stroke patient through patient-family groups

JUDITH GREGORIE D'AFFLITTI and G. WAYNE WEITZ

The intermediate service of the West Haven Veterans Administration Hospital is designed as a rehabilitative setting for medical patients who have completed the phase of diagnosis and early treatment. In our nursing and social work with recuperating stroke patients and their families on this service, we noticed that although many patients were engaged in a program of physical, occupational, and speech therapy, they and their family members were frequently having great difficulty with the emotional acceptance of the patients' disabilities. This was clear from the patients' depressive affect and inability to express their feelings about their illness, with the concurrent inability of families to exchange reactions with the patients about the stroke and the ways in which this was going to affect their family life. For example, patients were often very frightened that any disability would mean that they could not function at home again. Family members sometimes shared this fear, and families and patients could not communicate their concerns. Because of this poor communication, there often was a strained relationship between patient and family, and realistic discharge plans could not be made. In addition, the patients did not use the appropriate community supports that would have allowed the most effective community adjustment, i.e., rehabilitation centers, visiting nurse associations, and vocational retraining centers.

The importance of interpersonal relationships in the rehabilitation of chronic disease patients is noted in the medical and psychiatric literature. Litman[5] reported that 75% of his patients looked first to their families for support and encouragement and second to the hospital staff. Also, there are some indications that if patients can anticipate reentry into a functioning family unit, this influences their decision to engage themselves in a therapy program. Bruetman and Gordon[2] discuss rehabilitation in terms of a concurrent restoring of the patient's physiologic and environmental equilibrium. They see the family's having great impact on the patient's motivations and expectations. Robertson and Suinn[8] state that there is a relationship between between the stroke patient's rate of progress toward recovery and the degree of empathy between the patient and his family members. Specifically, they indicate that stroke patients improve more rapidly when there is predictive empathy, i.e., the ability of patients and family members to foresee each other's attitudes. Finally, Millen[6] states that optimum rehabilitation of stroke patients occurs only when there is physical and psychological stimulation. Frequently, stroke patients grouped together can influence one another

Reprinted from International Journal of Group Psychotherapy 25:323-332, 1974.

toward working out problems, while providing a mutual source of encouragement as well.

With these ideas in mind, we believed that we might be helpful to our patients and their families by having them participate in a patient-family group. It was hoped that the group process would facilitate communication so that the illness and feelings about it could be discussed more freely and that this would lead to a more realistic perception by the patient and his family of the amount of disability and the limitations imposed by it. Plans could then be initiated and implemented that would be consistent with these limitations, and the group could support individual members toward more independent functioning.

We began our group with two major goals: first, to encourage patients and families to talk and to share their feelings about the stroke in order to promote a constructive adjustment to the illness; second, to encourage the patient and his family to use the appropriate community resources and supports available to them. From our experience, it seemed that patients who had contacts outside the family after discharge were less likely to become depressed and regress in their physical and social functioning.

In order for the group to be viewed as part of the total rehabilitation effort of the Intermediate Service, our project needed the support of the director of the service and of the staff members. This was accomplished through our joint contact with the director, followed by his introduction and our presentation of the purposes and goals of the planned group at a staff meeting. This presentation enabled the staff to understand how the group would be structured and how its activities would complement rather than subvert or interfere with those of the medical, nursing, and rehabilitation staff.

There were four criteria for participation in the group: (1) The patient had to have had a stroke, although he might have additional medical problems. (2) He had to be competent mentally and verbally to participate

in a group. (3) He had to have a family member who was willing to participate. (4) His final destination from the hospital had to be his home.

These strictures were not intended to imply that the needs of the severely damaged patient or the patient without a family or the patient who would have to be placed out of a home setting were any less important than those of the group selected, only that the problems of such patients cannot be dealt with appropriately in a patient-family group and need to be approached by other methods of intervention.

The group met for an hour and half weekly for three months. Members were to participate for this time even if they were discharged. To date, four consecutive groups have been conducted. The authors worked as coleaders for the group sessions and shared the outside administrative responsibilities, i.e., referrals and contacts with community agencies, preadmission interviews, and contacts with staff members. Each group had three to five patients, each with his accompanying family participants. These included spouses, brothers, sisters, children, and sometimes friends. The selected patients were predominately male because the agency is a Veterans Administration Hospital. A variety of ethnic and cultural backgrounds were represented. There was a wide patient age range, 34 to 76 years. Most of the patients and family members approached the group with interest and enthusiasm; however, the group was not appropriate for all situations. For example, Mr. A. discontinued attending because no family member would join him, and he felt anxious and uncomfortable without family support. Mrs. C. showed her resistance by attending sporadically and arriving late; soon it became clear that she and her husband had marital problems which predated his stroke, and because she covertly planned placement of her husband in a nursing home, she had difficulty identifying with the other group members. Mr. C. felt uncomfortable about attending without her.

PROBLEMS OF GROUP ORGANIZATION

We encountered some unique problems organizing the patient-family group in a medical setting. Routine issues, such as selection of a meeting place and the physical preparation of the patients for the meetings, required special effort. We finally obtained the use of a quiet classroom. We needed the cooperation of the nursing staff on the units to have the patients up, fed, and toileted in time for the meeting. Although the staff verbalized interest in the group and a desire to help with it, their behavior sometimes indicated difficulty in accepting this new program. On some units, staff members continually forgot which patients needed to be ready and at what time. We tried to minimize this problem by keeping staff informed of the patients' group participation and progress. However, our patient-family group seemed to raise questions for staff members about their own involvement and competence with the patients. Since general medical ward atmosphere is often geared to the suppression of uncomfortable emotions, it was difficult for patients and staff members to accept such a group.

Another difficult organizational problem was the establishment of a contract with the patient and his family. Through trial and error, we learned that the patient should be approached first with an explanation and an invitation to join the group. Then if he expressed interest, permission to contact a family member was given to one of us or the patient would make the contact himself. If the patient was not first consulted and given the opportunity to be in control of the decision, he would be resentful and resistive to participating in one more thing being imposed upon him.

In meeting with the patient and his family to discuss the group contract, we discovered that they could not accept the view that the illness produced a family problem. This seemed too frightening at a time when the family was mourning and shifting roles. Their anxiety was bearable only if the patient's *stroke* was seen as the focal problem. Most people were willing to participate in a group which had as its purpose the sharing of problems and ideas related to the stroke and to the home care of the person with the stroke. The following is the statement of contract we found most successful in the initial meeting with patient and family, and in the initial group meeting:

It is often difficult for patients and their families to adjust their lives to a chronic disability, especially when it's time for the patient to come home from the hospital. We've found it can be helpful if people with these kinds of problems talk together about them. The purpose of this group is for discussion of the concerns you are and will be facing.

We experimented with an open and closed group structure, and found the latter more comfortable and apparently more productive. In the open group, as people left we replaced them with new members. This meant that the group was often disrupted by comings and goings and the issues of getting to know new members. Consequently, establishing a sense of group stability was particularly difficult. A cohesion developed in the closed group that allowed us to go further in the work of facing and living with the losses produced by the stroke.

In both types of group, we attempted to have patients continue participating in the group after discharge from the hospital. In most cases, however, people did not continue after discharge. They said it was too difficult physically to get the patient from home to the hospital. One patient did tell us he felt that "everything would be all right" once he got home, and he did not want to come back and tell us if things were not going well. We can only speculate that those first weeks at home are very difficult for the patient and family to face and share. Perhaps it is the first real confrontation with the change in physical and family functioning and the realization that everything is not "all right" in the sense that it is not the same as it was before the stroke. Additionally, the patients viewed the return to the hospital after discharge as a threat which seemed to heighten their fears and desires of being an inpatient again.

One last problem was in establishing a meeting time that was convenient for family participation. This varied with the composition of the group. If the participating family members did not work, they preferred meeting in the afternoon. If they worked, a time following the patient's evening meal seemed preferable.

GROUP ISSUES AND REACTIONS

Once the group was organized and group work begun, it became clear that the group members were mourning and trying to learn to live with their losses. The patient had lost some parts of bodily control and functioning. This resulted in loss of some independence, a change in self-concept, and a consequent loss of self-esteem. The patient feared total loss of control over himself, loss of his family because they might regard him, as he regarded himself, as an inadequate and useless burden, and the ultimate loss, death. The family also feared the total loss of a loved one as they had once known him and as he had once functioned in the family. The changes in the patient forced changes in the functioning of the rest of the family as they attempted to fill the places left vacant by the patient.

The patients and families struggled with their grief in the group, and this struggle can be seen in the framework of Engel's[3] process of grieving.

Shock and denial

In every meeting the group members expressed their disbelief and wished the loss away. "How could something like this happen so fast? What caused it? It can't be real. Some nights I'm sure when I awaken in the morning it will be gone as quickly as it came. I just can't believe it!"

"I'm getting better every day. Soon I'll be good as new. This arm will be fine if I just exercise it enough. You can do anything with will power, you know. I'll be back working and fishing in a few weeks."

"My husband's going to be fine, no problems. They're holding his job for him and he'll be back at work soon. I was worried when it first happened, but I'm not worried anymore."

Developing awareness

Although it did not often appear overtly, anger was expressed by the group members. "Why did this happen to me? What did I do to deserve it? Hospital staff don't take good care of me. The physical therapists don't tell me how to get this arm moving. The nurses wake me too early in the morning. The doctor never comes to check me." Occasionally, a patient would cry for the limbs that wouldn't move or the job he'd never work at again.

The family members felt resentment toward the patient for being ill and thus a burden, but guilt over this resentment prevented its direct expression. Instead, the family was often overprotective of the patient. "I wouldn't think of leaving him at home alone. . . ." "It took me three hours to get him dressed this morning" (patient able to dress himself on the unit in the hospital).

Restitution and resolution

A great deal of group time was spent sharing together what life used to be like. This is the way in which they began to resolve the losses. The men shared tales of their military experiences, of their work and pastime activities. The family members talked of the things they used to enjoy together and do for each other. There was a feeling of trying to recapture the "good old days." Sometimes this reminiscing led to an attempt to reconcile the past and present. "I know we won't be able to go out as much, but do you think we could go out to dinner sometimes?"

"Maybe I can't do my old job, but there are some things around the house I could manage."

"I can't fish anymore, but the boys could put me in the boat and take me with them anyway."

In the first stage, reminiscing can be seen as part of avoidance and denial; in this stage, it is adaptive and part of the resolution of the loss. The patients and their families moved in and out of these phases and feelings of grief throughout the three months of group participation. Although phases exist concurrently, the overall movement is toward resolution. Engel says that successful mourning takes a year or more; however, in these three months, the work was well begun.

The group members also spent a lot of time discussing the more concrete aspects of being at home again. What kind of equipment was needed in the house for the patient to live comfortably? Could he get up a flight of stairs to the only bathroom? How do you manage to get the patient in and out of a car? Can the patient be left alone in the house at any time? The group supported one another in facing problems, and such focusing on concrete details served the function of decreasing anxiety and allowing families to deal with the emotional aspects of restructuring their lives.

PROBLEMS AND REACTIONS OF LEADERS

It was difficult to lead a new kind of group in a somewhat nonsupportive setting. Although the literature reports a few group experiences with medical patients *or* their families (Strauss et al.;[9] Piskor & Paleos;[7] Bardach;[1] Heller[4]) we could find no precedent for a patient–family group of this nature.

We had the supervision of a psychiatrist whose expertise is group work and this was most useful. He helped us examine our structure and process, and encouraged us to experiment with new tactics when necessary. Most importantly, he supported us in our reactions to the helpless-hopeless feelings in our patients. A stroke is a catastrophe. The damage is highly visible. We found that we had strong wishes to "do something" for these patients and their families in a concrete way. These wishes made us vulnerable to their complaints that we were not doing enough and susceptible to their feelings of helplessness. In the beginning we tried to compensate for these problems by being active and directive leaders. We initiated conversation in most silences and often focused on individuals instead of allowing group involvement with issues raised by individuals. Both of these techniques served to supress anger from group members about not being helped to recover permanent losses. Also, we often responded directly to questions for which there was no answer that could resolve the real issue for the patient. For example, members repeatedly asked for information about the specific causes of a stroke and specific cures. Our concrete answers seemed unsatisfactory because the real questions were: "Why me? What did I do to deserve this? Am I going to have to live this way?" With experience and supervisory support, we came to understand that the real work of the group was in the patients' experiencing these hopeless-helpless feelings. Our role was to be less directive and more supportive of the group members so that, through our empathy and acceptance, they could express their feelings and work with them toward a more productive and independent emotional state.

OUTCOMES

There were several important outcomes of the group meetings. First to a greater or lesser extent, nearly all patients and their families shared difficult feelings. Through such openness, the participants often recognized that negative feelings about the stroke were not so frightening or threatening. For example, Mr. J. often felt depressed about his damaged body and inability to work at his former place of employment. At times, he started to cry, but his wife became anxious and made statements such as, "We can only think cheery thoughts." When Mr. J. was encouraged to express more of what he really felt to the group, he experienced a sense of relief, and the group helped his wife to tolerate her husband's tears and depression.

As the lines of communication became more open, families and patients began to be more realistic about their expectations. For example, Mrs. R. was secretly frightened that she would be tied to a life of drudgery once her husband was discharged from the hospital because she thought he would need constant supervision and care. When Mr. R. began to plan rehabilitation activities for discharge, she saw that he was not as helpless as she had thought. Other wives supported this idea through their experiences.

At other times, the outcomes were much more concrete and often revolved around decision making. Mr. and Mrs. L. had a two-level house which was inconvenient for Mr. L. because his wife worked and the facilities he needed were on both floors. After several group discussions, they were able to make the decision that they no longer needed the large house. They sold it and rented a ground-level apartment before Mr. L. was discharged.

As medical and rehabilitation evaluations became known to the patients and their families, they often shared the information with the group. From these discussions came the guidelines for using community supports. Mr. and Mrs. W. had lived a life of near isolation for eight years after Mr. W.'s first stroke. Both were unrealistically frightened of the stroke and remained in their third-floor flat almost constantly. Although they were never able to resolve their fears completely in the group, this time they were able to make more realistic community plans for discharge. Mr. W. was able to involve himself for several hours weekly in a work activities program of the local rehabilitation center, thus allowing Mrs. W. some time of her own.

A final outcome was perhaps less tangible, but certainly no less important. This was the increased knowledge and sensitivity of ourselves and floor staff to the reactions of stroke patients and their families to this illness. Although the floorstaff were sometimes resistive to our group, they could see that there were changes in pa-tients and families which could be related to their involvement in the group. For example, some patients were less withdrawn on the units and some families were more willing to accept the patients on weekend pass. We saw directly the negative and positive influences a family can have on the acceptance and adjustment a stroke patient makes to his limitations.

CONCLUSION

We have described a group method for helping stroke patients and their families adjust to this chronic disability through a shared mourning of their losses. The purpose of the article is to describe the methodology and technique of such a group so that others might be encouraged in similar endeavors. Although research needs to be done to evaluate such groups, we feel that the patient-family group described has been a positive force in the rehabilitation of stroke patients and their families toward a more independent and satisfying adjustment.

REFERENCES

1. Bardach, J. L. Group sessions with wives of aphasic patients. *International Journal of Group Psychotherapy* **19:**361-365, 1969.
2. Bruetman, M. E., & Gordon, E. E. Rehabilitating the stroke patient at general hospitals. *Postgraduate Medicine* **49:**211-215, 1971.
3. Engel, G. L. Grief and grieving. *American Journal of Nursing* **64:**93-98, 1964.
4. Heller, V. Handicapped patients talk together. *American Journal of Nursing* **70:**332-335, 1970.
5. Litman, T. J. An analysis of the sociologic factors affecting the rehabilitation of physically handicapped patients. *Archives of Physical Medicine and Rehabilitation* **45:**9-16, 1964.
6. Millen, H. M. The positive approach to the care of the stroke patients. *Michigan Medicine* **69:**887-890, 1970.
7. Piskor, B. K., & Paleos, S. The group way to banish after-stroke blues. *American Journal of Nursing* **68:**1500-1503, 1968.
8. Robertson, E. K., & Suinn, R. M. The determination of rate of progress of stroke patients through empathy measures of patients and family. *Journal of Psychososmatic Research* **12:**189-191, 1968.
9. Strauss, A. B., Burrucker, J. D., Cicero, J. A., & Edwards, R. C. Group work with stroke patients. *Rehabilitation Record* 30-32, nov.-Dec., 1967.

25

Emotional reactions in a renal unit

MORRIS GELFMAN and EMILEE J. WILSON

In the growing field of organ replacement, where psychiatrists are being called on to help deal with the complex emotional reactions of this type of patient, recent literature tends to stereotype this behavior by placing emphasis on the patient's denial of his illness and the fear of death which is said to haunt him.[1-5]

While in no way denying that these mechanisms are at work, we feel that advancement in the field would progress further if psychiatrists would consider that the fear of death may be a much stronger dynamic factor in the patient's family and in those of us responsilbe for his care than it actually is in the patient, and that more emphasis be placed on the importance of the personality pattern of the patient prior to the development of the physical illness (stress).

Let us discuss first the fear of death in hemodialysis and renal transplant patients. It would seem natural to assume that patients faced with an extremely stressful life situation and with a precarious future would have this primal anxiety and have to defend against it with denial; but do they? Beard[6] stresses the basic conflict of the hemodialysis and kidney transplantation patient as being between his marked enslavement to his restricted, at times, agonizing existence, on the one hand, and his fear of death on the other. With the first, we most heartily agree. This is truly what the patients say and their actions indicate. Abram[2] touches the crux of the matter when he discusses "the problem of living rather than dying." He points out that during this time some patients come to ask, "Is it worth living?"

Since some authorities[7] feel that a person cannot psychologically fear death, how can one account for the obvious anxiety and turmoil (as well as irrational behavior) experienced by the renal patient when his life is in the balance and the outcome unsure? Most medical personnel in a renal unit have been puzzled by instances where medical advice has been flaunted and the patients have behaved in a manner that would not in any sense be to their best interest if they wish to live (if they wish to avoid death.) They go on fluid and dietary binges that jeopardize their lives and realistically endanger the possibility of transplantation.*

---

*It may help the reader if he understands how the renal unit at Milwaukee County General Hospital is set up. It is primarily a transplant unit, accepting patients from dialysis units all over the state for transplantation. An attempt was made to bring all these patients in during dialysis for workup so that they would be acquainted with personnel and the unit. Frequently, a cadaveric match would be obtained before they were known to the unit and our first contact with them was postoperative. In addition, patients with complications of dialysis came in from all over the state so that our incidence of stress reactions was probably higher than in most units. Simultaneously, a short-term dialysis program capable of handling up to 18 patients was in operation, and many of these patients were awaiting cadaveric transplants. Now that a national matching system is in operation, the number on semichronic dialysis should be sharply reduced.

Reprinted from Comprehensive Psychiatry 13:283-290, 1972. Reprinted by permission of Grune & Stratton, Inc., and the authors.

We would feel that the answers lie primarily in the various and complex life forces and dynamics of the individual.

To illustrate our opinion that the fear of death need not be a pervasive dynamic, let us cite the following cases.

Case 1

This 30-year-old married man had been transferred to our hemodialysis unit for kidney transplantation. His major problem had been controlling his weight fluctuations due essentially to excessive fluid intake (which he totally denied). Communication with his previous dialysis unit revealed that they had similar difficulties with him. Despite numerous complications, most of them due to his own indiscretions, he was unable to maintain the state of physical health deemed essential for successful transplantation. He showed no understanding that his fluid indiscretions could jeopardize his transplantation despite many hours by many people explaining the mechanisms involved. Since he had three donors, his reaction was that if one did not work, he had two others to fall back on. In addition, he demonstrated no concern for other patients, although most of our patients watch each other's progress eagerly and become dejected when others are in difficulty (especially true for transplant patients).

From what has been described, one might expect that he had always been a rebellious person. Such, however, was not the case. His scholastic record in school was average. He was a big boy who wanted to play football, but instead worked to pay tuition at a high school where he felt the education superior. He missed many of the pleasures that most of his peers enjoyed but felt this would be compensated for if he could excel in the field he had chosen. Following graduation, he settled down and within a relatively short period of time worked his way up to an important, responsible position in a company where he was in charge of a large unit. He enjoyed his self-reliance and the importance his position afforded, and felt

his sacrifices had been worthwhile. He married a rather mature girl and his marriage had been a good one.

His "regression" and rebelliousness began after his illness became quite severe. His salary had been continued during his illness, and he had received added financial assistance from various members of his family, so that economically he had done well, and emotionally he had received great satisfaction from the attention showered on him. However, he was excessively demanding at home and on the renal unit. He denied that he feared death, but stated that the one thing that was most disturbing to him was that "I had always been able to get anything that I wanted for myself without having to rely on other people." He stated that the frustration of relying on others to bring him the things upon which his life literally depended was almost intolerable. This seemed to account for an outstanding feature of his illness, i.e., his attempts to manipulate medical personnel so that he could take control of medical management of his illness. We saw in him an unwillingness to make concessions to his illness and its treatment that had brought him literally to death's door. He refused to assume responsibility for his condition in areas which were his alone to control. (He failed to assume even the responsibility for keeping a record of his fluid intake.) He seemed to feel that he would eventually drive the renal unit to doing transplantation with his brother's kidney because there would be no other way for him to live.

Although we cannot deny that his kidney disease with its concomitant therapies was an almost overwhelming stress, we were nonetheless convinced that he was reacting to this stress in accord with his basic psychology. The drive which brought him rapidly upward in position and financial success was now misdirected towards getting what he wanted (transplantation) without regard for others (brother, wife, children) and without all the inconveniences experienced by other patients. We feel his difficulty was directly related to the type of life he had to lead with his illness and the manner in which he attempted to gain mastery over it. In this case his adaptive mechanisms failed because of their inappropriateness.

Eisendrath[8] makes the observation that rather than fearing death, a patient may welcome death (if he feels abandoned by family or other meaningful interpersonal relationships). We recently had the unfortunate opportunity of corroborating this thesis.

Case 2

The patient (from another dialysis unit) had previously received a kidney transplant which was rejected within days. He was returned to our unit about 6 months later for another transplant. Unknown to any of the personnel, his wife had started divorce proceedings and he told no one of this during the first four weeks after transplantation. Three days after transplantation, he became convinced that he was rejecting the kidney although there was no evidence for this. He became even more convinced as time went on and began refusing his immunosuppressive drugs on the grounds that they had caused the previous rejection. In all other spheres, he was oriented and in contact with reality. With coercion he did take this medication and his behavior was viewed as an attempt to gain attention. When he finally started talking about the fact that his wife was divorcing him, it was unknown whether this was real or hallucinatory since his wife and children had visited frequently with no indication of family difficulties. While the family, living some distance away, was being contacted to clarify the marital situation, he expired suddenly. No cause of death was found at autopsy and there was a good take of the graft. Unfortunately, we had no contact with this patient prior to transplantation and therefore cannot speculate as to why this occurred, based on his psychodynamics, other than he lacked the will to live. In the following case the outlook was more hopeful.

Case 3

This 25-year-old male began demanding immediate kidney transplantation. He had been on hemodialysis for 1 year and his condition had always been unstable. He developed bilateral thrombophlebitis of the upper extremities. With conservative medical management, the shunt was preserved. In spite of his insistence for transplantation, when not in the hospital he still indulged in water and dietary indiscretions and had been known to gain 15-20 lb in weight overnight. On these occasions he had to be brought back to the hospital for further dialysis. Was this man attempting suicide? Maybe; but why? We felt this behavior was the result of overlying, distressing psychological factors.

His past history revealed these pertinent facts: The youngest child in a family of three, he had never been happy or content living at home. (The older children seemed to be well on the road to failure so one questions how good the home situation ever was.) As an adolescent, there was a great deal of conflict between him and his mother. His school record was satisfactory but not too remarkable, although his capabilities were higher than his performance. Finally, he decided to enter college, but because of the financial situation, he had to work, instead of going to school, alternate semesters. It was while attending college that his renal disease was discovered. His nephritis was very acute and renal decompensation quickly ensued. He now found himself completely dependent upon his family, which precipitated a variety of ambivalent feelings. At the same time he discovered that he was receiving much solicitude from his mother which he had not experienced before. He obviously enjoyed the attention he received while on the dialysis unit. With this he had in many ways utilized his illness in the service of perpetuating this solicitude. Another painful dynamic factor occurred when it was discovered that his most suitable donor would be his mother toward whom he had marked ambivalent feelings (which she reciprocated). At the same time that he found he was receiving attention from her which he had not had before, he markedly resented the fact that his future well-being might very well depend upon her generosity in donating her kidney. In addition, his mother had the sole care of his sister's children and no arrangements for their care had been made for the period his mother would be in the hospital as donor. For the first year, his reaction to this situation was uncooperativeness which only prevented transplantation.

We attributed his dietary acting out to the numerous ambivalences he had failed to resolve. With the development of the thrombophlebitis, it became necessary that he give up his gain from his illness, and he then demanded transplantation even though it was clear to all that his physical condition would not permit it.

The decision was made to offer cadaver transplantation as opposed to psychotherapy (for resolving long-standing conflicts with his mother), because with life-threatening complications, we might not have had time to resolve those conflicts, and the mother seemed to have been actively perpetuating these conflicts, perhaps because of her own ambivalence toward her son and/or fear of the surgery for herself. Again, we felt time was too short and she was too unworkable. With the possibility of a cadaver transplant, his behavior became much more reasonable and the family completed arrangements for care of the children in the event the final decision was to use his mother as a donor.

The mechanisms here may seem obvious at first glance, but when reviewing the literature, one finds that there is a fairly constant tendency to view this as denial of illness and to direct therapy towards facing reality. This patient knew he was ill, he wanted to be well (if only to help care for his niece and nephew whom he had come to love). When he and his mother could strike a satisfactory relationship, all was well. When they were at odds, he did not want anything from her except to be left alone.

By offering the possibility of a cadaver transplant, he no longer needed to view her as his sole hope for survival (and she no longer could view herself this way) and he did become more able to face reality. On the other hand, when the mother was told she no longer needed to donate if this would present too many problems, she offered freely and voluntarily to remain a donor if needed. We interpreted this activity as evidence of her basic inauthenticity.

The complications of the illness and its treatment (hemodialysis) do gradually force the patient to face, at least partially, the reality of his situation. However, it must be kept in mind that unresolved conflicts can cause the patient to attempt solutions that are in conflict with reality and it is only by helping him resolve or bypass those conflicts that he can be brought into control.

GENERAL CONSIDERATIONS OF STRESS

In order to more completely understand the dynamics in these types of cases, the authors felt it necessary to investigate other known areas in psychiatry to correlate previous knowledge of reactions of human beings in situation of extreme stress and threat to life. The now classic volume *Men Under Stress*, by Grinker and Spiegel,[9] consistently emphasizes the fact that before any interpretation of a soldier's behavior under stress can be made, one must be knowledgeable of the underlying personality of this person. For example, a person who has been unable to establish group loyalties, who has been too overprotected and unemancipated from his parental ties prior to combat, may have severe difficulties when asked to perform responsibly and with self-reliance in the face of stress. Glass[10] has emphasized that modern techniques of treatment of combat reactions are aimed at preserving group cohesiveness and meaningful identifications for the combat soldier in the face of threat and danger. The fact that such techniques do work to alleviate anxiety in combat, suggests to us that the fear experienced in combat is due more to the loss of accustomed control and other meaningful relationships than to a fear of death per se. This anxiety can be equated to the threat to man's first Ur defense.[7] Because the person in these circumstances has lost the belief in his own invulnerability, he calls upon the collective strength of the group, placing his trust for his own welfare in the hands of the aggregate.

We feel that some such mechanism must have been at work in the preceding cases. All three patients had lost long-term control over their lives, one in the area of work where he received much gratification, another in the loss of a love object and possible supplier of narcissistic needs, one having to cope in a different manner with long-standing ambivalences. When, in the renal patients, fear of death becomes a pertinent feature, our observations would indicate many times that this is the result of the wish for the ultimate escape because the patient has lost faith in his own invulnerability, as well as his capacity to turn to significant others for a feeling of protection. Such dynamics are similar to those of suicide as stated by Masserman[7] who does not view suicide as a wish to die per se, but rather as a means of attaining the ultimate escape with a further reawakening and a means of retaliation towards those who have disappointed the patient the most.

EVOLUTION OF NEUROTIC (IRRATIONAL) BEHAVIOR

To understand overt psychiatric symptomatology of this type of patient, we must borrow from the known dynamics of neurotic behavior and apply them to this field. With the risk of sounding banal, we note that many theoreticians regard the psychoneuroses as ever desperate measures on the part of an individual to bring a semblance of control and certainty, however distorted, back into a person's life when his usual modus operandi has failed him. Many times such measures appear markedly irrational, but such measures, conscious or not, are not originally devised as such by the patient. Similarly we postulate that overt psy-chiatric symptomatology of the fear-driven renal patient is of the same order. In spite of the fact that his behavior may appear irrational to the observer, it serves as an adaptive mechanism of the afflicted person in an attempt to bring a sense of order back into his life when his usual and accustomed means of control have been lost. It is therefore of vital importance to understand the unique, underlying personality structure of this person before the significance of such behavior becomes meaningful. An example of this is the following case.

Case 4

This is a 32-year-old married woman with no children. Her past history revealed that she had been raised in a disrupted family situation which ended in divorce of the parents when she was 5 years old. Although the father was alcoholic, he had always been especially attentive and indulgent to his only daughter. He died when she was 10 years of age. The mother and older brothers had to run the family business and had little time for her genuine needs for guidance, but more or less let her have her own way in order to placate her, from which evolved a strong cynical attitude toward others. Later, although required to work in the family business, she was not expected to handle too much responsibility. At this time her adolescent interpersonal relationships were rather poor. Although realistically rejected most of her life, she managed to demand attention from others by creating minor crises. For example, she would do poorly in school, threaten to quit, and thus solicit a great deal of concern momentarily from the family and teachers. After graduating from high school, she continued to work in the family store where she was overprotected, with no realistic pressure put on her for maturity. While attending a downtown social function at the "Y," she met her husband. He was a man 10 years her senior. At first, the mother objected to this relationship, stating that her daughter was too young to marry, although at this time she was already 25 years of age. During her courtship, it was discovered that she had kidney disease, that her life would have to be curtailed, and that she should avoid pregnancy as long as possible. In spite of these restrictions her husband-to-be desired marriage to her. All her wedding plans were managed by the mother, and the marriage itself was one in which the husband and mother constantly catered to her needs. When her kidney disease grew worse, members of the family had to assume most of the responsibility for her care. It was her husband who insisted that she start hemodialysis. Finally, it was the husband who made the decision regarding transplantation.

During the time of active medical intervention (prior to transplant), she did not exhibit severe emotional problems, although occasionally she felt slightly depressed. There were no acute anxiety symptoms or any feeling that she was going to die. At all times she had husband, mother, and friends in attendance. However, following transplantation she found herself in a much different situation. The nursing personnel were unwilling to wait on her in the exaggerated and unrealistic degree her family had accepted. Since the family had also become tired of her excessive demandingness, they eagerly adopted and reinforced the recommendations of the staff that she become more self-reliant and assume the responsibility for much of her care (i.e., bathing, recording fluid intake and other simple routines). She responded with more demandingness. Shortly thereafter, she was placed in isolation because of a minor infection. The pressure for her to do things for herself continued. When her basic psychopathological pattern was disrupted, she, having lost her usual means of control, became extremely anxious, and psychosis with rather marked paranoid features and delusions of grandeur, ensued. This was handled with drugs and psychotherapy which not only returned her to her previous level of functioning, but she seemed to gain some insight and to function at a more mature level.

Thus far the patient has been able to leave the hospital and function in a more realistic manner. She remained somewhat grandiose and self-centered, seemingly a feature of her premorbid personality, fostered by a manipulative, alcoholic father who saw her infrequently, and continued by her mother and brothers after his death. Her husband probably married her for these same features, recognizing how well she would adapt to his style of living, and may have fostered them after marriage.

REACTIONS OF A "NORMAL" PERSONALITY

It is our impression that those patients who were previously well-adjusted, although realistically anxious about their condition, do not usually suffer the upheavals described above. The following case is used to demonstrate.

Case 5

This is a 31-year-old married woman who was successfully transplanted, whose emotional reactions to her illness were minor. She is one of the middle children in a family of seven. The home situation had always been stable and relatively happy, although there were always financial difficulties. The patient had a part-time job as an adolescent, but this did not interfere with her school record. Although she met her husband while in high school, they were not able to marry for several years because of his entry into military service. Her marriage had been stable, with little difficulty on the part of either of them in adjusting to marriage and the arrival of the children.

During her last pregnancy her kidney disease was diagnosed and she was given a poor prognosis for life. Instead of brooding about her physical condition, however, she participated as actively as she could in the raising of her children so that they would be as self-sufficient as possible when she was gone. Fortunately, dialysis became available to her, and during dialysis she remained actively involved in her children's lives.

Her early emotional course on dialysis was rather stormy because she was not adequately prepared, and her husband was absent. She was frightened of the dialysis apparatus, and the dialyzing process was not as successful as had been hoped. In addition, her husband, being a career army man, could not always be with her. Although the service attempted to be as cooperative as possible, there had been times when she had to face much of this turmoil alone.

Eventually she was transplanted, but the first transplant was immediately rejected. Interestingly, the medical personnel caring for her were more upset than she, and she ended up comforting them. She continued on dialysis with much greater success. Both of her own kidneys had been removed at transplantation, and her blood pressure returned to normal levels so that she felt physically much better after her surgery. On the day she was transplanted the second time, she had been downtown shopping with visiting relatives. Because of the haste necessary in the second transplantation, she did not have sufficient time to adequately prepare her children for the fact that she would be away from home. Fortunately, the second transplant took and was operant in 24 hours. Her major concern at this time, however, was for her husband and children's welfare. When reassured all would be taken care of, she was able to relax. Our impression of this woman was that she was one of the most stable people we had seen in the dialysis unit. In spite of extremely realistic distress to which she had been subjected, she was able to mobilize her considerable strengths to carry her through most remarkably and is able to contemplate future transplants, if needed, with equanimity.

SUMMARY

We feel that the basic cause of severe distress and psychiatric symptomatology of the patient facing hemodialysis and transplantation is that, of necessity, he must evolve a markedly constricted, agonizing existence over which he has lost a very serious degree of accustomed control. Further, the patient brings into the situation his own unique personality with its inherent strengths and weakness. Lastly, the patient must rest pretty well on his past interpersonal relationships, as well as previous accomplishments and skills without much room left for maneuverability and improvement.

The combination of all of these factors will in our opinion determine the individual's behavioral and emotional reactions to his illness. There is a marked urgency, expectancy of doom, and uncertainty, which telescopes all the personality strengths and weaknesses into one acute, agonizing, and intense stress and crisis situation. When the fear of death appears to be a clinical factor in the hemodialysis patient, the authors are convinced that this is a secondary issue, as well as a distraction from the realistic stresses described above. It is toward these stresses that the psychiatrist must direct his attention.

REFERENCES

1. Abram, H. S.: The psychiatrist, the treatment of chronic renal failure, and the prolongation of life: I. Amer. J. Psychiat. 124:1351, 1968.
2. —: The psychiatrist, the treatment of chronic renal failure, and prolongation of life. II. Amer. J. Psychiat. 126:157, 1969.
3. Lazarus, H. R., and Hagens, J. H.: Prevention of psychosis following open heart surgery. Amer. J. Psychiat. 124:1190, 1968.
4. Kemph, J. P.: Psychotherapy with patients receiving kidney transplant. Amer. J. Psychiat. 124:623, 1968.
5. Short, M. J., Wilson, W. P.: Roles of denial in chronic hemodialysis. Arch. Gen. Psychiat. (Chicago) 20:433, 1969.
6. Beard, B. H.: Fear of death and fear of life. Arch. Gen. Psychiat. (Chicago) 21:373, 1969.
7. Masserman, J. H.: The Practice of Dynamic Psychiatry. Philadelphia, Saunders, 1955, p. 468.
8. Eisendrath, R. M.: The role of grief and fear in the death of kidney transplant patients. Amer. J. Psychiat. 126:381, 1969.
9. Grinker, R. and Spiegel, J. P.: Men Under Stress. Philadelphia, Blakiston, 1945.
10. Glass, A. J.: Psychotherapy in the combat zone, Amer. J. Psychiat. 110:725, 1954.

26

A gynaecological experience

This account of an hysterectomy took the patient six hours to type because she is a severely disabled spastic. It makes very revealing reading and has something to teach everyone who reads it. The patient had lived with her disability for 31 years but some of the staff assumed that they knew more of her conditon than she did herself.

After 20 years of painful periods, which had not been relieved very adequately by Panadol, Ponstan or, latterly, Gynovlar 21, over a span of two years, I decided to ask whether it would be worth considering a D and C or a hysterectomy. At the somewhat early age of 31 I had to give adequate reasons for the latter, and adequate assurance that marriage and childbearing was not likely to occur.

As a handicapped person with an eye to the future of life without a cycle of monthy pain, and a realistic view of the sociological problems posed by marriage and child-rearing, I was able to give the assurance required. With this, the specialist said that a D and C was pointless—within three months the situation would return to the state before the operation. So a hysterectomy was decided upon, subject to a final decision by me.

I had heard that this operation could have depression as an after-effect, and as I had already had quite bad bouts of depression, the specialist suggested that I saw the consultant psychiatrist as an extra check. Before this psychiatric appointment Gynovlar 21 was discontinued. The psychiatrist's

Reprinted from Nursing Times, pp. 927-928, July 19, 1973.

opinion was that the operation would have no adverse psychological effect and, basing my final decision on this opinion I was put on a short waiting list.

At 10:15 am on a sunny Sunday I was admitted to the ward. Fortunately I had had minor abdominal surgery before, as well as several other admissions to hospital, so I was fairly familiar with the technique. I was accompanied by my father and two sisters, and I had asked them to refer all the inevitable questions to me, since I am the only one who knows the extra nursing care required. Despite this, the admitting nurse insisted on my sister getting me undressed and ready for bed, although I said that my sister was not used to coping with me. However, we managed. Fortunately the bed was of an adjustable height and it was a simple matter to swing from my wheelchair on to the bed with help from two nurses. (Throughout my stay, I insisted on there being two nurses at least for lifting; more for the sake of the nurses.) As soon as I was in bed, I was faced with two problems: keeping in an upright position, and sore heels. My knees have permanent contractures and for that first day I was permitted the use of a pillow under my knees which kept me upright for a fair length of time. The sore heels were prevented by sheepskin bootees.

Feeding in bed is not possible for me so a nurse came to give me my last meal. Before this a staff nurse came to shave me, a procedure I had been rather dreading because of the jumpiness of my legs and my generally uncontrolled movements. However, she was quick, and very patient, and I was able to immobilize my top half by grabbing the bed rail. Following the after-lunch rest the routine of medical examinations and other preoperative procedures continued. The admitting doctor left me until last as I was bed-fast, and wisely only did a chest and heart check. I was then asked to sign the consent form (the nurse told me that my father said I could sign, to which I replied, 'Not in bed') so I managed to initial it.

The next question was drugs and catheters. The problem of postoperative pain and the inability to use a bedpan were paramount. I wanted reassurance on both these points. The admitting doctor said I would be seeing the house surgeon and the surgeon performing the operation before I went to theatre, so I had to be satisfied with that.

OPERATION DAY

I was woken with a cup of tea and Valium 2 mg and Librium. The former was my normal drug régime, the latter I was told would 'calm you down, dear'. I found this attitude of giving patients drugs without specifying what they are for demoralizing.

Sister was on duty in the morning so I badgered her about: catheterization; cot sides; adequate splinting for my arm if a drip was going to be used; drugs; premedication; requests that the drip should go into my right arm, blood samples to be taken from the back of the hand as this avoided the danger of a broken needle and syringe if the attempt was made in the elbow.

Fortunately sister was understanding enough not to think I was trying to teach her nursing, but only trying to foresee the difficulties that beset the disabled in a hospital where gynaecology is the speciality. As will be seen later this proved quite a postoperative problem.

POSTOPERATIVE ARRANGEMENTS

Just before lunch (nothing for me) the surgeon came round and we discussed all the points just mentioned. Initially, the Valium was raised from 10 mg (my normal total daily dose) to 15 mg. He agreed to catheterize me in theatre, the process being more easily done when under the anaesthetic. Cot sides were already in position, and he saw by my involuntary movements that splinting was necessary for the drip and noted that, as I was left-handed, the drip would have to go into my right hand (which is unusable).

In the early afternoon the pre-operative medication was given. As well as having the desired effect of drying up secretions, for me it has the effect of removing what control I have over my movements. I explained this to the staff and instead of curtaining me off they left the curtains open and the specialling nurse kept a reassuring eye on me. Noise was kept to a minimum as, in this state, even a slight sound makes me jump.

After about an hour I was rolled on to the theatre trolley canvas by six people, asked about drug hypersensitivities, slipped on to the trolley, had my identification checked, and was taken to theatre. Finally the surgeon came in to the anteroom, reassured me about the IV drip and catheter, and then I was away.

As I regained consciousness I heard the surgeon say it was a 'piece of cake—only 40 minutes'. I then 'came to' again to see the drip nearly yanked out of my hand, and the surgeon muttering about splints! Between the waves of pain I was mercifully injected into oblivion; only to wake up every hour through the night to have my blood pressure taken. I remember vaguely trying to grab the cotside in an effort to keep my left arm still enough for the nurse to take it.

The next morning I really 'came to' and they ceased the injections and instituted a mixture of pethidine and Aspirin instead. Aspirin makes me sick if I take it over any length of time, so on my second day this was stopped and Panadol took its place. Unfortunately I developed a urinary infection to add to my discomforts. The pain of the operation was severe because I was unable to control the muscle spasms in my abdomen and by the fifth day these were so severe that I couldn't be touched without jumping. All nursing care was carried out with extreme gentleness but even washing my face was torture for my tummy.

I was exceptionally lucky with the nurses and physiotherapists; both tried to put themselves in my place. My only criticism is that basic bedside nursing, bed-bathing, attention to pressure areas, and so on—seemed to be in the background. I had to ask ward nurses for things to be done that were second nature to the very good agency nurses that we had in the ward.

Despite my entreaties to the house surgeon that the muscle spasm might be helped by an increase of Valium, nothing was really done for the pain until the evening of the fifth postoperative day when an enterprising staff nurse had me written up for Fortral. This eased me over the weekend, but on my eighth postoperative day I was still in severe pain, though by now my temperature had stopped 'yo-yoing'. That day, the surgeon did his second round and seemed surprised to see that I was still in pain. I explained that I thought it was my disability that was making it more difficult for me to recover. He asked me how long I had been taking Valium, and doubled the total dosage immediately. This, coupled with Fortral, hastened my recovery and by the end of the second week I was sitting up in my chair for periods of time. Unlike other patients who were up all day by this time (but resting on their beds) I got up for two, three and then four hours at a time, so that there was not too much lifting to be done.

CONVALESCENCE DIFFICULTIES

All along there had been a difficulty about convalescence. Patients undergoing hysterectomy were offered places in the hospital's own convalescent home on the coast. This, for me, had one or two snags. Patients leaving the hospital were rehabilitated to doing practically everything for

themselves. By the time they left the nursing supervision was minimal. With me, basic nursing had to be continued, and either a downstairs bedroom or a place with a lift was essential. Other non-essential factors would include adequate facilities for a general bath. This last was offered to me at the beginning of my third week, but I looked at the bath and estimated that although it would be possible to get in, getting out would be a major hazard both to the nurses and to me, so we left this exercise to later. (Bath heights were the problem.)

With the assistance of the medical social worker department, arrangements were made for me to spend a fortnight in a holiday home for the severely disabled, with convalescent facilities. This proved the answer, but I could not be accommodated for a further 10 days after the hospital fortnight was up. However, the doctors agreed that it would be best for me to remain in the hospital for the extra time.

PHYSIOTHERAPY A HELP

The removal of clips and the catheter assisted my mobility somewhat, for it was now a question of using a commode chair. Happily, this was able to be slid over the lavatory seat as, for a considerable time, I found it impossible to sit upright without side supports. I really began to feel we were getting somewhere when I could stand with support enough to change from bed to chair and from chair to lavatory. Immobility in bed concerned me because of the known dangers of thrombosis, but the physiotherapists did passive leg exercises from quite early on.

Any action on my part brought on massive muscular spasm. For this reason feeding myself when I was up was only reinstituted on my return home from convalescence. Of all the activities I can do, this is the most difficult, the most tiring and the one which involves the maximum of control. I felt justified in requesting to be fed in such circumstances.

For most patients after a hysterectomy, lifting is not advised for about a month afterwards. I use an overhead hoist—a monkey pole—for turning in bed as a normal process, and no one could really tell me with clarity whether the 'reach' was going to be too much. The physiotherapists had one idea and the doctor had another. I had no desire to do any damage to my operation site, so I took the longer of the two. On my return home I checked with my general practitioner who advised a further fortnight of turning assistance and assisting me into bed.

Looking back, the main things that struck me were:

1. The necessity for a two-way confidence in the doctor-patient relationship, when the patient has a marked physical disability. This means that the doctor must be able to trust the patient where the patient's experience of disability is greater than the doctor's. Perhaps there is something missing in medical curricula if a postgraduate surgeon has not come across adult cerebral palsy patients or those with other central nervous system disorders and is reluctant to take this into account in prescribing. And if the doctor for any reason cannot prescribe sufficient analgesia he should be able to tell the patient why. There is nothing less reassuring or more frightening than uncontrolled pain.

2. In specialist hospitals fuller notice could be taken earlier than admission of any problems likely to crop up where cerebral palsy patients are being considered for abdominal surgery. This would be particularly important where there is marked speech defect. I felt that I was having to be one jump ahead, for instance, before surgery I had to try and anticipate the need for catheterization as an alternative to the bedpan and not because catheterization was a normal part of surgical procedure for that operation.

3. Some sort of questionnaire could well be developed for the use of disabled patients (to be filled in by the patients or persons closely associated with each patient) indicating their pre-surgical ability, so that nursing deployment can be correct on admission. It should be stressed to the patients that they may bring in their own apparatus, for example, straws, wheelchairs, although some idea of ward equipment might be indicated. (These three points are useful for 'cold' admissions. Emergency admissions would virtually have to get by.)

Finally, for me, the operation was a complete success, giving me more opportunities of getting out and around without relying on nursing assistance. Freedom from cyclic pain is an added bonus. One disadvantage is residual incontinence, but these are early days yet and this may clear up spontaneously. The surgeon who did my operation runs a clinic for stress incontinence, and if this trouble does not improve I plan on being referred back to him for investigation.

27

Adjustment problems of the family of the burn patient

GENE A. BRODLAND and N. J. C. ANDREASEN

Patients who have been severely burned experience an intense and varied trauma involving catastrophic injury, severe pain, possible cosmetic or functional deformities, and a threat to their sense of identity and worth. Hospitalization is usually prolonged. During this time, the family of the burn patient often remains with him to comfort and console him. Because most of the attention of the medical staff is focused on the suffering patient, the family members remain in the background and few people are aware of their suffering and emotional needs. Yet, just as the patient himself must adjust to his injury, so the family must go through a completed process of understanding, accepting, and adjusting to the illness and distress of the loved one.

The adjustment problems of the adult burn patient have been the subject of only a few studies, and the problems of his family have drawn still less attention.[1] Studies done in England have examined the grief reactions of parents of fatally burned children and pathology in the parents which may have contributed to behavioral problems in surviving children.[2] One follow-up study of 10 children and their parents, an average of 4½ years after injury, discovered recognizable psychological disturbance (usually depression) in 8 of the mothers and none of the children.[3] This morbidity is

high, and it suggests that further examination of the reactions of families is needed.

The observations presented in this article are based on a study done over a period of approximately 1 year on the burn unit at the University Hospitals in Iowa City. A total of 32 adults and their families were evaluated psychiatrically on admission and were interviewed daily thereafter until the time of discharge. Initial evaluation was based on complete psychiatric and social histories and mental status examinations. The patients ranged in age from 20 to 59 with a mean of 36, in total body surface burn from 8% to 60% with a mean of 29%, and in duration of hospitalization from 2½ weeks to 3 months with a mean of 1 month. Patients outside the age range of 18 through 60 or with severe mental retardation were excluded.

The relatives of the burn patient appeared to go through an adjustment process, similar to that of the patients, involving two stages. The first stage was one of acute shock and grief analogous to the acute physical and emotional trauma experienced by the patient himself. In the second or convalescent stage, the relatives had overcome shock and disbelief; they rationalized and accepted the fact of the injury and its accompaniments and began to assist the patient in the process of recovery.

INITIAL REACTIONS OF RELATIVES

The family's first reaction on arriving at the hospital is usually relief that the patient

Reprinted from Social Casework 55:13-18, 1974. Published by the Family Service Association of America.

has not died or been burned more severely. Rationalizations that "it could have been worse" provide an affirmative basis from which to begin coping with the stress that they face. In this first stage, the relatives express little concern about the potential scarring that might take place. Their primary concern is for the recovery of the patient, no matter what his appearance on recovery. The following case history illustrates the initial reaction of many families in the first stage of hospitalization.

Mr. S, aged 23, was severely burned in a car-truck accident. Having been pinned in the truck cab which caught fire, he sustained third-degree burns over 45% of his body. He was transferred to the burn unit 2½ weeks after being burned and remained hospitalized for 2½ months. His wife, who visited him daily, expressed her feeling that the scarring which might result was not important. She said she "would be happy if he could get well no matter what his condition is, so the kids will have a father." She demonstrated a considerable amount of quiet desperation; tears were often evident when she expressed her feelings.

Despite expressions of relief that the patient has not died, the fear that the injury might ultimately prove fatal lingers with many relatives. Sometimes this fear is expressed overtly. Interwoven with these feelings is a well-repressed wish by some relatives that the patient would die and thereby avoid the pain and frustration that lie ahead of him. Relatives of patients who die as a result of burns support this idea; when informed that a love one has died, they often comment, "It is probably a blessing for he won't have to suffer any more now." Such feelings are usually suppressed because of the guilt they could arouse. The case of Mrs. K illustrates this reaction.

Mrs. K, aged 24, was burned in a natural gas explosion in her home. Her husband suffered more severe burns and subsequently died. Her comments following his death indicate a degree of relief. She said, "I will miss him and it will be hard without him. He won't have to suffer for months and months. I'm glad God took him

soon. I know he wouldn't want to live being terribly burned as he was. His death was a blessing." Mrs. K probably would not have said this before his death but as she rationalized in an attempt to face reality, these feelings were allowed to come to the surface.

During this early period, the relatives and the patients form feelings of trust or mistrust toward the medical staff. When a patient suffers from pain and fear, he and his relatives have to decide whether everything is being done medically to insure his comfort and recovery. Occasionally, patients and relatives question the competence of the staff and feel that the patient is the object of experimentation. The extended waiting period prior to skin grafting is often seen as abandonment and may lead to feelings of mistrust. Such feelings were expressed to the psychiatric social worker more often than to the medical staff. Relatives were concerned that by expressing angry feelings toward the staff they might jeopardize the patient's relationship with the staff.

Mr. L sustained a steam burn while working on a construction job. After skin grafting failed to take, the patient became suspicious and remarked that the resident doctor was practicing on him as if he were a "guinea pig." He requested that the social worker arrange for a transfer to a private doctor or to another hospital. He did not want to talk to the nurses or the staff doctor about his change, because it might cause hard feelings. It was determined later that his problem centered on the lack of communication between the resident and the patient. The problem was resolved when the resident made conscientious efforts to explain the treatment procedures more fully to the patient.

Soon after admission, a number of extensively burned patients experience confusion and disorientation as a result of an acute brain syndrome that often accompanies burn trauma. Many relatives found this reaction stressful. Sometimes a patient was verbally abusive or assaultive, and relatives had a difficult time in deciding whether this behavior represented his true feelings or whether it was the result of delirium. Relatives were frightened by this sudden "mental illness" and needed reassurance that delirium is a common occurrence in burn patients and that once the burn begins to heal, the delirium passes.

Mr. R, a 28-year-old farm hand, was burned over 60% of his body in a natural gas explosion. About a week and a half after admission to the burn unit, he became delirious. During his periods of confusion, he thought of a period during his second year of marriage when his wife had had an extramarital affair. Mr. R. angrily expressed the belief that this affair was still going on. His bewildered wife thought that this problem had been resolved 8 years before. Mr. R needed reassurance that his accusations were a result of his delirium. After Mr. R recovered, he denied any feelings of suspicion toward his wife.

Another source of difficulty for relatives is the psychologic regression that is often observed among the burn patients. Patients who have been quite self-sufficient in the conduct of their daily lives before being hospitalized often become complaining, demanding, and dependent during hospitalization. The family, unaccustomed to this behavior, becomes alternately confused and angry. They want to respond to the patient's needs but are confused by demands that seem so out of character. Relatives become angry when the patients do not give them credit for their efforts and continue with their childlike behavior.

REACTIONS AFTER INITIAL CRISIS

During the second phase of adjustment, the family is assured that the patient will survive and begins to consider the process of getting well. The family members begin to recognize that they and the patient still have many weeks in the hospital ahead of them. The patient and his relatives usually have no prior knowledge of the treatment and procedures required for recovery; now they begin to ask questions of physicians and nurses about the process of healing, dressing changes, grafting procedures, and so on. Often relatives of other patients on the ward are important sources of information, just as they are sources of reassur-

ance. The family of the patient must prepare themselves psychologically for an extended stay in the hospital. From a practical standpoint, family members must make arrangements for their own physical well-being during this period and establish "a home away from home." This often involves spending days at the hospital and nights in a nearby motel.

The pain the patient suffers is a primary problem at this time, and it often results in a sense of helpless frustration in the relatives. The patient seems to become increasingly cognizant of his pain once the threat of death has passed. He then begins to verbalize the pain, at times in tones of desperation. The helplessness which relatives feel in handling this pain produces conflict. On the one hand, they try to do everything within their power to aid the patient by making him physically comfortable and providing emotional support. On the other hand, relatives sometimes feel the staff could relieve pain more adequately by the administration of analgesic medication. The relative often is in a precarious position, trying to maintain a good relationship both with the patient and with the medical staff. Few persons understand fully the principles followed in the use of pain medication. The following example illustrates the development in one relative of mistrust of the staff.

Mrs. B was burned when she and her family were trapped upstairs in their burning home. She broke her arm when she jumped from a second-story window to escape the flames. Because of the burns, the staff were unable to put her arm in the correct cast. The arm was very painful. Because of her complaints of pain and her mother's frustration in attempting to alleviate the pain, the mother confronted the nurse with the accusation that the staff was neglecting her daughter by not giving her enough pain medication. Once the problems inherent in using potent analgesics for long periods of time were explained in detail, the patient's mother was much relieved and could again be supportive to the patient.

Another source of pain occurring during this period is the process of autografting.

The donor site, from which the skin of grafting is taken, often is more painful than the burn site itself, causing great distress to the patient. Further, the patient must lie quietly after the grafts have been placed, increasing the sense of helplessness felt by both patient and relatives. The fear of doing something that might disturb the graft is a significant cause of anxiety.

The frequent trips to the operating room for skin grafting are yet another source of anxiety. The fear of anesthesia must be faced each time the operative procedure approaches; the patient is anxious about being put to sleep and having to relinquish control. This anxiety is often sensed by the relatives.

REACTIONS DURING RECOVERY

Still later in the recovery period, the problem of pain is supplanted by one of itching, which creates a problem for the relatives who try to help the patient to tolerate each new stress. It often seems that total recovery will never arrive and that one discomfort is simply succeeded by another.

Another major problem faced during the recovery phase is fear of deformity. Most families initially expect grafting to restore fairly normal appearance. What medical personnel consider an excellent job of skin reconstruction is often viewed by the lay person as almost grotesque. Thus, patient and family tend to be disappointed by the results of grafting and to find a gap between their expectations and those of medical personnel. During this stage of recovery, the patient begins to prepare himself for facing the outside world by realizing that scarring and deformity may have made him unattractive and unacceptable to others with whom he has previously associated. He becomes hypersensitive to initial reactions and wonders what reactions he will find himself meeting the rest of his life. Relatives have similar fears.

The relatives' reactions are the first ones that the patient observes, and his distress is increased when he sees revulsion. A fairly typical case of family reaction was noted in a follow-up study of burn patients.[4] A young mother who had been hospitalized for 3 months eagerly anticipated seeing her children. She was greeted by her 5-year-old with "Yuk, Mommie, you look awful." Adult family members, on the other hand, tend to recognize intuitively that they need to be supportive and to help the patient establish a denial system. Yet, providing a reassurance that they do not always sincerely feel is often quite stressful for them. Only with time and thoughtful support on the part of doctors, nurses, and relatives can the patient resolve his feelings about disfigurement and come to realize that angry red scars eventually fade and that his appearance will gradually improve.

Sometimes relatives carry an additional burden because of their feeling that they have contributed to or caused the accident in which the patient was injured. Even when the relatives have had nothing to do with the injury, some feel guilty; they explain this feeling on the basis of not having foreseen the possibility of the accident and not having taken steps to prevent it. Eventually, the relative resolves his guilt feelings and achieves a rationalization that relieves him of full responsibility for the accident—for example, that the accident happened because it was God's will, because it would draw the family together, or because of the carelessness of others.

Notable throughout the recovery period is the difficulty that relatives have in dealing with the patient's need to express his feelings. They find it difficult to strike a balance between letting the patient describe his feelings about being burned and possibly handicapped and providing adequate emotional support. Sometimes relatives attempt to discourage the patient from expressing feelings of grief or fear and try to be constantly supportive and optimistic. In preserving their own comfort, they sometimes unwittingly deprive the patient of a necessary safety valve.

There are also relatives who become overwhelmed   by the emotional stress of sitting at the bedside of a loved one and sharing his suffering. Many are reluctant to leave the bedside in the early stages of recovery, fearing that something might happen while they are gone. Occasionally, relatives become too depressed or anxious and must be asked to leave the ward temporarily to regain their emotional equilibrium. Remaining at the bedside of a burned patient is an unusually draining experience for his relatives. Much like a young child, the burn patient tends to focus only on himself and provides little support in return, leaving little opportunity for relatives to converse or receive support from others.

RECOMMENDATIONS FROM THIS STUDY

A burn injury is a traumatic experience for the uninjured relatives, as well as the patient himself. The families of the burn patients face multiple stresses and adjustment problems. They go through essentially the same phases of adaptation as the patients, for they must cope with anxiety about death, communication difficulties with the medical staff, fear of deformity, and the boredom of a prolonged hospital stay, as well as enduring the trauma of watching a loved one suffer. In some respects, their suffering may be greater than that of the patient. Although they do not suffer pain directly, they must stand by in helpless frustration, their guilt over the fact that the injury occurred at all further enhanced by their guilt about the anger which they must inevitably feel sometimes. Although they do not fear death or deformity for themselves directly, they must face these threats more immediately than the patient. Few patients are informed of their prognosis soon after admission and, if they were, their minds would be too clouded by trauma to comprehend it fully; however, relatives cannot be shielded from this information, and they must receive it when their minds are usually in a state of heightened sensitivity and alertness.

Relatives may provide valuable assistance on wards by helping to feed the patient, by providing companionship for

him, and often by encouraging and assisting him with exercise and physical therapy. Nevertheless, nurses and physicians provide primary care, and the role of relatives must inevitably be simply a supportive one. This role is a difficult one to fulfill in such an emotionally draining situation unless the person providing the support receives support from others for himself. On the burn unit, this need was often met by the relatives of other patients. Although there was no formal effort by the staff to enhance such relationships, relatives often pooled their information about treatment methods, compared notes on the condition of the patient, and consoled one another when things were going badly.

Hospital burn units could learn a lesson from this phenomenon and formalize it in several ways. Relatives could be helped greatly if hospitals prepared a simple pamphlet to be given to them on arrival, explaining simple facts about injuries from burns and the operation of the unit. It should state the visiting hours established and describe the daily routine, the purpose of unfamiliar treatment methods such as the use of silver nitrate and sulfamylon, the rationale behind the use of milder and preferably oral analgesics, the usual course of recovery from a burn injury, the nature of the grafting procedures usually done, and so forth. A glossary of unfamiliar terms— *autograft, zenograft, debridement,* for example—should be included. Because of the complex nature of this type of injury, burn treatment units are often run quite differently from other hospital facilities, and relatives cannot carry over any prior hospital experience. For example, they find it difficult to understand the infrequent use of potent analgesics, although this practice usually becomes acceptable when they realize that the long-term use required in a burn injury might lead to dependence or addiction. On the affirmative side, on some burn units, rules about visiting hours are flexible and most relatives are permitted to remain with the patient as long as they wish.

A second way of providing communication and understanding among relatives would be the establishment of group support meetings. A group composed of family members or close friends of patients currently on the burn unit could meet at a regularly scheduled time once or twice weekly. The group would remain in existence, although the membership changed as the patient population changed. Ideally, this group would be conducted by a pair of group leaders—a psychiatric social worker and a nurse or physician who are members of the burn unit treatment team. A physical therapist, a dietitian active on the burn unit, and a psychiatrist familiar with the problems of adjustment to chronic illness would be other potential members or guest visitors.

The establishment of such a group would serve several purposes. It would demonstrate to the beleaguered relatives the interest and concern of the hospital staff, sometimes prone to leave relatives out of the picture because of their concern for primary patient care; regular group meetings would make efficient use of the professionals' time and experience. The meetings would also serve to educate relatives about problems of burn trauma, particularly when discharge draws near. Family members often take on primary responsibility for the patient at discharge and they greatly need adequate information about wound care, the need for continuing physical therapy, and the problems of emotional and social adjustment. The group discussions would provide relatives with an open forum for raising questions and for airing complaints. They would provide emotional support by strengthening the bonds formed between family members and alleviate some feelings of fear, frustration, futility, and boredom. Such a group would not be designed as therapy, but as a means of sharing strength and information. Limited experience with such group meet-

ings on burn units indicates, however, that often staff members also receive information and support from them.

A final way for social work staff to be effective on a burn unit is perhaps the most obvious. Families of patients often suffer significant financial expenses, and even after the patient is discharged the period of rehabilitation is prolonged. Family members and patients need to receive information about funds available to assist in the high cost of hospitalization, funds for care of dependents, and opportunities for vocational rehabilitation. An experienced and sensitive social worker can often provide subtle emotional support by demonstrating his concerned involvement as he offers his resources of information and interest to the family.

REFERENCES

1. Andreasen, N. J. C., Noyes, R., Hartford, C. E., Brodland, G. A., & Proctor, S. Management of emotional problems in seriously burned adults. *New England Journal of Medicine,* **286,**65-69 (January 13, 1972); Hamburg, D. A., Artz, C. P., Reiss, E., Amspacher, W. H., & Chambers, R. E. Clinical importance of emotional problems in the care of patients with burns. *New England Journal of Medicine,* **248,**355-59 (February 26, 1953); Hamburg, D. A., Hamburg, B., & deGoza, S. Adaptive problems and mechanisms in severely burned patients. *Psychiatry,* **16:**1-20 (February 1953).
2. Martin, H. L., Lawrie, J. H., & Wilkinson, A. W. The family of the fatally burned child. *Lancet* **295:** 628-29 (September 14, 1968); Martin, H. L. Antecedents of burns and scalds in children. *British Journal of Medical Psychology,* **43,**39-47 (March 1970); Martin, H. L. Parents' and children's reactions to burns and scalds in children. *British Journal of Medical Psychology,* **43,**183-91 (1970).
3. Vigliano, A., Hart, L. W., & Singer, F. Psychiatric sequelae of old burns in children and their parents. *American Journal of Orthopsychiatry,* **34,**753-61 (July 1964).
4. Andreasen, N. J. C., Norris, A. S., & Hartford, C. E. Incidence of long-term psychiatric complications in severely burned adults. *Annals of Surgery,* **174,**785-93 (November 1971).

28

Sex and serious illness*

BERNIE ZILBERGELD

Although there are some articles scattered here and there in the medical and psychologic literature on the sexuality of seriously ill patients, the subject has not received nearly the amount of attention it deserves. Until very recently the bulk of the literature on sex and serious illness focused primarily on the limitations of sexual expression in people with various medical conditions, noting, for example, that high proportions of patients with a certain disease were impotent or nonorgasmic or had a lower rate of sexual activity than before becoming ill. The articles said little about what these people could do to improve the situation or how health professionals could be of help, and they said even less about the desirability and importance of sexual expression for seriously ill people.

While it is true that patients with serious medical problems are concerned about many things besides sex, it is also true that many such patients are interested in their sexuality. They wonder how much of a man or woman they still are; if they are still attractive and desirable, and how their performance will be affected by their condition and treatment—in short, just what they can and can not do sexually. Because these issues are important to many patients, they should be important to health care professionals, at least insofar as we are committed to dealing with people rather than diseases.

Some people have little or no interest in sexual activity, and others find it so burdensome or boring that they are only too happy to have a medical reason for giving it up altogether. It goes without saying that we should not put any pressure on people who feel this way to do other than what they want. For the rest of this discussion, however, I want to focus on the large number of patients who feel otherwise: those who are interested in sexual expression.

Good sex is essential to the sense of well-being of these people. It helps them feel more like whole men and women still able to give and receive pleasure. It is also a way for them to remain close to their partners and feel comforted at a time when much in their lives is bleak and painful. Having sex can be a temporary escape from the harsh realities of a difficult situation. In brief, sex can bring pleasure and help patients feel good about themselves.

Nevertheless, if sex becomes a problem either because the medical condition makes a patient and/or partner afraid to engage in it or because a dysfunction develops, not only are that patient and partner deprived of the potential joy and sense of well-being, but there is now another prescribed activity, another failure, another bit of misery with which to contend. Frustration, unhappiness, and strife in the relationship between patient and partner can result.

*Serious illness, while not a precise term, refers to any medical condition more serious than a cold or flu. I use this term to indicate that the points in this presentation apply not only to patients with cancer and heart disease but also to those with other medical problems, for example, arthritis, diabetes, blood pressure abnormalities, cerebral palsy, spinal cord lesions, as well as major surgery of almost any type.

Sex is important for another reason. Many people in our culture believe that it is inextricably tied to physical affection, or touching, and that they should not touch or be touched unless they are ready and willing to go on to sexual activity. They fear leading their partners on or as one man put it, "I don't want to start anything I can't finish." Yet touching is extremely important in its own right. It is, at least potentially, a powerful means of comforting and being comforted, of caring for and feeling cared for, and of maintaining a sense of connection with loved ones. During times of stress and illness, it can provide a tremendous amount of solace.

We need to bring up touching and sex in order to separate the two, so that patients can do whatever is most appropriate for them; so that, for example, a patient can feel free to enjoy physical affection without feeling compelled to go on to sex.

The following case illustrates what often happens with sex and serious illness.

Jack is a 43-year-old man with testicular cancer. Seven months before coming to see me he had had two operations in which one testicle and the retroperitoneal lymph nodes were removed. Subsequently he was treated with radiation and chemotherapy. Before the surgery he had enjoyed an active sex life with his fiancée, Marti. They had also done much nonsexual touching, and, although their communication patterns had not been as well developed as they might have been, the couple had done enough talking to deal with most of the important issues in their relationship.

After the surgery, Jack was unable to have an erection. He was quite depressed about this; in fact, the lack of erections caused him much greater concern than the cancer. His whole relationship with Marti was in trouble.

She was completely turned off to sex. It was difficult for her to express herself for fear of hurting Jack, but she was gradually able to give voice to her complaints. She was bothered by Jack's significant loss of weight during and after his hospitalization

and annoyed that he always wore a hairpiece to cover his baldness (a result of the medical treatment). She was hurt and angry that he was no longer interested in touching and that he seemed to have only one thing on his mind since his surgery—sex. She said that his sex drive had increased tenfold since his return from the hospital. He never got an erection, but that didn't stop him from trying, and Marti was tiring of the whole show.

I saw Marti and Jack four times during a period of 5 weeks. At first I just helped them to talk to each other and clear the air. A number of important things had gone unsaid for a long time. Jack could not do anything about his weight loss, but he could at least understand that Marti liked it better when he was heavier. He had not realized how much his wig offended her, how much she missed the touching they used to do (when he thought about it, he realized that he also missed it), and how much she resented his constant demand for sex (actually, he had not been aware of just how often he was asking for sex). Marti seemed relieved just to get her feelings out in the open. Both of them learned something important about Jack's increased sexual desire: It really had nothing to do with sex. Rather it was an attempt to prove that everything was back to normal. In response to a question from me during our first meeting, Jack answered that erections and sex "would prove that I'm really okay, that I'm normal, as good as any other guy, that everything is going to be fine."

I asked them to continue their talking at home and suggested that Jack start to differentiate between his desire for sex and his desire to prove himself. When he felt the latter he could tell Marti about it if he wished, but he should not try to have sex. I also suggested that they resume nonsexual touching.

As the weeks went by, Jack and Marti started getting along better. They developed a greater understanding of themselves and of each other; they could say what they thought and felt, and they were doing things that felt good to both of them. They even started talking about their fears of the future, a subject that had been neatly camouflaged by the constant go-arounds about sex. During one of the touching exercises I had asked them to do, they both became highly aroused and went on to a satisfying sexual experience.

Jack's erections returned and his sexual desire decreased to its prehospitalization norm. Marti's sexual interest returned when the touching was reinstated and when Jack stopped trying to have sex all the time.

I knew something important had happened the last time I saw them—Jack was not wearing his wig and they seemed more in tune with each other than before. I called approximately 2 months later to see how things were going and was told that they were getting along well and sex was fine.

I don't want to end this presentation on a note of false optimism. Jack still has cancer and his future is uncertain. That is the hard reality of the case. But he and Marti are enjoying each other, and their relationship is not in danger of disintegrating because of sexual difficulties.

Let us take a closer look at some of the salient points of this case.

First, both Jack and Marti were overwhelmed by feelings they did not know how to handle. Jack feared for his life (with good reason) and desperately tried to use his hypersexuality to prove there was nothing to fear. His fears and frenzied attempts to have sex only served to block effective sexual response. Marti had similar fears, felt cheated (by the lack of touching and talking), and also felt perplexed and angered (by Jack's increased sexual demands). Further she had some negative feelings about Jack's physical appearance and felt guilty for having them. After all, Jack was seriously ill and what happened to his body was not his fault. How could she justify her negative reactions?

Second, both Jack and Marti and their relationship were suffering. Neither partner felt they were getting what they wanted, and Marti had several times considered breaking the engagement. The sexual problem was having serious ramifications and could hardly be called trivial.

Third, no medical authority in the hospital or out, had said anything to Jack or Marti about touching, sex, or the feelings that might occur as a response to Jack's illness and treatment. Jack's doctor talked to him in detail about many other aspects of recuperation (for example, diet, medication, and return to work) but said nothing about any personal, emotional, or sexual issues. No one talked to Marti about anything either, even though she visited Jack in the hospital every day and accompanied him to most of his follow-up appointments.

The tragedy of this case is that the problems Jack and Marti presented to me could easily have been prevented had one of the health professionals treating Jack talked to the couple about possible emotional reactions, touching, and sex. If someone had spent as few as 30 to 60 minutes discussing these issues with Jack and Marti, I doubt that they would have needed to see me.

Why didn't anyone take the time to talk to this couple or, more generally, why aren't the emotional and sexual lives of patients given serious consideration? It is difficult to say with certainty, but several possibilities suggest themselves.

In the first place, most people consider surgery, medication, nutrition, and exercise to be subjects that are more or less objective, medical, and essential, whereas they view feelings and sex as complex issues that are not necessarily vital to recovery. The most important concern apparently is to ensure the patient's survival and physical well-being. Anything else is a luxury not worth bothering about.

In addition it takes time to deal with sex and feelings, and time is always in short supply. Most health workers find it acceptable to spend time discussing treatment (although some believe that even this is a necessary evil), whereas they consider it a waste to spend any time dealing with the emotional and sexual responses to an illness and its treatment.

All of this is compounded by the fact that many health professionals are not comfortable dealing with sexual issues. Neither their personalities, experience, nor training equips them to resolve problems in this area.[2,5,6] Even those who have some interest and are comfortable with the subject voice the concern that they would soon be out of their range of competency. It is as if they believe that, since they are not sex experts or fully trained sex therapists, there is no point in raising the issue at all.

A last possible reason for health care personnel not confronting sexual issues is the depressing array of ideas, presented in medical schools and the medical literature, regarding sex and serious illness. One could easily get the impression, and many health professionals certainly have, that certain types of people (for example, older persons, diabetics, paraplegics and quadriplegics, those with heart disease, and those with some kinds of cancer) can not or should not engage in sex. This belief is so widespread that it deserves further discussion.

It is true that many people with serious illnesses do have problems with sex, but the conclusion that the illness causes the sexual problem is often erroneous. In reality, the illness or condition is usually *not* what causes the sexual difficulties. As Jaffe[4] points out:

Loss of sexual function due to medical factors in terminal illness is less extensive than is often assumed. Nonetheless, a self-fulfilling prophecy persists on the part of the patient, spouse and care-giver: a terminally ill individual will neither be interested nor able to function effectively in sex. This assumption may have evolved from people's association of cancer with pain, such that significant others try to spare their loved ones any additional discomfort. Yet this belief is not necessarily valid, for severe pain occurs in less than 15 per cent of cancer patients. Thus, emotional reactions of the patient, family, and care-giver are as important in precipitating sexual dysfunction as is the illness itself.

My own experience and that of others who have worked with seriously ill patients support Jaffe's statement as far as it goes. I would go even further, however, and argue that the emotional reactions of patients and those around them are far more important in the precipitation of sexual problems than the illness itself. What is true for terminally ill patients is even truer for patients with serious though not terminal conditions.

Patients with serious illnesses are usually depressed, afraid, confused, and perhaps angry as well. All of these feelings can interfere with sexual interest and functioning. In addition, these patients no longer fit our culture's prototype of sexuality, if indeed they ever did. All of us have learned that sex is for the young, the healthy, and the agile, and further that sex should be spontaneous and passionate with no room for special considerations or needs. Sex should be, in the words of novelist Erica Jong, a "zipless fuck," where not even clothing offers any obstacle.

But what of people who have real obstacles and needs? Where is there room in this picture for a woman with only one breast, or for a man or woman whose body has been ravaged by disease or treatment, or for a person who has to take medication before engaging in sex or has to keep some handy in case it is needed during sexual activity? What about a woman who is no longer confident of her ability to lubricate or respond in some other way or a man who isn't sure he'll have an erection? What about patients who find certain postures and positions painful and are no longer agile? What about persons who fear that too much excitement or movement will cause themselves or their partners pain or a need for medication?

Forced to confront their own mortality and the realization that they no longer meet the cultural standard of sexual desirability and being anxious about sex as well as many other things, seriously ill or disabled persons not surprisingly often have trouble with sex or give it up altogether. But it does not have to be that way. Results that I and others have achieved with seriously ill or disabled patients strongly suggest that no matter what the disease or condition, if a patient desires to be sexually expressive, some degree of satisfaction is almost always possible. It probably will not be a "zipless fuck," but it nonetheless can be enjoyable to patient and partner, a source of well-being, warmth, and pleasure.

WHAT CAN BE DONE?

The suggestions that follow are intended only as general guidelines. Obviously, different institutions and situations require different emphases. It makes little difference who actually deals with patients' sexuality; it could be a doctor, a nurse, a nurse practitioner, a social worker, or anyone on the staff who is comfortable with the subject and has some skills in the area. Whoever it is, however, there is no need for him or her to be a fully trained sex therapist.

1. It is essential to educate health care staff about the sexual needs and problems of patients: Sex is important to many patients. They want help in this area, and without such help they are likely to develop problems. As examples of these assertions, the results of two studies are instructive.

In a study of long-term patients, Sadoughi and associates[8] found that more than half said they would have liked to discuss sexual issues prior to discharge. In a survey of cardiac patients by Tuttle,[9] two thirds of the group reported a significant and lasting reduction in sexual activity. Tuttle's analysis is particularly interesting:

Having received little or no advice from their physicians, these patients set their own patterns which represented a considerable deviation from their previous activity. Our interviews suggested that this change in behavior was based on misinformation and fear.

2. In planning treatment, consider sexual consequences and discuss them with the patient. Certain procedures and medications are more likely to cause sexual difficulties than others. The patient has the right to know about possible consequences so that he or she can make the decision that is most appropriate. A patient with little or no interest in sex may agree to a radical procedure, whereas another patient to whom sex is important may elect a treatment that has less chance of interfering with sexual functioning even though it may not be what the physician would recommend.

3. Include the patient's sexual partner in discussions and decisions about sex whenever possible. The partner's understanding and cooperation are crucial. Leaving the partner out is almost certain to result in problems. If a patient does not have a partner, this fact should form part of the discussion about sex. Masturbation and other forms of self-pleasure can be explored, as well as the patient's plans for finding partners in the future (assuming, of course, that the patient desires to be sexual with a partner). Some patients without partners believe that no one will want them now that they are sick or disabled. Dealing with this issue often takes some time, as well as therapeutic skill, and a referral may be required.

4. Give patients and their partners some ideas about possible emotional reactions to the illness and treatment. It is important for patients and partners to know that the illness and treatment might cause them to feel depressed, angry, or whatever; this awareness can help dispel any guilt they might develop about their feelings. It is important that they have some understanding of how they may react to their feelings. Some patients try to prove their health and deny their feelings of depression and helplessness by becoming hypersexual, whereas others are so overcome by their feelings of unattractiveness and fear of failing that they avoid sex altogether. Giving patients some information about what to expect will help them deal with whatever reactions they have. Recall that Jack and Marti were given no information about their possible feelings and reactions; their problems were a direct result of this oversight.

If a patient or partner needs someone to talk to in detail about his or her reactions, it is helpful if someone on the staff can either serve this function or make a referral to someone who can.

5. Include touching and sex in any discussion with patients about other aspects of their illness and recuperation. The caregiver needs to determine what the patients' interests in these areas are and how they may best be served.

Dispensing accurate information and correcting erroneous beliefs is especially important. As one example, many cardiac patients and their partners fear that sexual activity will precipitate another heart attack and that the patient will die in the midst of intercourse. The available data do not support this contention. Sexual activity is not dangerous for most cardiac patients provided that they follow a few rules, for example, have sex with a long-term partner in familiar surroundings and restrict the amount of food and alcohol consumed before sex.[10]

6. Encourage patients to be physically affectionate with their partners throughout their hospitalization and treatment to whatever extent possible, not only because of the support and warmth touching supplies but also because its continuation will make possible a smoother transition to sexual activity when that is appropriate.

7. Instruct the patient or couple to return gradually to sexual activity in ways that permit a maximum of comfort and enjoyment and a minimum of pressure and anxiety. Remind them that sex may not be as it was before (obviously it is helpful to have some information on their previous pattern of sexual expression), at least not right away. It might be helpful to suggest some of the graduated exercises used by sex therapists. For example, rather than trying to have intercourse the first time, a couple could give each other full body massages or take turns giving each other sexual pleasure by hand or mouth with no pressure for lubrication, erections, or orgasms.

In general the principles for resuming sexual activity are no different from those governing the resumption of other activities. Even athletes understand that they cannot go out and run 5 miles at a fast pace immediately after surgery or treatment for a serious illness. They have to get back into running gradually by first taking short walks, then longer ones, then jogging a bit, then longer but still slow runs, etc. The same principle applies in sex.

Health workers can help a patient understand that sex is not an all or nothing activity. The patient should do whatever feels comfortable at the moment and stop whenever stopping seems advisable. This is often difficult to carry out because of the patient's desire to satisfy his or her partner and because of the fear of misleading or frustrating that partner. The caregiver can help by pointing out that there are many ways to satisfy a partner (for example, intercourse is not always necessary) and that the long-range sexual interests of both partners will be served best if the patient does only what is comfortable. The importance of including the partner in such discussions is obvious.

8. Follow sexual issues just as you keep track of other issues. When the patient returns for follow-up visits and examinations, the health professional should inquire about sex and make suggestions when appropriate. The rule is: Let the patient know you have a continuing interest in his or her sexuality.

9. If serious problems develop or if you as a caregiver realize that you do not have the time, interest, or skill to take patients as far as they want to go, give them other resources to which to turn. Reading is a valuable aid for many patients. Although most of the medical literature is too technical or depressing for most patients, many health associations (for example, cancer, heart, ostomy, diabetes) have useful pamphlets on sex. There is still a large need for better quality and more readily available manuals for patients with different illnesses and conditions, a need that I hope will be filled in the near future. A model for such books is the fine manual for paraplegics and quadriplegics recently published by Mooney and associates.[7] Some women patients will benefit from reading *For Yourself*[1] or *Becoming Orgasmic*,[3] even though these books do not deal in detail with illness;

Male Sexuality[11] will be useful to some men.

Other patients will need referrals to competent sex therapists. Fortunately there is a sufficient supply of such therapists in most metropolitan centers.

10. Finally something must be said about the hospitals in which so many of the patients we are talking about spend so much of their time. While many of these institutions are marvels of technologic efficiency, hardly any are organized to meet the personal and psychologic needs of their patients. Little thought has been given to the patient's need for privacy and intimacy. Aside from prisons and military installations, I cannot think of another institution for adults in which it is normal practice for authorities to come into a room without knocking. It seems contradictory to talk about touching, emotional expression, and sex in such a situation.

If we take the sexuality of chronically or terminally ill people seriously, we must do whatever we can to ensure that our patients have the privacy to meet their needs, whether these be having an intimate conversation with a partner, touching a partner, masturbating, enjoying sexual activity with a mate, or just having time to be alone and think.

REFERENCES

1. Barbach, L.: For yourself, New York, 1975, Doubleday & Co., Inc.
2. Ebert, R., and Lief, H.: Why medical students need sex education. In Lief, H., and Karlen, A., eds.: Sex education in medicine, New York, 1976, Spectrum.
3. Heiman, J., LoPiccolo, L., and LoPiccolo, J.: Becoming orgasmic, Englewood Cliffs, N. J., 1976, Prentice-Hall, Inc.
4. Jaffe, L.: The terminally ill. In Gochros, H., and Gochros, J., eds.: The sexually oppressed, New York, 1977, Association Press.
5. Lief, H.: Medical students' life experiences and personalities. In Lief, H., and Karlen, A., eds.: Sex education in medicine, New York, 1976, Spectrum.
6. Lief, H., and Ebert, R.: A survey of sex education in U.S. medical schools. In Lief, H., and Karlen, A., eds.: Sex education in medicine, New York, 1976, Spectrum.
7. Mooney, T., Cole, T., and Chilgren, R.: Sexual options for paraplegics and quadriplegics, Boston, 1975, Little, Brown & Co.
8. Sadoughi, W., Leshner, M., and Fine, H.: Sexual adjustment in a chronically ill and physically disabled population: a pilot study, Archives of Physical Medicine and Rehabilitation, **52:**311-317, 1971.
9. Tuttle, W., Cook, W., and Fitch, E.: Sexual behavior in post-myocardial infarction patients, American Journal of Cardiology. **13:**140-153, 1964.
10. Wagner N.: Sexual behavior and the cardiac patient. In Money, J., and Musaph, H., eds.: Handbook of sexology, Amsterdam, 1977, Elsevier.
11. Zilbergeld, B.: Male sexuality, Boston, 1978, Little, Brown & Co.

29

Understanding the psychologic factors in rehabilitation

HERBERT G. STEGER

As the number of individuals surviving into old age increases, the number of elderly persons being treated in comprehensive rehabilitation programs also increases. Rehabilitation care, in contrast to acute medical care, typically requires a holistic approach to the patient[1] and an understanding of the psychologic and social factors that influence him, his disability, and the rehabilitation process.

Understanding the psychologic factors in rehabilitation of the physically disabled elderly patient is especially significant for two general reasons. First, the elderly patient is in a markedly different life-cycle period than younger patients. The life-cycle issues confronting the elderly patient affect his adjustment to disability and his involvement in rehabilitation activities. Second, rehabilitation is largely concerned with restoring the maximum independent function possible, to allow the patient to overcome or compensate for functional losses. Such rehabilitation efforts rely heavily on the patient's learning new skills—from simple motor skills to the complicated social skills necessary to establish and maintain successful "positive dependence."[1] However,

Reprinted from Geriatrics © 1976 (May) by Harcourt Brace Jovanovich, Inc.
This work was supported in part by project grant 44-P-45065/9-14 from the Rehabilitation Services Administration, Office of Human Development, United States Public Health Service.

the elderly patient may be seriously hampered in acquiring new learning in the rehabilitation setting because of problems with motivation, sensory loss, emotions, memory loss, or intellectual deficits that can be associated with illness and disability.

IMPACT OF DISABILITY AND THE LIFE CYCLE

Sudden onset of severe physical disability is a life crisis with great psychologic impact.[1,2] In many ways, the disabled patient is confronted with a psychologic task similar to that of coping with certain impending death or with the death of a loved one. He must grieve through, accept, and adjust to permanent physical, functional, psychologic and social losses.

The typical reaction to sudden, permanent disability is denial of its significance, seriousness, or permanence. Such a denial phase may serve to temporarily protect the patient from the full, terrible impact of his injury; however, denial also may reflect either his relative ignorance about or inexperience with his disability and its implications or his previous experiences of recovery from acute, reversible illness. A patient who is able to progress from denial typically experiences a period of depression, which is interpreted as mourning for the actual and potential losses resulting from the disabilty. This period appears to be an important component in becoming able to accept the losses and the changes they

243

have brought. Full acceptance of the disability is often accompanied by a transition in the patient's orientation—from losses to potential, from the past to the present and future, and from being a sick person to being a different person.[2] The process of giving up the past and accepting the reality and potential of the present and future, which is so important for resolution of sudden physical disability, also seems to describe a significant existential task for all human development.

This is an idealized model of the impact of disability and the process of adjustment, based primarily on observations of adults who have had a sudden, irreversible disability. However, a number of variables, including both the type of onset of disability and the patient's age, can influence the impact of disability.[3] For example, gradual onset of functional losses allows a patient to make gradual physical and psychologic accommodation to the changes and imposes less strain on his coping skills than does sudden disability. Similarly, the impact of disability differs according to the patient's life-cycle stage and the development tasks influenced by the disability.

The elderly are in a life-cycle period characterized by significant and manifold personal losses.[4] Comfort[5] has described this period as one in which "Our most cherished performances, mental, sexual, and social; the esteem of our fellows; and our own sense of identity will deteriorate. This process is even more bitter than death." Coping with these losses presents significant developmental tasks. The elderly person has to accept and adjust to a deteriorating body, reduced sexuality, a dependent pattern of living, reversal of the child and parent roles, receiving more than he is capable of giving, and a reduction in extent and complexity of social group involvement, with an eventual return to the simpler, face-to-face relationships[6] that also characterize the world of the infant. Resolution of the problem of dying is another major task confronting the elderly.[4]

Successful performance of develop- mental tasks can enhance and lead to further development of the aged person's personality. For many disabled elderly patients in rehabilitation programs, however, the primary issues of physical deterioration and adjustment to their losses remain unresolved and are the source of considerable maladaptive coping, which adversely affects the rehabilitation process. Physical illness, for example, has been frequently associated with depression[7,8] and suicide[9,10] in aged patients. Goodman[11] and Zarit and Kahn[12] have suggested the significance of depression in reaction to serious physical illness and disability. Many elderly persons perceive serious illness and disability as being developmentally "overdue," foreshadowing serious physical deterioration and death. Elderly persons without significant cortical dysfunction are less likely than younger persons to deny their condition and are more depressed. Thus, they are less likely to experience a problem with denial in postdisability adjustment, possibly because the implications of disability are much more apparent and foreboding and may even be expected.

THE DEPRESSION CAUSED BY LOSSES

The depression in disabled elderly patients is somewhat different from that in younger persons,[7,8] although it appears quite similar to the depression or mourning that is experienced by younger disabled patients. External reality losses, particularly the losses associated with physical disability, play a more significant role in depression in the elderly than do guilt and covert, unexpressed hostility, which usually underlie depression. Dovenmuehle[8] found that his disabled elderly patients often became depressed when attempting to perform some previously gratifying behavior that had been part of their ordinary daily life. The patient's inability to dress himself after a stroke, for example, can prove to be not only a hindrance to independent living but also a cause of continued depression. Fordyce[13] has pointed out that such behaviors, which previously were useful but which no longer result in the desired positive consequences, not only contribute to the patient's depression but also may cause him to withdraw from rehabilitation because of the punishing effects of failure and the pain or discomfort that result from his efforts.

A traditional psychotherapeutic approach to management of this mourning depression in the disabled elderly person may not be helpful, since the physical disability is so frequently the basis for the patient's emotional symptoms. In describing such a situation. Dovenmuehle[8] said, "Since neither the psychiatrist nor the patient had any immediately effective alternatives to personal suffering, the end result was destructive in that it associated relationship with the psychiatrist with destructive emotional experience." Fordyce[13] has suggested attempting to deal directly with what appears to underlie the patient's depression or grieving: the sudden ineffectiveness of his behavior and the deprivation of positive reinforcers that results from the disability. Rehabilitation efforts should maximize the positive results of the patient's behavior by assuring him that he can successfully achieve the treatment task and expected performance increments, by providing large amounts of positive reinforcement for his rehabilitation efforts, and by minimizing failure or criticism. This approach attempts to alleviate depression by focusing on behavior rather than to treat the depression as a way of influencing behavior. It appears to be an appropriate method of working with the disabled elderly person whose depression is related to reality losses, who may not respond favorably to traditional psychotherapeutic efforts, and for whom the long-term benefits of achieving the goals of the rehabilitation program provide questionable motivation.

As previously mentioned, disabled elderly patients must be understood in the context of the large number of losses that characterize their life period. For many such persons, the losses resulting from disability only add to a long list of accumulated dep-

rivations. Aging already has stripped them of family, companions, vocation, recreation, finances, belongings, prestige, and social roles, as well as physical health. Disability often is the final blow to tenuously maintained independent living, so that acceptance of a dependent, institutionalized status becomes unavoidable. Such losses are significant in rehabilitation, since they not only affect the patient's emotional status but also make it difficult for natural rewards to maintain and extend the behavioral and functional gains achieved during rehabilitation. For a younger patient, improvement in mobility opens a variety of rewarding activities and naturally serves as a basis for still further functional gains. It is thus unnecessary to focus on continual reinforcement of ambulation, even though this may have been necessary during rehabilitation training. However, for the elderly disabled person in a nursing home or even in a private residence, there are few rewarding involvements that serve to maintain self-care skills or other functional gains achieved in rehabilitation. In fact, competing responses characteristic of the dependent patient role are often rewarded by family or institutional care, and the elderly person's efforts at self-care and independence frequently meet with frustration and failure if not outright punishment and rejection.

PHYSICAL DETERIORATION AND THE SICK ROLE

Disability in the elderly occurs during a life period when chronic health problems are likely to be an additional major concern. In fact, identifying oneself as "old" appears to be not so much a matter of chronological age as an association with sickness, disability, or physical weakness.[14] A common feature of old age is "body monitoring,"[15] a vigilance about bodily functions that previously required little or no attention but that now demand time, attention, and effort. Such monitoring can become a hypochondriacal way of life when chronic disease or disability is present. Preoccupation with physical functioning and care may serve as a compelling way for an elderly person to avoid loneliness, a feeling of failure, anxieties, and depression over losses.[16] Thus, the involvement in the chronic sick role[17] can serve as a socially approved, even expected way for the elderly to escape the stresses of aging and also can provide a substitute social role during a time when role losses have deprived them of social identity, at a time when "individual old people must forge their own roles—when and where they can."[15]

When the chronically ill or newly disabled elderly patient enters a health care setting, he quite likely will find the sick role or patient role to be rewarding because of the staff's attention. This is particularly true if he has been experiencing social and interpersonal deprivation and isolation.[18] Unfortunately, such professional concern and attention in acute medical settings typically depend on the patient's illness and on his expression of the appropriate sick role behaviors. In helping the patient abandon the sick role to assume the more active, participating role required in rehabilitation, the staff should remember that the patient's previous alternative to the sick role may have been loneliness, unhappiness, and isolation. Withdrawing staff attention and concern because of sick role behaviors can result in an increase in his physical complaints, dependence behaviors, or depression in an effort to recapture the staff's interest.

The staff must provide sufficient support and incentive for the elderly patient to abandon the sick role, especially if it was his major social role before hospitalization. Alternative, rewarding roles should be available for the patient in the hospital during rehabilitation. He should be involved, when appropriate, in activities such as decision making, determining therapy goals and schedules, personal housekeeping, disposition planning, self-medication, and providing senior functions[4] for the younger patients. Such activities, with relinquishment of the passive, dependent sick role,

can help the elderly patient effectively come to grips with the developmental task of accepting and adjusting to a deteriorating body[6] or achieving a body transcendence rather than a body preoccupation.[19] However, because the sick role focuses attention away from an empty life, loneliness, and losses and provides a meaningful social role and powerful social reinforcement from medical institutions and professionals, the elderly person may find it difficult or even impossible to give up, particularly since few viable alternatives are available in our society.

In aged persons, personal interests and goal orientation typically undergo an alteration away from family, career, achievement, and success and toward more existential concerns, greater orientation to internal and personal issues,[20] and a greater need for personal safety and security. This reorientation and the manner in which it is realized, together with situational factors such as illness and losses and lifelong personality and coping patterns, to a large extent determine an elderly person's behavior. An individual's successful adaptation to life-stage tasks can result in continued personality growth and potential, just as failure to cope successfully can mean maladjustment, stagnation, anxiety, and despair.[4]

Because the increased depression, isolation, and dependence on the sick role resulting from physical disability can contribute to maladaptive coping, rehabilitation efforts should include helping elderly persons to resolve regressive developmental tasks[6] and, when possible, the problem of death. These are critical issues for the future of these patients—just as significant for rehabilitation as vocational and educational concerns are for disabled adolescents and young adults. The common failure of rehabilitation programs to deal with these issues may reflect young rehabilitation workers' belief in a lack of potential in the aged, the rejection and fear of the elderly[5] that pervade our society, or perhaps the legacy of a cultural perspective that growth and development in the life cycle are childhood phenomena, preparing one for maturity, and that the later years represent merely the deterioration and dissolution of that full-bloomed maturity.

LEARNING DURING REHABILITATION

During and after rehabilitation, the elderly are confronted not only with psychologic adjustment to disability but also with a variety of learning tasks directed at attaining a degree of functional independence. Even though research has shown that *healthy* elderly persons are intellectually normal and do not fit the cultural stereotype of senility, elderly persons with physical illnesses, especially chronic conditions, are likely to have intellectual, memory, and learning problems. The learning problems of brain-damaged patients, particularly stroke patients, and the approaches to their rehabilitation management have been well documented.[21] However, an actual deficit in the learning ability of elderly persons without brain damage has not been documented. They have not proved to be rigid and untrainable. The difficulties encountered appear more likely to be a result of the motivational, task, and performance factors that confront them in learning situations.

Elderly patients have numerous motivational problems that can hinder learning in the rehabilitation setting. For example, they tend to be quite cautious and are likely to avoid situations that present a risk of failure or embarrassment.[22,23] This may be reflected in their lack of involvement in rehabilitation activities or in tentative involvement only when they are sure of success, which contributes to their greater number of errors of omission than of commission.[24] Approaches that can be valuable in adapting rehabilitation training to overcome the cautiousness of the elderly include maximizing patients' opportunities for success, avoiding criticism or other negative reinforcement, allowing them to select a task and set performance goals as much as possible, and avoiding involving them in childish tasks in which a failure to perform would cause embarrassment. Posi-

tive reinforcement helps to assure the most effective rehabilitation learning and helps in maintaining a supportive environment for these patients. Although underinvolvement and apathy about task performance might be expected in the elderly, some research has suggested that patients can become overinvolved and overaroused.[24] Emotional overarousal tends to interfere with task performance and can cause difficulty in learning and retaining the skills necessary to accomplish the task. For example, evaluation situations can pose considerable difficulty for elderly patients. In these situations, they are particularly vulnerable to the stress of failure, because participation usually is not a matter of choice, they are not able to select the tasks, and they cannot avoid failure since tasks are presented to demonstrate deficit areas. A supportive atmosphere can be established during the assessment by interspersing success with failure, using either liberal time standards or none at all, reducing competitive implications of the patients' performance, and finishing the evaluation with tasks the patients can accomplish.

The personality and developmental changes with aging that lower competitiveness and desire to achieve success also reduce the importance of subjecting the present for future gain. The merits of hard work or postponing gratification in order to attain future reward are much less motivating for elderly individuals than for younger ones.[25] Thus, it is difficult to expect that the promise of abstract future benefits from rehabilitation will generate much active involvement in treatment. Instead, the outcome and benefits of treatment presented to patients should be fairly concrete, utilitarian, and related to their immediate life situation.

Learning tasks themselves can inhibit the elderly patient in acquiring new learning. The rate of speed at which task materials are presented can have a significant effect, since an elderly person tends to respond more slowly than a younger one.[23] When material is presented too quickly, the patient will have difficulty in mastering the task. However, if he is allowed to set the pace himself, he will show much less deficit in his performance. Learning tasks in which materials are presented in novel fashion also tend to cause problems. Therefore, innovations in rehabilitation therapy or procedures, to which a younger patient adapts readily, can cause difficulty for an elderly patient. It is important to attempt to discover whether the patient has preferred learning styles or techniques and any areas of particular vocational or avocational interest that can aid him in rehabilitation. For example, the staff can modify a patient's hobby of stamp collecting to provide for training in memory, perceptual accuracy, perceptual motor skills, and socialization, as well as for motivation and reward for rehabilitation performance.

The meaningfulness or the relevance of a rehabilitation task plays an important role in the elderly patient's involvement and performance. Rehabilitation tasks related to his daily care activities have a high degree of meaning and relevance. However, a considerable number of tasks may appear to be irrelevant, demeaning, and even infantile; indeed, many have been developed for use with infants. In evaluation and treatment activities, maintaining as much relevance as possible to the patient's daily life should insure greater involvement and better performance.

COMMENT

A wish to avoid reminders of their future and mortality, pervasive social rejection of the elderly, and the lack of rewarding outcome in work with elderly patients may prevent some rehabilitation professionals from discovering the level of interest, challenge, and attraction in working with the aged that they find in involvement with younger patients. Certainly, rehabilitation efforts, no matter how intense or motivated, cannot be expected to change a lifelong pathologic personality pattern, compensate for devastating losses, slow the process of aging, or prevent eventual death. However, helping the elderly disabled patient to ac-

tively cope with the psychologic problems of aging and disability—behavioral, developmental, and existential—during the process of rehabilitation will enable him to benefit more from treatment and assure him of a better opportunity to realize the emotional and behavioral potential of advancing years.

ACKNOWLEDGMENT

Dr. Daniel J. Feldman contributed significantly to my awareness and understanding of the human response to illness and disability through seminars on somatopsychiatry conducted at the University of California, Irvine.

REFERENCES

1. Feldman, D. J. Chronic disabling illness: A holistic view. J. Chronic Dis. 27:287, 1974.
2. Adams, J. E. Lindemann, E. Coping with long-term disability. In Coelho GV, Hamburg D. A., Adams, J. E. (Editors): Coping and Adaptation. New York, Basic Books, Inc., Publishers, 1974.
3. Safilios-Rothschild, C. The Sociology and Social Psychology of Disability and Rehabilitation. New York, Random House, Inc., 1970.
4. Butler, R. N. Toward a psychiatry of the life-cycle: Implications of sociopsychological studies of the aging process for the psychotherapeutic situation. Psychiatr. Res. Rep. Amer. Psychiat. Assoc. 23:233, 1968.
5. Comfort, A. What price longevity? Med. Wld. News: Geriatrics/1971, p. 18.
6. Barrett, J. H. Gerontological Psychology. Springfield, Ill., Charles C Thomas, Publisher, 1972.
7. Gordon, S. K. The phenomenon of depression in old age. Gerontologist 13:100, 1973.
8. Dovenmuehle, R. H. The relationship between physical and psychiatric disorders in the elderly. Psychiatr. Res. Rep. Amer. Psychiat. Assoc. 23:81, 1968.
9. Kiev, A. Treating depression in the elderly. Chronic Dis. 8:2, 1974.
10. Weiss, J. M. A. Suicide in the aged. In Resnick, H. L. P. (Editor): Suicidal Behaviors: Diagnosis and Management. Boston, Little, Brown and Company, 1970.
11. Goodman, M. N. Age and adaptation to acute illness (myocardial infarction). Proc. Am. Psychol. Assoc. 7:657, 1972.
12. Zarit, S. H., Kahn, R. L. Aging and adaptation to illness. J. Gerontol. 30:67, 1975.
13. Fordyce W. E. Psychological assessment and management. In Krusen, F. H., Kottke, F. J., Ellwood P. (Editors): Handbook of Physical Medicine and Rehabilitation. Philadelphia, W. B. Saunders Company, 1971.

14. Riley, M. W., Foner, A. Aging and Society, New York, Russell Sage Foundation, 1968.

15. Butler, R. N., Lewis M. I.: Aging and Mental Health: Positive Psychosocial Approaches. St. Louis, The C. V. Mosby Company, 1973.

16. Busse, E. W., Pfeiffer, E.: Functional psychiatric disorders in old age. In Busse, E. W., Pfeiffer, E. (Editors): Behavior Adaptation in Late Life. Boston, Little, Brown and Company, 1969.

17. Kassebaum, G. G., Baumann, B. O. Dimensions of the sick role in chronic illness. J. Health Hum. Behav. 6:16, 1965.

18. Granick, S. Psychological study in the management of the geriatric patient. In Chinn, A. B. (Editor): Working with Older People: A Guide to Practice. Clinical Aspects of Aging. U. S. Public Health Service Publication No. 1459. Washington, D. C. U.S. Government Printing Office, 1971, vol. 4.

19. Peck, R. C. Psychological developments in the second half of life. In Andersen J. E. (Editor): Psychological Aspects of Aging. Washington, D. C., American Psychological Association, 1956.

20. Neugarten, B. L.: Perspectives of the aging process. Developmental aspects. Psychiatr. Res. Rep. Amer. Psychiatr. Assoc. 23:42-48, 1968.

21. Diller, L.: Perceptual and intellectual problems in hemiplegia: Implications for rehabilitation. Med. Clin. North Am. 53:575, 1969.

22. Donahue, W.: Psychologic aspects. In Cowdry, E. V. (Editor): The Care of the Geriatric Patient. St. Louis, The C. V. Mosby Company, 1968.

23. Schaie, K. W.: Translations in gerontology—from lab to life: Intellectual functioning. Am. Psychol. 29:802-807, 1974.

24. Botwinick, J.: Aging and Behavior. New York, Springer Publishing Company, Inc., 1973.

25. Stotsky, B. A.: Coping with advancing years. In Brown, L. E., Ellis, E. O. (Editors): Quality of Life: The Later Years. Acton, Mass, Publishing Sciences Group Inc., 1974.

PART VII

The chronically ill child

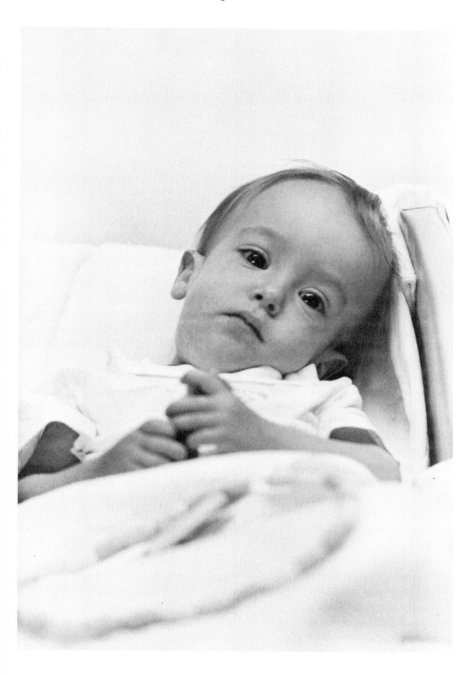

30

Long-term physical illness in childhood: a challenge to psychosocial adaptation

AKE MATTSSON

Robert Louis Stevenson, a victim of pulmonary tuberculosis, once wrote, "Life is not a matter of holding good cards, but of playing a poor hand well." Children with a chronic physical disorder who have successfully mastered the physical, social, and emotional hardships associated with their illness well illustrate his point. This paper intends to review the common forms of emotional stress experienced by the child with a long-term illness and by his parents. It also describes the major adaptational techniques enabling the sick child and his family to achieve a satisfactory psychosocial adaptation.

Long-term or chronic illness refers to a disorder with a protracted course which can be progressive and fatal, or associated with a relatively normal life span despite impaired physical or mental functioning. Such a disease frequently shows periods of acute exacerbations requiring intensive medical attention. Long-term childhood disorders may cause significant and permanent interference with the child's physical and emotional growth and development. This is in contrast to acute non-life-threatening illnesses in which both physical dysfunctioning and attendant emotional up-

set usually are of a limited duration and do not as a rule interfere with the child's overall development.[1,2]

The prevalence of chronic conditions in childhood is staggering if visual and hearing impairments, mental retardation, and speech, learning, and behavior disorders are included. Such a scope yields an estimate of 30% to 40% of children up to the age of 18 suffering from one or more long-term disorders.[3] Even if only serious chronic illnesses of primary physical origin are included, American and British surveys still report that 7% to 10% of all children are afflicted.[4,5] The most common physical conditions are asthma (about 2% of the population under age 18), epilepsy (1%), cardiac conditions (5%), cerebral palsy (5%), orthopedic illness (5%), and diabetes mellitus (1%). Less frequencies pertain to cleft palate, bleeding disorders, anemias, blindness, and deafness.

The following classification of long-term childhood disorders is based on consideration of ontogenetic stages and nature of pathogenic factors:

1. Diseases due to chromosomal aberrations (e.g., Down's syndrome, Klinefelter's syndrome, Turner's syndrome)

2. Diseases as results of abnormal hereditary traits (e.g., spherocytosis, sickle cell anemia, hemophilia, cystic fibrosis, muscu-

Reprinted from Pediatrics **50**:801-811, 1972. Copyright American Academy of Pediatrics, 1972.

253

lar dystrophy, osteogenesis imperfecta, diabetes mellitus, inborn errors of metabolism; certain forms of "congenital malformations" such as microcephaly, clubfoot, cleft palate, dislocation of the hip, blindness, and deafness)

3. Diseases due to harmful intrauterine factors (e.g., infections such as rubella, congenital syphilis, and toxoplasmosis with their attendant malformations; damage from massive radiation, various drugs, prenatal hypoxia and blood type incompatibilities)

4. Disorders resulting from perinatal traumatic and infectious events including permanent damage to central nervous system and motor apparatus

5. Diseases due to serious postnatal and childhood infections, injuries, neoplasms, and other factors (e.g., meningitis, encephalitis, tuberculosis, rheumatic fever, chronic renal disease; physical injuries with permanent handicaps; tumors and leukemia; orthopedic diseases; convulsive disorders; atopic conditions; mental illness and mental retardation of organic etiology)

PSYCHOLOGIC IMPACT OF LONG-TERM ILLNESS

Children with long-term physical disorders are subjected to a multitude of emotionally stressful situations, often of a recurring nature. Acute illnesses pose similar psychologic threats which usually prove less harmful due to their shorter duration.[1,2,6-10] The common causes for emotional stress associated with long-term illness are:

Malaise, pain, various physical symptoms, and reasons for illness

Uncertainty as to why pain and suffering occur is a psychic stress to anyone. The preschool child in particular has little ability to comprehend the causality and nature of an illness and tends to interpret pain and other symptoms as a result of mistreatment, punishment, or "being bad." In a child's mind nothing happens by chance, and he looks for reasons for an event such as an illness in the immediate past.[11,12] Children up to the ages of 8 to 10 often attribute illness and injury to recent family interactions, e.g., they got sick because of their disobedience or because the parents failed to protect them. They might then blame themselves or other family members for causing the disease. These distorted interpretations of their bodily changes often become perpetuated by their reluctance to ask questions and vent their irrational fears about why they became ill. Other examples of children's crude cause-and-effect reasoning relative to illness are: A young colitis patient blamed his illness on having "eaten something dirty"; a child with cardiac disease had "run too much"; a diabetic girl had "eaten too much candy"; a hemophilic boy developed a hematoma because his "skin was so thin."

Young patients afflicted with a hereditary illness will usually learn of the likely genetic transmission before or during adolescence. Under whatever circumstances this knowledge is obtained by the child, it is potentially traumatic to the child-parent relationship. Many such children voice hostile accusations against their parents, as they try to master the anger, sadness, and anxiety aroused by their recognition of the hereditary nature of their disability.

Hospital admissions, nursing, and treatment procedures

The often frequent and lengthy hospital admissions, for the chronically ill child involve separations from his family, school, and set of friends. He is expected to adjust to an unfamiliar, regimented hospital environment, with a confusing array of health specialists and frightening, often painful medical procedures.[7,13,14] Again, it is the preschool child that tends to suffer most from these stressful separations from the trusted family setting. Such repeated episodes can be destructive to the child unless a strong "therapeutic alliance" between his parents and the medical staff provides him with a plenitude of visiting and care by the mother, a homelike ward setting, and ample information and preparations regarding procedures.[8,10,13,15]

Any ill person who receives nursing care at home or in a hospital experiences feelings of helplessness, embarrassment, and irritation. To be "treated like a child" during an illness is often more upsetting to a young patient than to an adult.[6,7,11] A bedridden child, unable to dress and feed himself and to use the bathroom without help, resents the loss of such recent gains in his development. The less ill he feels, the stronger his resentment. Anger, humiliation, and anxiety about the backward pull toward a state of helpless dependency are frequently observed, and the hospital staff and the parents may become targets of defiant protests. Some children regress to more babyish behavior without much protest and need considerable help to regain achievements in motor and social functioning after an illness.

Injections, infusions, immobilization, surgery, and other procedures arouse anxiety beyond the discomfort involved, because they reactivate the universal childhood fears of bodily mutilation and disfigurement and the illogical views of medical procedures as a punishment for actual or imagined misdeeds. Such fantasies generally cause less problems for the older grade school child, because his strides in cognitive development enable him better to comprehend the causal and temporal relationship of an illness or injury.[12] Most sick children find immobilization and restriction of activity emotionally stressful. They rely on freedom of movement to discharge tension, to express dissatisfaction and agression, and to explore and master the environment. Sudden or prolonged motor restraint of a young child can cause him to panic, develop temper tantrums, and become a serious management problem. At other times, he might show the opposite reaction of withdrawal into an apathetic, depressed state. The child with poor ability or lack of opportunity to verbalize his feelings is more prone to show marked behavioral reactions to forced restraints.

Changes in the emotional climate

Family members tend to change their attitudes toward their sick child and usually become more loving and indulgent, letting up on discipline and rules.[6] Changes in the opposite direction are rare but potentially more dangerous: Some parents reject their ill child, criticize him for causing much inconvenience, and even neglect his care. Any of these changes in family attitudes can be confusing to the child as, for instance, when he has to relinquish the secondary gains of being sick.

Stress factors related to special chronic syndromes

Certain aspects of causation, symptomatology, and medical care of many long-term illnesses pose special problems and fears to the child and his family. Some common examples of such situations follow.

Fluctuations in the control of *juvenile diabetes* frequently seem related to emotional factors.[16,17] The diabetic child, along with his family, may worry about attacks of hypoglycemia or acidosis as a result of highly emotionally charged family interaction. Some adolescents in rebellious, hostile, or depressed states abandon their diabetic regime as angry and self-destructive means to threaten or retaliate. This abandonment is often conscious, which indicates a far more serious maladjustment than the chronically ill person's common use of his ailment as an escape or a defense.

Similar to the young diabetic patient, the child with a *convulsive disorder* frequently fears loss of consciousness or uncontrollable strange behavior while suffering from a seizure. Seizures are socially stigmatizing especially when they take place at school and among peers. The epileptic teen-ager feels uniquely frustrated, as he cannot obtain a driver's license until after several years without seizures. This prolongs his dependence on the parents for providing transportation in regards to many school and leisure activities.

Children with *serious respiratory disease,* such as asthma[18-20] and cystic fibrosis,[21] commonly harbor fears of suffocation, drowning, or dying while asleep. The asthmatic child often finds that his wheezing will evoke anxious, indulgent, and sympathetic responses from his family, whose members may feel responsible for contributing to his attacks of labored breathing and discomfort.

The child with cystic fibrosis has to cope with such embarrassing symptoms as flatulence and stool odor, with the complex management of postural drainage and nebulization, and with the growing awareness that his illness is hereditary and progressive, carrying a poor prognosis.

Chronic bleeding disorders, such as hemophilia, often cause the young child to be concerned about fatal bleeding resulting from physical trauma and certain medical procedures, e.g., venous puncture. Emotional distress might increase the likelihood of bleeding in face of minor physical trauma or even lead to "spontaneous" bleeding episodes without apparent trauma.[22,23]

The child with a *chronic heart disease* of infectious or congenital nature often has minimal signs of a serious condition and may find it difficult to comprehend the nature of his illness and the reasons for restrictions, extensive work-ups, and surgery. Furthermore, the knowledge of an affliction of one's heart seems especially frightening due to the common ambiguous and symbolic references to "the heart" in everyday language.[24,25] An active psychoeducational preparation for heart surgery is of special importance since states of marked apprehension and depression may complicate cardiac surgery in childhood and adolescence.[26]

An increasing number of children with *chronic renal disease* are treated with hemodialysis and kidney transplantation. Several unique features pertain to these procedures.[27,28] The life-perpetuating kidney machine often creates frightening fantasies in the child, such as fears of bleeding to death or of the machine assuming control of him. The use of immunosuppressive drugs causes Cushingoid appearance and inter-

feres with the child's growth, already stunted by preexisiting uremia. Consequently, these young patients often feel isolated and apart. This may be particularly difficult for the teen-ager, seeking independence from his family and a sense of identity among his peers. After kidney transplantation, many children find their parents tending to overprotect them and to use threats implying possible failure of the new kidney as a means of controlling their activities. The occurrence of "kidney rejection anxiety" at times of minor physical symptoms has been observed in children as long as six years after a successful transplantation. In cases of actual kidney rejection, requiring a return to hemodialysis, the young patient, like the adult, usually responds with a depressed, withdrawn state. Children in particular then tend to blame themselves for "destroying" the kidney given to them as a special gift, often by a family member. It should be noted, however, that follow-ups on children who have undergone renal transplantation have found many of them showing growth spurts as long as five years after surgery and a good adjustment as young adults.[29]

Children with *ulcerative colitis* and similar conditions often have unrealistic fears of certain food items harming them. Their frequent inability to control defecations cause much embarrassment. The common family preoccupation with the ill child's diet and with his stools requires energetic pediatric counseling. These children and their families often have to be prepared for a temporary or permanent ileostomy when other treatment methods fail. Such a procedure entails many realistic problems which are particularly stressful to an adolescent as he is beginning to establish intimate heterosexual friendships.[30] The counseling assistance of an older person with a successful ileostomy can be useful in supporting the young patient's self-image and confidence.

The recent interest in children and teenagers of *short stature,* often complicated by delayed sexual maturation,[31] has shown that a major problem of the undersized child is related to his environments's tendency to baby him "as a dwarf" instead of treating him according to his chronological age. His sense of uniqueness may cause him to withdraw, leading to an inhibition of his cognitive and emotional development.[32] Some short youngsters cope by an excessive denial of their condition and become either good-natured jokers with few agressive strivings or spunky and overly assertive individuals.

The format of this paper does not permit further illustrations of specific emotional stress factors associated with many chronic handicaps and disorders in childhood, such as mental retardation,[33] brain dysfunction and cerebral palsy,[34-37] congenital amputees,[38,39] orthopedic conditions,[40] cleft palate,[41] and cryptorchism.[42] Helpful reviews of the psychological implications of long-term sensory, motor, visceral, and metabolic conditions in young patients are given by Prugh,[8] Apley and MacKeith,[10] Vernon et al.,[14] Kessler,[43] and Green and Haggerty.[44] The unique emotional burdens associated with fatal illness in childhood and adolescence have recently been reviewed by Friedman[45] and Easson.[46]

Additional psychologic threats

The child with a serious, chronic disease has to cope with threats of exacerbations, lasting physical impairment, and, at times, a shortened life expectancy. Other common concerns of his and his family relate to mounting medical expenses and the interference of his illness with schooling, leisure activities, vocational training, job opportunities, and later adult role as a spouse and a parent. In learning to live with a disability that demands continuous medical attention often away from home, the growing child is expected to assume responsibility for his own care and accept certain limitations in his activities.

The final outcome of the child's attempts at mastering the continuous stress associated with his disability cannot be assessed until young adulthood. Each progressive step in his emotional, intellectual, and social development changes the psychologic impact of the illness on his personality and on his family and usually equips him with better means to cope.[37,47] Changes in the disease process and in familial circumstances will also affect the adaptational process.

COPING BEHAVIOR AND ADAPTATION IN CHILDREN

Several authors have used the conceptual framework of coping behavior to describe the responses of children and parents to such severe stress situations as serious illness, separation, and the threat of death.[23,48-51] This term denotes all the adaptational techniques used by an individual to master a major psychologic threat and its attendant negative feelings in order to allow him to achieve personal and social goals. Coping behavior, then, includes the use of cognitive functions (perception, memory, speech, judgment, reality testing), motor activity, emotional expression, and psychologic defenses. (Defenses represent unconscious processes aiming at reappraisals and distortions of a threatening reality to make it more bearable.[48,52]) Successful coping behavior results in adaptation, which implies that the person is functioning effectively.

Many studies on long-term childhood disorders report a surprisingly adequate psychosocial adaptation of children followed to young adulthood.[7,8,10] These well-adapted patients have for years functioned effectively at home, in school, and with their peers, and with few limitations other than those realistically imposed by their disease and its sequelae. Their dependence on their family has been age-appropriate and realistic, and they have little need for secondary gains offered by the illness. From age 6 to 7, these children's use of such cognitive functions as memory, speech, and reality testing provided them with a beginning understanding of the nature of their illness. This allowed them to accept limitations, assume responsibility for their care, and assist in the medical management. This appropriate appearance of a sense of self-protection served the vital function of self-preservation and precluded the development of helpless, inactive dependence on their environment.[53] While slowly accepting his physical limitations, the well-adjusted child finds satisfaction in a variety of compensatory motor activities and intellectual pursuits, in which the parents' encouragement and guidance assumes great importance.

In addition to cognitive flexibility and compensatory physical activities, the appropriate release and control of emotions is an essential coping technique. The expression of anxious, sad, impatient, and angry feelings at times of exacerbations, and of confidence and guarded optimism during periods of clinical quiescence is characteristic of well-adapted children with a chronic illness.

In terms of psychologic defenses, most of these patients use denial as well as isolation in coping with their emotional distress caused by pain, malaise, and interrupted plans. They also show an adaptive use of denial of the uncertain future, which enables them to maintain hope for recovery at times of crisis, for more effective medical care, and for a relatively normal, productive adult life. Identification with other young and adult patients afflicted with a chronic handicap is a helpful defense for many children. Learning about and associating with others who are successful in dealing with similar problems can effectively support the development of a positive self-image as a socially competent and productive individual. Many of the well-adapted young patients display a certain pride and confidence in themselves as they become successful in mastering the ongoing stress associated with their illness.

The nature of the specific illness appears less influential for a child's successful adaptation than such factors as his developmental level and available coping techniques, the quality of the parent–child relationship, and the family's acceptance of the handicapped member.[8,10,12] Regarding the latter point, the parents' ability to master their initial reaction of fear and guilt,

and their tendency to overprotect the child, has received much emphasis.[8,23,54-57]

Children and adolescents with prolonged poor adjustment to their chronic disorder tend to show one of the three following behavioral patterns.[8,22,23] One group is characterized by the patients' fearfulness, inactivity, lack of outside interests, and a marked dependency on their families, especially their mothers. These youngsters present the psychiatric picture of early passive dependent states and their mothers are usually described as constantly worried and overprotective of them.

The second group contains the overly independent, often daring young patients, who may engage in prohibited and risk-taking activities. Such youngsters make a strong use of denial of realistic dangers and fears. At times their reality sense is impaired and they seem to seek out certain feared situations, challenging the risk of trauma. Since early childhood, many of these rebellious patients have been raised by oversolicitous and guilt-ridden mothers. Usually at puberty, they rebel against the maternal interference and turn into overly active, defiant adolescents.

A third, less common pattern of maladjustment is seen in older children and adolescents with congenital deformities and handicaps. They appear as shy and lonely people harboring resentful and hostile attitudes toward normal persons, whom they see as owing them payment for their lifelong sufferings.[58] Usually these patients were raised in a family that emphasized their defectiveness and tended to isolate or "hide" them in an embarrassed fashion. They came to identify with their family's view of them and developed a self-image of a defective outsider.

These illustrations of prolonged maladaptation to a chronic illness differ from more temporary situations, where the disease and its management become the vehicle for conflicts between the patient and his parents, siblings, friends, or school. Overt or covert refusal to cooperate in the medical regimen can be used as an effective weapon by a resentful young patient. Practically all children with a chronic disability will occasionally try to take advantage of their disease in order to avoid unpleasant situations, as for instance a disciplinary action or a school test.

EMOTIONAL STRESS AND COPING BEHAVIOR OF PARENTS

When a serious, long-term illness afflicts a child, the initial reaction of his parents usually includes acute fear and anxiety related to the possible fatal outcome of the disease. A closely associated stage is that of parental disbelief in the diagnosis, particularly if the obvious signs of illness have subsided.[55] The parents might then complain about being poorly informed by the physician and occasionally "shop around" for additional medical opinion, which will disprove the initial diagnosis. Beyond those denying, often uncooperative attitudes of the parents, feelings of mourning the "loss" of their desired normal child and feelings of self-blame in regard to their ailing child usually begin to emerge.[24,54] When the parents become aware of and can verbalize these feelings, they are able to accept the reality of the serious disability and its impact on the whole family.

A crucial factor in determining the parents' acceptance is their ability to master resentful and self-accusatory feelings over having transmitted or in some way "caused" their child's disorder.[23,54-57] Those parents who remain highly anxious and guilt-laden about their ill child tend to cope with their emotional distress by overprotecting and pampering him, and by limiting his activities with other children. Such prolonged parental overconcern, usually more prominent among mothers, can often be related to one of the following predisposing factors:[47,59] The child suffered a life-threatening condition at birth or as an infant, from which the family did not believe he would recover; the child is afflicted with a hereditary disorder present among relatives; the child's illness reactivates emotional conflicts in the parents stemming from the past death of a close relative; or the child was unwanted, causing a mixture of loving and rejecting feelings, particularly in the mother.

Any child being raised by oversolicitous, controlling, and fearful parents senses the parental expectation of his vulnerability and likely premature death.[59] He may either accept this tacit view and assume passive–dependent characteristics, or he may rebel against the parents' concerns and become a daring, careless youngster, who seems to challenge their notions of his fragile condition.

The factors mentioned here as common determinants of prolonged parental overconcern also may lead to parental rejection or neglect of a disabled child and to extreme parental denial of the severity of the illness. These latter types of reaction are infrequent compared to the former one of overprotection. Again, strong unresolved feelings of guilt for the child's illness are often present in such detached and uncooperative parents.[10,23] They may talk angrily about all the inconvenience their child's ailment causes the family, and they often blame crises and complications on the child or the medical staff. In addition, they frequently "forget" instructions about the home care and are inconsistent in guiding their child. Such a child, when sensing the parental rejection, will often respond with both despondent and defiant attitudes, which greatly jeopardize his clinical condition.

Parents who have successfully adapted to the challenge of raising a chronically ill child will enforce only necessary and realistic restrictions on him, encourage self-care and regular school attendance, and promote reasonable physical activities with his peers. These well-adapted parents use some common psychologic defenses in coping with the constant strain caused by their child's illness.[60] For example, they tend to isolate and deny their anxious and helpless emotions, especially during a medical crisis, which helps them to remain calm and assist effectively in the medical care. When the crisis is over, many parents experience a rebound phenomenon of feeling depressed and irritable, indicating that certain painful affects have been denied consciousness until that time when it is safer to experience them.

It is common among parents of handicapped children to show attitudes of critical superiority toward health specialists, particularly toward house officers. Some of this criticism may be valid, but one also senses that the parents are trying to ward off, by denial, their long-standing helpless feelings in this manner. They may also displace and project helpless and angry feelings about their child's condition onto various medical professionals and blame them for delays or mistakes in treating their child. Closely related to denial is rationalization, that is, the defensive use of rational explanations, valid or invalid, in an attempt to conceal some painful emotions from oneself. One commonly hears from parents of chronically ill children that the disorder has enriched the whole family, both emotionally and spiritually, and has developed their sense of compassion and tolerance. While indeed there may be some truth in such statements, these attitudes assist the parents—often the healthy siblings too—in hiding from themselves sad and resentful affects related to their unique burden.

All effectively coping parents, along with their sick children, use intellectual processes to master distressing emotions caused by the illness; that is, they rely on the coping technique of "control through thinking."[61] The parents often make it a point to learn all they can about the medical, physiological, and even the psychological aspects of the disease. Thus, they lessen their anxiety by familiarizing themselves with the likely future course of development of the child.

The association and identification with other parents of seriously ill children is helpful to many parents. Informally and in group discussions, at times conducted by a health specialists, they can share many of their distressing hardships and learn to adopt more realistic and relaxed child caring attitudes and also pass on their positive experiences to less knowledgeable parents.[33,60]

CONCLUSION

The successful psychological management of a child with a long-term physical illness and his family depends on two interrelated factors:[8,10,23,55,56,62] (1) the continuous "personalized" support and counseling by the physician, who should be alert to all the incompatible feelings with which both the the patient and his parents are coping; these affects are normal reactions, which often will subside if given time and verbal expression; and (2) the parents' acceptance of the disease with its uncertain course and impact on the family, which implies that they have gradually mastered their conflicting emotions aroused by their child's ailment.

The parents as well as their child require repeated, truthful, and comprehensible information about the illness, its etiology, and therapeutic concepts. Whenever possible, they should be prepared for procedures and likely changes in clinical manifestations. Such preparation helps to mobilize their intellectual functions and psychologic defenses to cope with the anticipated stress. The physician should make sure that his explanations and plans are understood by the parents and the young patient, and well coordinated with the collaborative efforts of his medical, nursing, and social service colleagues. The medical team and the parents can greatly assist the ill child by encouraging him to ask questions and to verbalize distressing feelings.

The parents need instruction to develop in their child an increasing responsibility for self-care and protection. The goal of raising the handicapped child as normally as possible may be achieved by promoting reasonable activities with other children and regular schooling, modified by individual needs. Overprotection and undue restrictions, both at home and in school, should be discouraged. The father's active involvement in the child-rearing can be fostered by his assuming major responsibility for helping his ill youngster to succeed in compensatory activities and interests. In terms of the healthy siblings, the physician should assess whether they are receiving needed parental love and attention as well as acceptance of their frequent feelings of anxiety, resentment, and guilt toward their ailing brother or sister.

The physician should tactfully call attention to parental attitudes of overindulgence, lenient discipline, or neglect which can endanger the child's emotional growth. He may suggest a psychiatric consultation when he notices many unresolved conflicts in the parents responsible for prolonged overprotective, inconsistent, or rejecting handling of the child. Psychiatric intervention can also be of value for some young patients with marked difficulties in adapting to their long-term illness, such as children showing defiant, risk-taking behavior, a fearful, passive dependence, or hostile, embittered attitudes toward their environment and life situation.

REFERENCES

1. Mattsson, A., & Weisberg, I. Behavioral reactions to minor illness in preschool children. *Pediatrics,* **46,** 604, 1970.
2. Carey, W. B., & Siblinga, M. S. Avoiding pediatric pathogenesis in the management of acute minor illness. *Pediatrics,* **49,** 553, 1972.
3. Stewart, W. H. The unmet needs of children, *Pediatrics,* **39,** 157, 1967.
4. Pless, I. B. Epidemiology of chronic disease. *In* M. Green & R. J. Haggerty (Eds.) *Ambulatory pediatrics.* Philadelphia: W. B. Saunders Co., 1968. Pp. 760-768.
5. Rutter, M., Tizard, J., & Whitmore, K. *Handicapped children. A total population prevalence study of education, physical, and behavioral disorders.* London: Longmans, 1968.
6. Freud, A. The role of bodily illness in the mental life of children. *Psychoanalytic Study of the Child* **7,** 69, 1952.
7. Langford, W. S.: The child in the pediatric hospital: Adaptation to illness and hospitalization. *American Journal of Orthopsychiatry* **31,** 667, 1961.
8. Prugh, D. G. Toward an understanding of psychosomatic concepts in relation to illness in children. *In* A. J. Solnit & S. A. Provence (Eds.), *Modern perspectives in child development.* New York: International Universities Press, 1963. Pp. 246-367.
9. Shrand, H. Behavior changes in sick children nursed at home. *Pediatrics,* **36,** 604, 1965.
10. Apley, J., & MacKeith, R. *The child and his symptoms.* Philadelphia: F. A. Davis company, 1968. Pp. 209-215, 216-240.
11. Jessner, L. Some observations on children hospitalized during latency. *In* L. Jessner & E. Pavenstedt (Eds.), *Dynamic psychopathology in childhood.* New York: Grune and Stratton, Inc., 1959. Pp. 257-268.
12. Freeman, R. D. Emotional reactions of handicapped children. *In* S. Chess & A. Thomas (Eds.) *Annual progress in child psychiatry and child development, 1968.* New York: Brunner Mazel, 1968. Pp. 379-395.
13. Robertson, J. *Young children in Hospitals.* New York: Basic Books, 1958.
14. Vernon, D., Foley, J., Sipowicz, R., & Schulman, J. *The psychological responses of children to hospitalization and illness. A review of the literature.* Springfield, Illinois: Charles C Thomas, 1965.
15. Mason, E. A. The hospitalized child—his emotional needs. *New England Journal of Medicine* **272,** 406, 1965.
16. Swift, C. R., & Seidman, F. L. Adjustment problems of juvenile diabetes. *Journal of the American Academy of Child Psychiatry* **3,** 500, 1964.
17. Tietz, W., & Vidmar, T.: The impact of coping styles on the control of juvenile diabetes. *Psychiatry in Medicine* **3,** 67, 1972.
18. Dubo, S., McLean, J., Ching, A., Wright, H., Kauffman, P., & Sheldon, J. A study of relationships between family situation, bronchial asthma, and personal adjustment in children. *Journal of Pediatrics* **59,** 402, 1961.
19. Purcell, K., Brody, K., Chai, H., Muser, J., Molk, L., Gordon, N., & Means, J. The effect on asthma in children of experimental separation from the family. *Psychosomatic Medicine* **31,** 144, 1969.
20. Purcell, K., & Weiss, J. H. Asthma. *In* C. G. Costello, (Ed.), *Symptoms of psychopathology.* New York: John Wiley & Sons, 1970. Pp. 597-623.
21. McCollum, A. T., & Gibson, L. E. Family adaptation to the child with cystic fibrosis. *Journal of Pediatrics* **77,** 571, 1970.
22. Agle, D. P. Psychiatric studies of patients with hemophilia and related states *Archives of Internal Medicine* **114,** 76, 1964.
23. Mattsson, A., & Gross, S. Social and behavioral studies on hemophilic children and their families. *Journal of Pediatrics* **68,** 952,1966.
24. Glaser, H. H., Harrison, G. S., & Lynn, D. B. Emotional implications of congenital heart disease in children. *Pediatrics,* **33,** 367, 1964.
25. Toker, E. Psychiatric aspects of cardiac surgery in a child. *Journal of the American Academy of Child Psychiatry* **10,** 156, 1971.
26. Barnes, C. M., Kenny, F. M., Call, T., & Reinhart, J. B. Measurement in management of anxiety

in children for open heart surgery. *Pediatrics, 49,* 250, 1972.

27. Abram, H. S. Survival by machine: The psychological stress of chronic hemodialysis. *Psychiatry in Medicine* **1**, 37, 1970.

28. Bernstein, D. M. After transplantation—the child's emotional reactions. *American Journal of Psychiatry* **127**, 1189, 1971.

29. Lilly, J. R., Giles, G., Hurvitz, R., Schroter, G., et al. Renal homotransplantation in pediatric patients, *Pediatrics*, **47**, 548, 1971.

30. McDermott, J. F., & Finch, S. M. Ulcerative colitis in children. Reassessment of a dilemma. *Journal of the American Academy of Child Psychiatry* **6**, 512, 1967.

31. Rothchild, E., & Owens, R. P. Adolescent girls who lack functioning ovaries. *Journal of the American Academy of Child Psychiatry* **11**, 88, 1972.

32. Money, J., & Pollitt, E. Studies in the psychology of dwarfism: II. Personality maturation and response to growth hormone treatment in hypopituitary dwarfs. *Journal of Pediatrics* **68**, 381, 1966.

33. Mandelbaum, A. The group process in helping parents of retarded children. *Children,* **14**, 227, 1967.

34. Birch, H. G. *Brain-damage in children. The biological and social aspects.* Baltimore: Williams & Wilkins Co., 1964.

35. Gardner, R. A. Psychogenic problems of brain-injured children and their parents. *Journal of the American Academy of Child Psychiatry* **7**, 471, 1968.

36. Chess, S., Korn, S. J., & Fernandez, P. B. *Psychiatric disorders of children with congenital rubella.* New York: Brunner Mazel, 1971.

37. Minde, K. K., Hachett, J. D., Killon, D., & Silver, S. How they grow up: 41 physically handicapped children and their families. *American Journal of Psychiatry* **128**, 1554, 1972.

38. Gurney, W. Congenital amputee. *In* M. Green & R. J. Haggerty (Eds.), *Ambulatory pediatrics.* Philadelphia: W. B. Saunders Co., 1968. Pp. 534-540.

39. Roskies, E. *Abnormality and normality: The mothering of thalidomide children.* Ithaca, New York: Cornell University Press, 1972.

40. Myers, B. A., Friedman, S. B., & Weiner, I. B.: Coping with a chronic disability: Psychosocial observations of girls with scoliosis treated with the Milwaukee brace. *American Journal of Diseases of Children* **120**, 175, 1970.

41. Tisza, V. B., & Gumperty, E. The parents' reactions to the birth and early care of children with cleft palate. *Pediatrics* **30**, 86, 1962.

42. Cytryn, L., Cytryn, E., & Rieger, R. E. Psychological implications of cryptorchism. *Journal of the American Academy of Child Psychiatry* **6**, 131, 1967.

43. Kessler, J. W. *Psychopathology of childhood.* Englewood Cliffs, New Jersey: Prentice-Hall, 1966. Pp. 332-367.

44. Green, M., & Haggerty, R. J. (Eds.). Part VII. The management of long-term illness. *In Ambulatory pediatrics.* Philadelphia: W. B. Saunders Co., 1968. Pp. 441-768.

45. Friedman, S. B. Management of fatal illness in children. *In* M. Green & R. J. Haggerty (Eds.), *Ambulatory pediatrics.* Philadelphia: W. B. Saunders Co., 1968. Pp. 753-759.

46. Easson, W. M. *The dying child. The management of the child or adolescent who is dying.* Springfield, Illinois: Charles C Thomas, 1970.

47. Mattsson, A., & Gross, S. Adaptational and defensive behavior in young hemophiliacs and their parents. *American Journal of Psychiatry* **122**, 1349, 1966.

48. Murphy, L. B. *The widening world of childhood.* New York: Basic Books, 1962.

49. Friedman, S. B., Chodoff, P., Mason, J. W., & Hamburg, D. A. Behavioral observations on parents anticipating the death of a child. *Pediatrics,* **32**, 610, 1963.

50. Chodoff, P., Friedman, S. B., & Hamburg, D. A. Stress, defenses, and coping behavior: Observations in parents of children with malignant disease. *American Journal of Psychiatry* **120**, 743, 1964.

51. Mattsson, A., Gross, S., & Hall, T. W. Psychoendocrine study of adaptation in young hemophiliacs. *Psychosomatic Medicine* **33**, 215, 1971.

52. Lazarus, R. S. *Psychological stress and the coping process.* New York: McGraw-Hill, 1966. Pp. 258-266.

53. Frankl, L. Self-preservation and the development of accident proneness in children and adolescents. *Psychoanalytic Study of the Child* **18**, 464, 1963.

54. Solnit, A. J., & Stark, M. H. Mourning and the birth of a defective child. *Psychoanalytic Study of the Child* **16**, 523, 1961.

55. Tisza, V. B. Management of the parents of the chronically ill child. *American Journal of Orthopsychiatry* **32**:53, 1962.

56. Green, M. Care of the child with a long-term life-threatening illness: Some principles of management. *Pediatrics* **39**, 441, 1967.

57. Findlay, I. I., Smith, P., Graves, P. J., & Linton, M. L. Chronic disease in childhood: A study of family reactions. *British Journal of Medical Education* **3**, 66, 1969.

58. Freud, S. *Some character types met with in psychoanalytic work: I. The "Exceptions."* (1916). London: Hogarth Press, standard edition, vol. 14, pp. 311-315, 1957.

59. Green, M., & Solnit, A. J. Reactions to the threatened loss of a child: A vulnerable child syndrome. *Pediatrics* **34**, 58, 1964.

60. Mattsson, A., & Agle, D. P. Group therapy with parents of hemophiliacs: Therapeutic process and observations of parental adaptation to chronic illness in children. *Journal of the American Academy of Child Psychiatry* **11**:558, 1972.

61. Bibring, G. L., Dwyer, T. F., Huntington, D. S., & Valenstein, A. F. A study of the psychological

processes in pregnancy and of the earliest mother-child relationship. Appendix B: Glossary of defenses. *Psychoanalytic Study of the Child* **16,** 62, 1961.

62. Solnit, A. J. Psychotherapeutic role of the pediatrician. *In* M. Green & R. J. Haggerty (Eds.), *Ambulatory pediatrics*. Philadelphia: W. B. Saunders Co., 1968. Pp. 159-167.

31

The child with heart disease

FLORENCE BRIGHT ROBERTS

Five-and-a-half-year-old Tommy Jackson is being pushed down the hospital hallway in a wheelchair. He is an attractive child—curly auburn hair, large blue eyes, and at least half a million freckles. But in place of a smile is a very unhappy, peevish frown, and a strained, pinched expression covers his face. His mother is pushing his wheelchair.

"You're pushing me too slow. Go faster. I want to go to the drug store."

"Mommy's awfully tired, Tommy—don't you want to eat your lunch now? We ordered a chocolate milkshake just like you wanted."

"I don't want chocolate—I want strawberry. I don't like chocolate any more. I want that red fire truck in the drug store."

"But Tommy, you just got the blue dump truck this morning."

"I played with it already. I want the fire truck. If you don't get it for me I won't eat any lunch."

"Now, Tommy, dear, you must eat your lunch. We can get you a strawberry milkshake if you want one. I tell you what, let's go down to the drug store and get the fire truck and a strawberry milkshake. We can have lunch there."

Hazel Jackson is a tired, frustrated mother and she can't understand why Tommy is never satisfied. He is an unhappy, frustrated little boy and he can't understand why the things he asks for are never as wonderful as he thought they'd be.

Tommy was born with a rather serious congenital heart defect which required a

Reprinted with permission from American Journal of Nursing **72**:1080-1084, 1972. Copyright American Journal of Nursing Co.

temporary shunt at birth. He progressed well physically but is a little smaller than average. He has just had corrective open heart surgery which the doctor has said makes him essentially a "well child." He should be physically recovered by midsummer and will be old enough to start first grade in September.

But how can Tommy start first grade? He has never played with other children. Though he can dress himself, he prefers his mother to do it. The only person he has ever stayed with when his mother was out of the house is his grandmother. Tommy may never be a "well child" emotionally and socially.

IMPACT ON LIFE-STYLE

The heart is recognized by even young children to be vital in sustaining life. I know of one boy with congenital heart disease who became very fearful as his exercise tolerance diminished. Finally, he told his nurse that he was afraid he would outgrow his heart. He said, "I used to be able to run around the house without stopping. Then I started getting bigger. Now I can walk only to the corner of the house before I have to rest."

Recent publicity on heart transplants has added a new dimension to the average person's awareness of his heart. And children, too, respond to the publicity. One little girl who had undergone open heart surgery became upset as her third postoperative week approached. She had heard on television that a heart transplant patient had died during the third postoperative week and she was convinced that she, too, would die then.

One problem in working with heart patients is that their prognoses are difficult to determine and may change from time to time. Although life and health are uncertain for all people, most assume their own death or the likelihood of illness to be distant or even irrelevant until they are faced with a condition such as heart disease. Then, frequently they say that the uncertainty of their condition is the hardest aspect to bear.

Another problem faced by most heart patients, and one that is of particular importance in working with children, is the chronicity of the condition. Often this results in the whole family's living in a state of chronic anxiety. It is well documented that anxiety is highly communicable, especially in the parent-child relationship. This anxiety, besides using energy needed by the child for physical recovery from disease, can cause severe developmental problems. Shirley says:

From the long-term point of view, the harm is that the anxious child is afraid to grow up. Instead of becoming increasingly independent and self-reliant, the chronically anxious child finds his security in maintaining his dependence on others.(1)

Anxious children have a natural tendency toward dependence and, in addition, often have dependency fostered by parents, especially by mothers who frequently cope with their own anxiety by overprotecting their children.

Another characteristic of heart disease which affects the life-style of the child is the often necessary isolation or partial isolation of the child from normal contacts with his peers. This can cause many problems in social and emotional growth.

Medical care can be expensive in money, time, and energy. Fortunately, many of the children are covered financially by the federally funded Crippled Children's Services, but the inconvenience, extensive travel, and interrupted family routines which even free care demands, are heavy burdens for parents.

THE TEAM

Three aspects of care for children with any chronic disease are crucial to consideration of the specific problems faced by children with cardiac disease. To begin, those who are working with chronically ill patients must function as a team—their communication must be frequent and complete so that the parents and child are not confused by apparent inconsistencies in the treatment plan. I have seen a mother extremely disturbed merely because different physicians used different words to explain their therapeutic plan for her child.

The parents must have complete confidence in their medical team. This team, of course, includes more than the hospital personnel who see the patient only in the acute phases. The parents and even the child himself, if he is old enough, need to participate in planning the care. Others who should also be included are the visiting nurse, school teachers, social workers, and, in many instances, clergymen, who often have a continuing and sustaining relationship with these families.

THE FAMILY

Secondly, one cannot treat any child successfully unless that child is viewed as a member of a family—not its center, but a member of it. The child's interaction within his family has more influence upon his subsequent development than any other experiences. Let those of us who work with children not deceive ourselves; the lasting influence that we as professional persons have upon the child can come only if we work effectively with the family unit, particularly the parents.

The most important aspect of care of the chronically ill child is meticulous, and sometimes frustrating, work with the child's parents, particularly with their feelings and attitudes. The actions of most people, though they like to see themselves as rational beings, are influenced more by feelings and attitudes than by reason. A parent may know that Johnnie should receive penicillin prophylaxis but if that parent believes that all drugs are addictive and harmful if taken over a long period of time, he may not give the medication beyond the acute crisis of an infection. Or, if the parent sees his child as an invalid, the child comes to see himself this way, too.

Another problem to keep in mind is that strong feelings, particularly anxiety, interfere greatly with communication skills, and failure to follow instructions may be a result of distorted perceptions. Many times parental anxiety must be reduced before care can even be discussed.

Most parents, however, do everything in their power to provide the best possible care for their children. Failure to produce desired results is more often due to a lack of effective health teaching than to a lack of parental concern. Parent education is *our* problem, one which needs careful thought and action.

Most parents of chronically ill children need help in seeing their own needs and in meeting them. Too often the care of the child consumes so much time and attention that parents, especially mothers, forget their personal needs and the needs of each other. A person or a couple who is emotionally and physically exhausted cannot continue to give to others in a healthy way. Many parents will feel guilty about using time or other resources to meet their own needs, and they need help in understanding the vital importance to the family of their doing just that.

Other members of the family also need to be considered. Brothers and sisters of the sick child often live in his shadow. Of necessity, parents must use a large portion of their resources for the sick child, but all too often he becomes their consuming interest. Other children may be either ignored or expected to become adult long before they are able to do so. They need not suffer irreparable damage because of illness in the family—but they may, if everyone forgets that they exist.

THE CHILD

The third major point to keep in mind in working with chronically ill children is to find out how the child sees his situation. The child needs to be listened to and encouraged to express, either verbally or through play or drawings, what he thinks is happening to him. The feeling tones the children express come primarily from their parents. Older children, siblings, significant adults outside the family, and peers may also influence their reactions.

Children have been asked in studies why they are sick. The usual answer is that they have been bad(2). Where this idea comes from is not certain, but many times parents inadvertently convey an unspoken threat in trying to get their children to wear sweaters or rubber boots or to slow down and not play so hard. As a result of these admonitions, children may feel very guilty about being sick. In conjunction with this guilt, many children feel that medical care itself is a punishment.

Some parents use doctors and hospitals as overt threats in order to maintain behavioral control over their children. Anna Freud says that a child is not able to differentiate pain caused by disease processes within his body from that inflicted in the course of medical treatment(3). It is well documented that injections, rectal temperatures, and the various pokings and proddings a child experiences during illness are frequently perceived as hostile attacks(4). There are numerous examples also of children perceiving medical personnel as enemies. Laboratory technicians, for example, may be seen as vampires of a sort.

Death and fear of death are not uncommonly sources of anxiety in children. Often this fear is communicated unwittingly by anxious parents, but some believe that most children over three years of age are aware of death sufficiently to fear it(5).

Often associated with fear of death is fear of general anesthesia, as many children, particularly young ones, confuse death and sleep. The child may also fear that some harm in the form of body mutilation may come to him while he is under anesthesia. Careful and honest preparation for procedures or hospitalization or both can prevent many of these misperceptions. But the child must be encouraged to communicate his perceptions; otherwise one can never be sure what he is thinking about his experiences.

RESTRICTION OF PHYSICAL ACTIVITY

Piaget indicates that for preschool and young school-age children, spontaneous movement is equated with life, while death and lack of movement are seen as synonymous(6). To restrict physical movement according to Spitz, is to take away the child's best defense against frustration and anxiety (7). Mastery over one's body is a developmental task of childhood and it requires motor activity in large quantities. It may be helpful to remember that decreasing the child's level of anxiety and frustration will decrease his need for motor activity and that those motor skills most recently acquired are the ones the child is most reluctant to give up. This is why sick toddlers are frequently found standing in their cribs even when exhausted(8).

For the older child, the restricted activity more often is perceived in terms of loss of peer contact and normal activities. Shirley believes that a child's feeling that he is losing out in the process of living is often more prominent in his field of awareness than the fear of physical ill health or death(1). The typical child will resent such restrictions to some degree. Explanations of why they are necessary will help, but firm limits may also be necessary. If a child welcomes the sick role, he may be using it as an escape from his inability to relate satisfactorily to his peers or to meet other demands of daily life successfully. He will need help in giving up this role at the appropriate time.

There is one aspect of heart disease which needs to be considered in viewing children's perceptions: body image. A child's perception of his body and his ability to control and use it has a great influence upon his self-concept.

Cyanotic heart disease may result in severely stunted growth and abnormal skin color. Rheumatic heart disease is often treated with steroids, resulting in obesity. More than one little girl has become severely depressed over her increased appetite and weight gains as a result of steroid therapy. It is amazing to hear the unkind comments and teasing that these children must accept from hospital personnel.

DAILY LIFE

Maintaining as high a degree of normalcy as is possible and continuing treatment routines are two major goals in rearing children who have heart disease. Perhaps the greatest problem for parents in relation to these goals is the consistent use of discipline and limit setting for the sick child.

Because of parental feelings of guilt and anxiety over the child's condition, parents tend to try to compensate the child for his being ill. Often this results in the parents trying to satisfy the child's every wish. Unfortunately, children are naturally demanding creatures and their desires may become insatiable, particularly if they are encountering frustration as they will when ill. Needs, however, are different. Needs must be met. But trying to pacify the child and "keep him happy" may, in fact, interfere with meeting his real needs.

Parents who try to fulfill the child's every wish will not only find they have set an impossible task, but also may discover that they are causing the child actual harm. In the process, the parents become frustrated. The natural sequel to frustration is anger—often expressed by parents as general irritability and inconsistency in dealing with the child's behavior. As the parent becomes aware of his irritability toward the child, his feelings of guilt and anxiety increase and he tries even harder to "be nice" to the child, and thus becomes even more frustrated.

A child needs consistent limits to make his world predictable and therefore nonthreatening. This is particularly true for ill children whose bodies are playing tricks on them. As the child experiences his parents' inconsistency and irritability, his own anxiety increases. One way he deals with anxiety is to attempt to control his environment by increasing his demands. As his demands increase, so do his parents' irritability and inconsistency, perpetuating the cycle.

This vicious cycle can be prevented more easily than it can be corrected. The key factors are anticipatory guidance of parents at the time of diagnosis and continuing guidance throughout the course of the illness.

In working with new parents of a handicapped baby, one must remember the meaning of that baby for the parents and what the birth of a less-than-perfect child represents. Since these parents almost always feel guilty, helping them to handle their guilt constructively is especially important in preventing later relationship distortions.

One scheme that seems to be useful in considering discipline and limit setting is behavior-modification theory which is based on the reward system. Social rewards, such as a smile or a "thank you," are the most valuable in the long run, but sometimes a more concrete reward such as candy or a toy is used briefly to begin the shaping process. The important point to remember is that behavior which is rewarded is reinforced and that which is ignored tends to be extinguished.

We need to help parents, as well as ourselves, to begin to see what behavior we are actually rewarding. If a parent gives a child a toy to make him stop whining and pleading, then the parent is actually rewarding the whining and pleading, and instead of doing away with it, he is really strengthening it. In the same way, we often reinforce regressive behavior whereas we fail to notice or reward steps toward independence and growth. Many times, also, we have to teach a child what behavior is appropriate as well as what is not. Then we must be sure to continue to reward the behavior we desire.

Closely allied with limit setting is the control of activities. Children with cyanotic heart disease will usually limit their own activities to a level of comfort. This is usually quite sufficient. They do need at times, however, to have encouragement to use their energies to develop skills for activities of daily living.

Children with rheumatic fever or rheumatic heart disease present a different management problem: they often have to have external limits set for them because they do not feel sick. One should emphasize what the child *can* do and point out his progress. Here, perhaps more than any other place in the treatment program, involvement and cooperation of the child is necessary.

He should be taught enough about his disease to understand why his activity must be limited and to take a responsible part in limiting his own activities. Sometimes standard concepts may need to be modified. For instance, bed rest, which is frequently prescribed, might not be so restful for a child as playing quietly at a table would be. Craft activities should be encouraged and, as soon as possible, the child should resume schoolwork. The American Heart Association distributes a booklet called *Have Fun . . . Get Well* which is often helpful to parents in suggesting inexpensive activities.

Education is especially important for all cardiac children, as their future job security may depend upon it. They cannot usually compete physically for unskilled jobs(9).

DIET

Infants with serious cardiac defects frequently have feeding problems. Because of reduced oxygenation of the blood, they often tire before feedings are completed and may show mild to severe cyanosis during feedings. Subsequently, they fail to grow and thrive as they should. Since one component of mothering is feeding, successful feedings and growth of the baby are very important to a mother's self-concept.

The frightening cyanotic episodes and the failure of cardiac children to grow often convinces the mother that she is a "bad" mother—a perception most damaging to her own self-esteem and eventually harmful to the mother-child relationship. It is especially desirable for a nurse to visit in the home to demonstrate and supervise feeding techniques until the mother becomes comfortable. Periodic re-evaluations are helpful so that solid foods may be introduced successfully and other changes made as needed.

For the child with rheumatic fever or rheumatic heart disease, a restriction in sodium is occasionally necessary. This can be accomplished without too many inconveniences if the child is helped to understand the necessity. The mother needs to be aware of certain high sodium foods, such as milk and some cola drinks. She needs to be taught also to read labels carefully and to avoid patent medicines, particularly laxatives because of the sodium they may contain. Again, the positive should be emphasized: what the child can eat. Anna Freud has said:

On the whole, considerably less harm is done by the necessity of withholding desired foods than by an anxious mother urging or even forcing unwelcome food on an ill child(10).

MEDICATIONS

Parental accuracy in administration of drugs cannot be assumed and careful teaching and follow-up are essential. A few years ago I briefly surveyed mothers' administration of medications to their chronically ill children. I interviewed 30 middle- and lower-middle-class mothers who were administering a total of 52 drugs. Although the sample was not large enough to be conclusive, I found that more than two thirds of the mothers were not administering the drugs strictly as prescribed. Some of the errors were minor, such as a change in the time of day the drug was given. In other instances, however, the errors included changes in the dosage, the number of doses

given per day, or a discontinuation of the drug—all, as far as I could tell, without the doctor's knowledge. Again, the child should, if at all possible, be made responsible for self-administration with parental supervision.

Let me close with a thought which, though it is not mine originally, summarizes for me the approach most helpful in working with any chronically ill children:

The handicapped child is first a child and, second, a child with a problem.

REFERENCES

1. Shirley, H. F. *Pediatric Psychiatry*. Cambridge, Mass., Harvard University Press, for the Commonwealth Fund, 1963, p. 528.
2. Beverly, B. I. Effect of illness upon emotional development. *J. Pediatr.* 8:534, May 1936.
3. Freud, Anna. Role of bodily illness in the mental life of children. In *Psychoanalytic Study of the Child*, edited by Ruth S. Eissler and others. New York, International Universities Press, 1952, Vol. 7, p. 69.
4. Erickson, Florence H. Helping the sick child maintain behavioral control. *Nurs. Clin. North Am.* 2:695-703, Dec. 1967.
5. Jackson, Nancy A. A child's preoccupation with death. In *ANA Clinical Sessions 1968, Dallas*. New York, Appleton-Century-Crofts, 1968, pp. 172-179.
6. Piaget, J. *Language and Thought of the Child*. New York, Humanities Press, Inc., 1959, p. 204.
7. Spitz, Rene. Anaclitic depression. In *The Psychoanalytic Study of the Child*. New York International Universities Press, 1946, Vol. II, P. 313.
8. O'Grady, Roberta S. Restraint and the hospitalized child. In *Current Concepts in Clinical Nursing*, edited by Betty S. Bergersen and others. St. Louis, C. V. Mosby Co., 1969, Vol. 2, pp. 192-202.
9. American Heart Association, Vocational Advisory Service. *Vocational Counseling for Children With Heart Disease or a History of Rheumatic Fever; a Pilot Study*. New York, The Association, 1961.
10. Freud, *op.cit.*, p. 73.
11. American Public Health Association, Committee on Child Health. *Health Supervision of Young Children*. New York, The Association, 1955.

PART VIII

Understanding pain and suffering

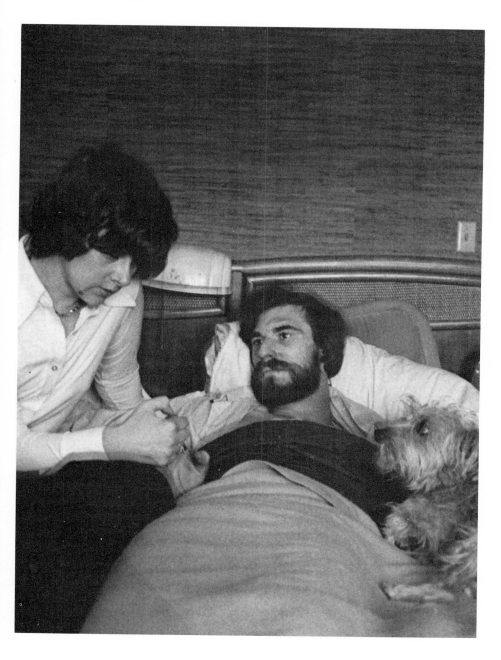

32

The world of the patient in severe pain of long duration*

LAWRENCE LeSHAN

In physical illness there are many situations in which the patient has severe pain of long duration which is impossible or inadvisable to control by chemical or surgical means. The psychotherapist has only very rarely seen this as an area in which his skills may be of use. Only in the use of hypnosis (particularly since its major scientific advances of the past few years) has he worked in this field on any large scale. Outside of this, such psychological help as has been given in an attempt to aid the patient in pain, has been left usually to the clergyman or to the physician. The intuitive understanding they provided has often been of great depth and efficacy, but the time and energy they could bring to bear on the problem has been limited. It would appear that the insights of modern psychology and psychiatry might make worthwhile contributions if applied to the problem.

In the course of a 10-year research program on the psychosomatic aspects of neoplastic disease [1–10] a good deal of time was spent by the writer with patients in severe pain, or facing the threat of severe pain. Certain impressions gained and observations made during this work, may, perhaps, be worth presenting. This paper is an attempt to describe these observations and to provide a tentative philosophical basis for future work in this area by psychotherapists.

Our understanding of pain is usually taken from our experience with acute pain—the toothache, the burn, the cut or bruise. This type of pain is conducted very rapidly in the nervous system, causes defensive reflexes and usually passes quite quickly. We are taught from childhood to regard this as a good and useful warning. We generalize from this to the severe, chronic pain causing genuine suffering which we see in an advanced cancer, a trigeminal neuralgia or a severe arthritis. This generalization leaves much to be desired and its validity is extremely doubtful. There are qualitative differences between the two types. They are apparently discontinuous. In this paper I shall be discussing the second type of pain, the severe chronic type which does not provoke defensive reflexes and which gives the patient no clue at all as to how to lessen it.

The amount of published material on the subject of the situation of the patient in chronic pain is surprisingly small. Buytendjick [11, p. 15], in one of the few serious works on the subject, has commented on this.

"Modern man regards pain merely as an unpleasant fact which, like every other evil, he must do his best to get rid of. To do this, it is generally held, there is no need for any reflection on the phenomenon itself."

Reprinted with permission from Journal of Chronic Disease 17:119-126, 1964, Pergamon Press, Ltd.
*This paper, and the research which led up to it, has been made possible by a grant from Frederick Ayer II.

We shall here be concerned with some aspects of the phenomenon and then attempt to draw some implications from these for the psychotherapist.

THE PERSON IN PAIN

If we observe the world with which we are concerned here—the *universe* of the patient in chronic pain—we can perceive a similarity to the universe of the nightmare. If we look at the terror dream, and ask what are its structural components, we see that there are three basic ones: (1) terrible things are being done to the person and worse are threatened; (2) others, or outside forces, are in control and the will is helpless; (3) there is no time-limit set, one cannot predict when it will be over. The person in pain is in the same formal situation: terrible things are being done to him and he does not know if worse will happen; he has no control and is helpless to take effective action; no time-limit is given. This aspect of the psychic assault upon the integrity of the ego that accompanies severe, chronic pain is a major one: the patient lives during the waking state in the cosmos of the nightmare.

This is further emphasized by the meaninglessness and inexplicability of pain. Mental suffering seems to follow naturally from our thoughts and actions; with the possible exception of some of the obsessive compulsive states, it is somehow organic to us, syntonic to our views of ourself. Chronic pain is alien; it seems to indicate an utter senselessness. It appears to be meaningless and so, since it is very hard for man to accept that real experience may be unreasonable, we attempt to give it meaning. Our ancient guilts and anxieties are aroused, and we try to assign our pain to these insufficient causes. Although this is a frequent reaction, it rarely leads, for individuals of our society, to a useful sense of meaning. Not only does the lack of a time-limit militate against this, but the concept of purgatory (in this world or the next) is not a part of the Zeitgeist. This attempt, however, further weakens the ego as is done, even more, by the returning concept that there *is no sense* to the pain. The meaning of pain has been approached by every great religion and philosophy. In our own anti-metaphysical culture it is largely ignored. This lack of a perceived meaning, of a culturally understood context, makes it much harder for the individual to deal with chronic pain. As the Nazis well understood and demonstrated, meaningless and purposeless torture is much harder for the person to accept and resist than is torture which the subject can place in a coherent frame of reference. A perceived senselessness in the universe weakens our belief that our efforts have validity and point. They appear to be essentially futile. This makes it much harder to continue these efforts, including those of coping with pain and stress.

It is common, in our generalization from acute to chronic pain, to assign to pain the idea of a warning; a signal that something is wrong and that we should do something about it. This orientation often makes it more difficult for the therapist to be clear about the problems involved. Scheler [12, p. 41] points out that the sensation of weariness says 'rest,' dizziness at the edge of an abyss says 'step back,' and hunger that one should eat. Chronic pain, however, indicates only a state of existence. It does not warn or tell us what to do. It does not help us act and may be so severe as to disrupt potentially useful activites and habits. The adequate expression of thirst is to drink. The adequate expression of this kind of pain is only a scream.

Another aspect of the psychic assault made by severe pain is implied in this. It is related to the fact that it is important to ourselves that we respond to strong stimuli; that we are connected to and react to the environment. With pain this is much more difficult; we are constantly pushed towards suffering rather than interacting. We cannot act, we can only bear. Time and space are the basic framework for our exchanging energy with the cosmos and thus replenishing the strength of our psychic coherence. Pain weakens our relationship with this framework. There is a pulling to the center, a centripetal force that brings our energies and our consciousness into ourselves and away from all else and all others. "It is a peculiarity of man," says Victor Frankl [13, p. 74], "that he can only live by looking to the future—*sub specie—aeternitis.*" When he has no real goals in time, the inner life decays. There is a real loss of time perspective in pain—we are pulled in the immediate. The intensity and duration of the stimulus binds us to it. Our libidinal energy is pulled back from its objects and used as a defensive wall against the pain. However this shift of the libido increases our focusing of attention on the pain and thereby makes it fill our life-space to a greater degree and reduces our ability to deal with it. The lost objects can no longer sustain us and help us maintain our inner integrity and sense of being, purpose and meaning. Pain permits personal existence to continue with little assistance from our usual orientations, defences, safeguards and associations. It attenuates our relationships with the outer world at the same time that it weakens the inner structure. In painless consciousness we are filled with images, associations, thoughts. In the loud loneliness of pain, only our existence is real. We float alone in space, conscious only of the suffering.

These reactions and the passive, helpless quality of being in chronic pain tend to press us strongly towards a psychic regression. Our dignity and our hard-won adult status is weakened. The body image—our sense of our physical aspects and a basis of our sense of being, our *persona*—is blurred as the pain seems to obliterate the rest of the body. We are conscious only of the area that is providing the overwhelming sensations. The ego strength is further weakened by this reduction of the complexity of the organization of the adult perception of the body. It returns us to the body-image (and, with this, the feelings, the helplessness and dependency) of childhood. This is further added to by the fact that when we are in severe pain we, as in childhood, have to depend on others to take the important actions in our lives.

This is one reason that pity for the person in pain is an extremely corrosive emotion and—when perceived by the patient—further makes less his ability to deal with the situation. The pity re-enforces the regression through its implication of a lower status. The strivings to retain dignity and adulthood can be re-enforced through empathy, emotional contact and respect. Pity only weakens them.

It is usual to view pain as an event. As the above comments indicate, it may sometimes be more usefully viewed as a situation, a weltanschauüng, a position in the universe. Its quality is determined by the total context. As E. Strauss puts it, "There are no such things as sensations in themselves, there are only sensitive beings." (Quoted by Buytendjick [11, p. 122].) Hebb [14] has pointed out that pain is felt when C-fiber nervous impulses disrupt a well-organized pattern of activity. However when these same impulses are assimilated into a well-organized neural action pattern no pain is felt. In discussing pain in cancer, Gotthard Booth has stated that ". . . pain is frequently more dependent on the moral than on the physical condition of the patient," [15, p. 317]. The football player who does not feel the pain of his bone fracture, the schizophrenic who severely mutilates himself with little or no pain sensation, the flagellant in ecstasy, are all too well known to need exposition here. There can be no pain without involvement of the higher nervous centers and it is how these centers handle, absorb and integrate the pain, that will determine its perception and the ability to resist it. In Tolstoi's magnificent existential novel, "The Death of Ivan Illytch" [16], it was only when Ivan realized the total meaninglessness of his life that he was overwhelmed by the pain of his cancer. As long as there seemed to him to be a valid meaning to his existence, he could resist it and retain control and dignity. Once he lost the sense of the meaning of his life, he could only start screaming and continue to scream until he died. The emotional state, the 'lebensgefühl,' determines in large part the perception of pain, and its power over a person. One woman who had had terribly severe pain for many years from an inner ear disorder, but who had continued her active, useful and ebullient life in spite of this, responded to the question of how she did it by saying, "When the pain is severe, I rise above it and look at it from a higher level." To dismiss this remark and technique as 'hysteroid' would be missing the entire point. She retained command over herself and the pain and so was not overwhelmed as a person by it. Her psychic structure remained intact and master of her fate.

We have discussed here the general situation of the person in pain. It may be worthwhile also to be aware of some specific aspects which may play a part in the total situation.

These special aspects are possibilities that it appears advisable to keep in mind before action against the pain is taken by means of drugs, suggestion, hypnosis or other methods.

Pain as communication

Szasz [17] in his discussion of this area has pointed out that pain may be used as attempt at communicating with another person. It can be a way of stating a psychic situation; an aggression or a cry for help. In studying the specific person who is in pain, it may be important to ask oneself, "Is he saying something by this?" "Is there a message in it?"

Pain as an answer to psychic needs

Engel [18], Cangello [19], and others have discussed in some detail the use of pain to fill an inner need; to maintain the psychodynamic structure of the person. We understand this in mental suffering. One patient on being reassured that she had not hurt others, cried out in real anguish, "Don't take away my guilt." An experienced psychotherapist will recognize the cry and the needs behind it. However, our cultural orientation towards pain that it is evil and must be immediately relieved is so strong that, in spite of our knowledge of the cases where chronic pain has been relieved, to be followed immediately by emotional breakdown or suicide, we often ignore this problem.

One patient, who had suffered severe pain for several months and was now free of it, spoke of her fear that she would not be able to maintain the 'real' feelings and relationships which had arisen during the pain. "I am afraid" she added, "that if I feel good, I'll go back to my phony ways of living again."

"I have discovered by experience," wrote Girolamo Cardano in 1575, "that I cannot be long without bodily pain, for if once the circumstances arises, a certain mental anguish overcomes me, so grievous that nothing could be more distressing" [20].

The questions should be asked: "Is there a purpose behind this pain in this particular patient?" "Does it hold off guilt?" "Does it provide him with a sense of being 'real' that he desparetely needs?" "Is it a conversion symptom and, if so, of what?" One ignores these questions at the risk of successfully answering the patient's conscious plea for relief and destroying his adjustment.

SOME GUIDELINES FOR THE THERAPIST

We have discussed briefly some general and some special aspects of the problem of pain. We now proceed to some of the implications these concepts may hold for the therapist who must help the patient with pain that cannot be relieved by physical means.

The hardest task for the therapist, and yet perhaps the most basic, is to help the patient arrive at a meaning, a making some sense out of what is happening to him. Here there can be no rules as to how this is done, only an orientation as to its importance. Each patient must be helped to the path most syntonic to *him*, to his own sense of meaning, not the meaning that makes sense to the therapist. His uniqueness is crucial and the knowledge of this, in itself, may be helpful. To know—to be reenforced in the knowledge—that one is unique and irreplaceable—as a loved one or one who loves, as one with special tasks, or in some other manner, gives much support to the psychic structure and the ability to handle the situation. (This is one reason why experiments with pain-relieving agents often have such positive effects on the control subjects who are receiving only placebos. Their participation in the experiment itself reenforces their status as individual persons, increases their ability to deal with the pain and thus decreases their perception of it.) One patient was able to understand the connection between her pain and the healing process; that the pain was an inexorable part of treatment. She said, "Now that I know there is a reason, I feel it much less and can keep doing things when it comes. It's like the difference between childbirth and the other pains. In labor you know something will be produced at the end. It's never as bad as when the pain doesn't produce anything."

It is perhaps important for the therapist first to be clear about his own feelings in this area before he can effectively help the sufferer. If he believes that there *is* a meaning, even if he cannot find it, he is in a much better position to help. Out of his great experience with pain, Victor Frankl wrote, "If there is a meaning in life at all, then there is a meaning in suffering. Suffering is an ineradicable part of life, even as fate and death" [13, p. 67]. Just as it is important that the psychotherapist who works with the dying patient has to come to terms with his own feelings about death [4, 9], so too, it is important for the psychotherapist who works with the patient in severe pain to have come to terms with his feelings about pain.

Some patients may be able to make sense of the perception that this experience has brought them fully face to face with themselves and their universe. That they are no longer 'metaphysically heedless'; that their knowledge of their own existence has been deeply increased. (Indeed, Buytend-

jick [11] and others have theorized that it is this very increase of self-consciousness that is the basic 'function' of chronic pain.) "Your pain," said Kahlil Gibran [21] in *The Prophet,* "is the breaking of the shell that encloses your understanding."

One patient who had suffered very severe pain for a long period, and still was in acute, physical distress, said, "Sometimes with a lot of pain, a person becomes 'verklart' (clarified) and all the trivial unimportant things become unimportant. You stop spending your life worrying about them."

Other patients can understand that the experience they have had can never be taken from them, that after it is over they will never need to fear anything again and that, as Nietzsche put it, "That which does not kill me, makes me stronger." Other patients may see the pain they have as *existing in itself* and *their* experiencing it saves someone else from the experience. Each patient must be helped to his own solution. The effectiveness of the psychotherapist depends, in large part, on his ingenuity in helping the patient to the best answer for him as an individual. It is the knowledge of the importance of this that is central for the therapist. Dostoïevsky said, "There is only one thing I dread, not to be worthy of my sufferings." In this dark and wise sentence we see the need for the emergence and maintenance of the self in the welter of pain.

A second major guideline for the therapist is to help the patient find ways to act and react to the situation: to help the patient take some semblance of control over his situation. In the act of control, much strength is given to the inner being: the person is strengthened. Sometimes the patient must be helped to understand that for certain tasks, the action that is called for is to do nothing but to wait and bear and that this can be an active, not a passive, process. This can be a very valuable insight to some patients.

Frequently the patient feels he can only 'be brave and heroic' or surrender. This can be an impasse which demands more than the patient has to give. The value of 'a stiff upper lip' is often vastly overestimated by both the patient and those around him. Sometimes just permission to cry ("some things are worth a few tears") reduces the rigidity and makes it possible for other responses to take place. This should not be done, however, with the patient with a rigid, brittle ego which may be overwhelmed and drowned by a passive-dependent flood. In these patients it is necessary rather to re-enforce the rigid defenses (often with obsessive-compulsive techniques) than to weaken them.

One can also help some patients to understand the concept that the facts, including the facts of our inner life, are not as important as our attitude toward them. In the old story where one soldier was reproached and ridiculed by another for feeling fear under shellfire, the first answered: "It shows we are different, but it does not show I am inferior. If you were one-half as frightened as I am, you would have run away long ago." The 'fact' of pain impulses is also less important to the person's ability to deal with them than his attitude toward them.

A third lead for the therapist sometimes may be to make the 'nightmare' conditions conscious. To understand clearly the psychic pressures on a person, sometimes makes them much easier to resist. Not only do we understand that the pressures and our reactions are 'natural,' 'expected,' but also that they are universal and not special and secret to us. Further, the more an emotion and its causes are looked at clearly and objectively, the weaker it tends to become. Booth [22] quotes Spinoza that "Suffering ceases to be suffering as soon as we form a clear and precise picture of it."

One major way of helping the patient in pain is to help him remove the focus of concentration from the pain to outside events. The pain is felt to be worse when it occupies the entire life field. Work, occupational therapy, relating to others; these things do much more than just 'pass the time.' They also diminish the pain. Both 'attention' and 'consciousness' are essential to the perception of pain. We can reduce one or the other, but the reduction of 'attention' can often be surprisingly effective.

In the demand the psychotherapist makes that the patient turn his energies outward from the pain and that he function as a person, the therapist should avoid being too 'soft' and gentle. He can make high demands; this indicates far more respect and consequently strengthens the person far more than over-concern. The same orientation that we have toward mental anguish in psychotherapy is called for here. To be loving and demanding is a difficult road to walk, but it is the road that gives the greatest support and help to the patient. Sometimes the therapist can be aided in this if he asks himself whether his goal for the patient is painlessness or if it is composure, dignity and mastery.

CONCLUSION

Each of us lives in a unique, existential universe. The effectiveness of the psychotherapist who would relieve suffering is related to his understanding of, and empathy with, the universe of the sufferer. This is as true for the person with severe chronic pain as it is for those whose anguish is felt in the emotional sphere. It is also true, however, that the universes of those in pain tend to have common trends and pressures which appear to have implications for the therapist. This paper has been an attempt to describe some of these commonalities.

REFERENCES

1. LeShan, L. and Worthington, R. E.: Loss of cathexes as a common psychodynamic characteristic of cancer patients. An attempt at statistical validation of a clinical hypothesis, *Psychol. Rep.* **2**, 183, 1956.
2. LeShan, L. and Worthington, R. E.: Some recurrent life history patterns observed in patients with malignant disease, *J. nerv. ment. Dis.* **124**, 460, 1956.
3. LeShan, L.: A psychosomatic hypothesis concerning the etiology of Hodgkin's disease, *Psychol. Rep.* **3**, 565, 1957.
4. LeShan, L. and Gassmann, M. L.: Some observations on psychotherapy with patients with neoplastic disease, *Amer. J. Psychother.* **12**, 723, 1958.

5. LeShan, L., Marvin, S. and Lyerly, O.: Some evidence of a relationship between Hodgkin's disease and intelligence, *Arch. gen. Psychiat.* **1,** 477, 1959.

6. LeShan, L.: Personality states as factors in the development of malignant disease: a critical review, *J. nat. Cancer Inst.* **22,** 1, 1959.

7. LeShan, L. and Reznikoff. M.: A psychological factor apparently associated with neoplastic disease, *J. abnorm. soc. Psychol.* **60,** 439, 1969.

8. LeShan, L.: Some methodological problems in the study of the psychosomatic aspects of cancer, *J. gen. Psycho.* **63,** 309, 1960.

9. LeShan, L. and LeShan, E.: Psychotherapy and the patient with a limited life span. *Psychiatry* **24,** 318, 1961.

10. LeShan, L.: Some statistical evidence of the effect of psychological factors on the cancer mortality rate, *Arch. Psychiat.* **6,** 17, 1962.

11. Buytendjick, F. J. J.: *Pain; Its Modes and Functions,* University of Chicago Press, 1962.

12. Scheler, M.: *Vom Sinn des Leides,* Moralia, Leipzig, 1923.

13. Frankl, V.: *From Death Camp to Existentialism,* Beacon Press, Boston, 1959.

14. Hebb, D. O.: *Organization of Behavior,* Wiley, New York, 1957.

15. Booth, G.: Disease as a message, *J. Religion & Hlth,* **1,** No. 4, 309, 1962.

16. Tolstoi, Leo: *The Death of Ivan Illytch and Other Stories,* New Library of World Literature, New York, 1960.

17. Szasz, R.: *Pain and Pleasure,* Basic Books, New York, 1957.

18. Engel, G. L.: 'Psychogenic'. Pain and the pain prone patient, *Amer. J. Med.* **26,** 899, 1959.

19. Cangello, V. W.: Hypnosis for the patient with cancer, *Amer. J. clin. Hypnosis,* **4,** 215, 1962.

20. Cardano, Girolamo: *De Vita Propria Libra.* (1575). Trans. by Stoner, J., Dutton, New York, 1930. Quoted in *The Portable Renais Reader,* p. 519. Ed. by Ross, J. B. and McLaughlin, M. M., Viking Press, New York, 1958.

21. Gibran, K.: *The Prophet,* p. 60, Knopf, New York, 1936.

22. Booth, G.: Values in nature and in psychotherapy, *Arch. gen. psychiat.,* **8,** 38, 1963.

33

The foundation of bioethics

MILTON D. HEIFETZ

What is the ethical basis of decision-making in medicine? Human tragedy raises ethical problems that must be faced openly and honestly. The fundamental principles determining the resolution of these moral dilemmas should apply to all areas of bioethics.

Ethics are the societal principles underlying human behavior. Since they are a human contrivance, they are only as absolute and as rigid as a society wishes to make them.

The ethical base of the western world and more specifically of American society is unique: The United States has with great wisdom postulated a strong separation between church and state, but it has also derived its ethical base from doctrines with strong religious overtones.

The fundamental axiom underlying the American ethic is the axiom "Do not to others as you would not have others to do you." This axiom carries within it the concept that, if people wish to be absolutely free, they have to grant the same freedom to others. But unrestricted freedom could be harmful. This unacceptable drawback is resolved by the corollary that freedom is inviolable as long as the exercise of that freedom does not bring harm to others.

The basic premise of freedom (including the right to privacy and the right of self-determination) constitutes the substructure of the United States judicial system. Ideally absolute freedom should be inviolable.

This principle is tempered by the doctrine of *parens patriae* (state paternalism), which postulates that a truly civilized society should protect those who are weak and innocent from the possible misuse of freedom by those who are more competent or more powerful.

These two fundamental principles, of which the right of self-determination remains the most honored, underlie western social behavior in every biologic phase of life.

The right to die originates in the same principles as does the right to live. It is fundamentally the right of self-determination, the right of free choice.

In 1928, Supreme Court Justice Louis Brandeis stated:

The makers of our Constitution . . . sought to protect Americans in their beliefs, their thoughts, emotions, and their sensations. . . . they conferred . . . the right to be left alone . . . the most comprehensive of rights and the right most valued by civilized man.[1]

The right to be left alone refers not only to the right to act wisely, but also to the right to be foolish.

In complex medical situations we sometimes cannot see, or psychologically do not wish to see, how this basic principle applies, and we may therefore attempt to solve bioethical problems through secondary ethical concepts such as the sanctity of life, economic priorities, the meaningfulness of suffering, or the thought that only God can determine the course of life. There is undoubtedly some validity to all such ethical factors, but never in a secular free society should any of these secondary concepts be given the same weight as the right of self-determination—the basis of individual dignity, the hallmark of a free person.

The difficulty in understanding the ethical basis of a given situation should not lead us to invoke new or secondary ethical concepts. Ethical values do not change just because medicine is enlarging its technical skills. Value judgments of what is right or good rarely arise out of changing circumstances. On the contrary, changing circumstances demand a better understanding of the basic law, not the use of new or lesser ethical concepts.

How do these ethical precepts apply to the right to refuse therapy—the right to die, especially if medical judgment attests that the refusal of treatment would be foolish?

The most important consideration is not what the physician would or would not wish to do, but the patient's rights. The physician has no rights in such circumstances. He has only a role to play. That role is to inform, advise, recommend, and persuade. It is the patient who has full power. The patient who is competent has the right to know the most important details of his or her illness; the right to refuse treatment; the right to be informed of that right; and the right to direct, manage, live, and die if he or she wishes, as long as no one else is harmed in the process.

This fundamental right of the patient who is competent to say "no" to a doctor and thereby refuse treatment must be preserved. If the refusal of treatment results in death, then that is the individual's prerogative. The physician may try to persuade the individual to do what is medically wise, but to persuade does not imply the right to coerce, as long as the individual is a competent adult.

To evaluate properly this basic right of patients, medical professionals may have to realign their own psyches regarding the meaning of life and the fear of death.

The platitude that as long as there is life there is hope and therefore we must prolong life regardless of its quality can be cruel.

There are humane qualities in death. Life is precious and awesome. To hold it lightly dehumanizes it, but to divorce it from the dignity of personal choice debases it.

Those who would aggressively treat a dying subhuman patient with no hope of recovery contrary to the patient's request—especially when they would not wish to be treated if they themselves were in that condition—act hypocritically. They masquerade safely under a facade of morality because society rarely blames physicians for prolonging life.

How many men or women would want to live if recovery of human qualities were impossible? Many, if not most, would beg to be allowed to die. If this is true, how moral is that man or woman or that society who would prevent an individual's right to make that decision? Those who would deny that right of self-determination to others fall into the trap of doing to others what they would not have others do to them.

When a physician permits a competent patient to die who wishes to do so, there is no break in morality. There is a facing of responsibility through adherence to the individual's right of self-determination.

Although there have been occasional judicial decisions to the contrary, the courts have repeatedly upheld the right to refuse medical treatment. In 1962 Judge Bernard S. Meyer, Jr., refused to force a competent adult member of the Jehovah's Witness faith to accept a blood transfusion under the doctrine of self-determination. He said:

It is the individual . . . who has the final say, and this must be necessarily so in a system of government which gives the greatest possible protection to the individual in the furtherance of his own desires.[2]

In another ruling 2 years later this right of self-determination was overruled. The case involved another member of the Jehovah's Witness faith. A 25-year-old mother of a 7-month-old child was seriously ill and in need of blood. She refused a blood transfusion. A court order sought by the doctor and hospital was approved by Circuit Court

Judge J. Skelly Wright, who overruled a lower court decision.[3] He rightfully invoked the doctrine of *parens patriae*—the right and obligation of the state to protect those unable to care for themselves—on the basis that the death of the mother would have been tantamount to the abandonment of her child contrary to the child's welfare. This doctrine of state paternalism reflects the value a civilized society places on the mutual concern its members should all have for each other. But this concern must not become distorted self-righteousness and interfere with the right of self-determination when the exercise of this freedom would not harm others.

Judicial support of the right of self-determination as it applies in medicine has also been tested for the incompetent.

In 1972 in Allentown, Pennsylvania, Mrs. Maida Yetter refused to undergo surgery for the removal of a breast cancer. At the time of this refusal Mrs. Yetter was alert and competent. Approximately 1 year later Mrs. Yetter's fear of possible surgery caused her to become delusional. At the time of her delusional state, when she was obviously incompetent, her brother asked the court to appoint him guardian so that he could authorize the surgery. The court rejected the brother's request, noting that "the Constitutional right of privacy includes the right of a mature, competent, adult to refuse to accept medical recommendation that may prolong one's life." The court ruled that she was competent at the time of the initial decision and added that:

> . . . balancing the risks involved in our refusal to act in favor of compulsory treatment against giving the greatest possible protection to the individual in furtherance of his own desires, we are unwilling now to overrule Mrs. Yetter's original . . . competent decision.[4]

The court upheld the important principle of her right of self-determination even though it meant her death.

This case gives legal support to the concept that the wish of an individual made while competent must be respected even if that individual subsequently becomes incompetent.

The fact that a competent patient has the right to refuse any treatment—and thereby to choose death—means that the individual has the right to die. This right to die has existed throughout our nation's history.

Why is this right so frequently ignored? Why do physicians hesitate to inform patients of their right to say no? Why do doctors so often treat when such treatment only debases the process of dying? I am inclined to reject the often-stated opinion that physicians refuse to accept the death of their patients because of their own fear of death or because physicians simply cannot accept defeat. The reality of the situation probably lies in a mixture of the tradition to continue to treat and a hidden fear of unwarranted criticism or legal action by survivors if treatment is stopped.

It is important to understand this heritage if we are to protect the right of the individual to refuse treatment, especially during a possible future state of incompetency. To respect the individual's wishes it is necessary to protect the physician for obeying those wishes. A properly written, precisely worded statement to the physician, which places the physician in jeopardy for disobeying it, is the best means of satisfying this prerequisite. The following is a sample of such a directive.

DIRECTIVE TO MY PHYSICIAN

This directive is written while I am of sound mind and fully competent.

I insist that I have complete right to refuse any medical and surgical treatment unless a court order affirms that my decision would bring undue or unexpected hardship on my family or on society.

Therefore:

If I become incompetent, in consideration of my legal rights to refuse medical or surgical treatment regardless of the consequences to my health and life, I hereby direct and order my physician or any physician in charge of my care, to cease and refrain from any medical or surgical treatment which would prolong my life if I am in a condition of:

1. Unconsciousness from which I cannot recover
2. Unconsciousness over a period of 6 months
3. Irreversible mental incompetency

However, although mentally incompetent, if conscious, I must be informed of the situation, and if I wish to be treated I am to be treated in spite of my original request made while competent.*

If there is any reasonable doubt of the diagnosis of my illness and the prognosis, consultation with available specialists should be obtained.

This directive to my physician also applies to any hospital or sanitarium at which I may be at the time of my illness, and it relieves them of any and all responsibility for the action or lack of action of any physician acting according to my demands. If any action is taken contrary to these express demands I hereby request my next of kin or my legal representative to consider, and if necessary, to take legal action against those involved.

I hereby absolve my physician or any physician taking care of me from any legal liability pertaining to the fulfillment of any of my demands.

Signed _____

---

*It is important to understand this apparent paradox. These instructions specify the only time a request or demand made while incompetent can override one made while competent. The possibility that next of kin might attempt to take advantage of a state of incompetency by too readily following a prior directive ordering cessation of therapy makes these instructions necessary.

There has been much discussion of the need for a law outlining the right to die. This is unfortunate. There is no law stating that a patient must accept treatment, unless refusal of treatment would either be contrary to public health laws (such as those requiring vaccinations during a period of epidemics) or bring harm to others. There is no law that gives the physician the right to treat without consent except in an emergency or with specific court authorization. Therefore there is really no need for a law granting people the right to die. That right exists as does the right to live; both originate in the freedom of decision, which reflects our constitutional right to privacy and its corollary, self-determination.

What is needed to protect the individual's right is not a new law, but generally greater public awareness of patients' rights and specifically a strong written directive to the physician that forces him or her to obey the patient unless a court order is obtained to the contrary.

EUTHANASIA

What is the relationship between the right of self-determination, including the right to die, and euthanasia?

Translated literally from the Greek, euthanasia means "well" or "easy death," but since 1869[5] its commonly accepted meaning has been "the act of inducing an easy death." In our discussion "euthanasia" will designate the willful putting to death of an individual with the intent of preventing suffering—in other words, mercy killing.

The removal of a respirator from a patient who can no longer recover from a state of coma is not euthanasia. On the other hand, giving an injection of a massive dose of morphine that causes the death of the same patient would be euthanasia. The difference is simply that euthanasia interferes with life's natural course. The act itself, not natural processes, is the cause of death. By contrast, actions that cease treatment, whether by not starting the treatment (omission) or by removing the treatment (commission), allow nature to take its course, making the disease process itself the actual cause of death. There are those who would legalize euthanasia. This I believe is dangerous.

Euthanasia for a seriously deformed and retarded newborn (or, in rare cases, for an adult) is at times humane and correct, moral and right. Nevertheless the doctor or parent who overdoses an anencephalic monster is committing infanticide, a variant of euthanasia. To end the life of such an organism is humane, but to kill, regardless of circumstances, must remain subject to the scrutiny of our courts. Never should the taking of a life be free of court judgment.

In the United States, where motivation is not a defense in cases of homicide, consent or request for euthanasia is not legally acceptable. The law considers the deliberate and premeditated taking of life as murder in the first degree. However, the flexible *attitude* of the courts has been more reasonable. Altruistic motivation has been considered an extenuating fact in judging homicides. This gap between the written law and legal practice in the United States, as it pertains to mercy killing, is an embarrassment to the law and must be closed. We should modify our laws instead of surreptitiously bypassing them. We should pass laws that grant our courts the right to consider and honor motivation and intent in cases of euthanasia and the right to declare no penalty.

SUICIDE

The same principle that underlies the right of a competent adult to die by refusing medical care determines the ethical and legal right to suicide.

Three groups of people attempt suicide: (1) those suffering from transient or chronic emotional disorders; (2) those emotionally sound but aged, alone, and without a sense of purpose in life; and (3) those near death whose remaining days or weeks are not deemed worthy of the effort to live.

The first and second groups are in need of psychologic and sociologic support. We must encourage the development of suicide prevention centers and psychologic help for these two groups of people.

The third category—those physically devastated and near death—is another matter. People in this group, although under emotional stress, are frequently still capable of reasoned judgments. I believe that, if they desire to leave life through suicide, we should not only give them the courtesy of respecting their wish but also should provide them with medical assistance to commit suicide if they wish to have it.

At times death-dealing medication left by the bedside of a dying person can be a most sought-after blessing and a humane symbol to the person in this kind of need. It is illegal to do this in the United States. Maybe it is time to change the law, bearing in mind that any assistance to commit suicide must be tightly controlled. Only patients who are alert and competent, who are unequivocably near death, who do not wish to continue their dying state in spite of psychiatric help, and who specifically ask for this type of assistance should be able to receive it.

We must cease forcing decisions upon others because of our personal idiosyncrasies. At times we must look at death as a welcome release from an untenable life. It is part of life's pattern. At times it should be sought, not avoided. This is not a question of holding life less precious, but of considering death less terrifying. Nature frequently removes the fear of death from the elderly, the infirm, or the hopelessly ill and in fact often allows them to welcome death.

If life is a hopeless state of anguish to a coherent and understanding adult, does anyone have the right to insist that he or she live in that state against his or her will? What happened to free choice? Who is the transgressed if even the agonized is not? Certainly psychiatric help should be utilized to assist such people to adapt to their tragic lot, but to insist that life must be lived when all efforts to help have failed is a presumptuous imposition on a fellow human's right of self-determination.

Death is a natural process neither to be feared nor resented. What should be feared is the inability to feel the joy and serenity of life.

THE TRAGIC NEWBORN

How does the ethical base that we have evolved apply to the management of the tragically endowed newborn—the newborn who does not have the potential of achieving even near-normal human mental or physical qualities?

We speak of the right of self-determination, but the newborn cannot speak for himself or herself. Therefore any action or lack of action is not necessarily in accordance with the newborn's wish. This holds true even for children and adolescents who can (although not legally) speak for themselves. Their right to decide, their authority, is relegated to their parents, but this does not mean that parents have absolute control over their offspring. The parental right to decide is tempered by that same doctrine of *parens patriae,* which protects the weak and incompetent.

How do we balance this equation of parental right of decision and societal obligation to protect the weak? Let us apply this equation to the tragic newborn. These infants fall into three categories:

1. Those who are so damaged that nothing can keep them alive
2. Those damaged infants who will live without need of medical care
3. Those newborns who could not live without medical care and who, even with medical care, would live only a subhuman existence

I am discussing only children in the third category. Should these hopelessly damaged newborns receive the full benefit of medical science if that science can enable them to live only on a subhuman level? Should medical aid ever be withheld? What factors must enter into these decisions? First and foremost, parents must be *fully* informed about the degree, significance, and prognosis of the damage. Second, they must be informed of their legal right to give or withhold consent for treatment.

What should society, as reflected in the recommendations and actions of the physician, consider as pertinent factors in the exercise of its obligation to protect the weak when parents refuse to authorize life-saving medical or surgical treatment for their newborn? In general it is necessary to evaluate what can be coldly termed the "salvage value." This factor is vital in any decision to approve or withhold treatment. What kind of child will result? Can the child be relatively self-sustaining in the future? Will life be one continuous form of agony for the child? Will life be meaningful to any degree? What is meaningful, and to whom?

When evaluating the tragic newborn it is necessary to balance his or her present and future condition against the effect on parents and siblings. To do this we must better understand the value and significance of devastated life at the newborn stage. We must ask whether pregnancy and birth are so sacrosanct that all other factors become irrelevant in spite of the knowledge that women can almost always become pregnant again. We must weigh the validity of that future subhuman existence and the right to maintain that life against the sadness and cruelty imposed on parents and siblings living with such a child and against parental rights. What happens to the child and the family after all the doctors and other experts leave and those concerned with the problem must live with it alone?

Our society frequently and glibly invokes the doctrine of sanctity of life without trying to understand the rights of parents and the effect of the tragically endowed newborn on the family. Certainly some families are drawn closer together as their members cooperate to shield the child and find aid for him or her if aid is possible. Yet regardless of how family members work to help the mentally retarded and deformed child, the parents inevitably ask, "What will happen to the child when we are dead?" Many families disintegrate under this kind of pressure. The anguish experienced by the family of a newborn who is drastically deformed and/or mentally damaged without hope of recovery to even a near-normal state, and yet who is alive in the physiologic sense of the word, is one of the most heartbreaking dilemmas I know.

It is not uncommon for physicians to recommend and for parents to authorize that every effort be made to save the child although the parents intend to put the child into an institution—never to see him again. Is this humane?

In one case, a baby was born hopelessly and completely paralyzed from the waist down by a severe myelomeningocele, but there was no evidence of mental retardation. The parents had two normal children, ages 3 and 5 years. They asked me not to operate to prevent the chance of meningitis. I agreed. The child developed meningitis and died.

Even though there may be a normal brain and therefore normal intelligence, I do not believe that newborns with predictably devastating deformities should be treated.

The late Donald D. Matson, a respected pediatric neurosurgeon of the Children's Hospital Medical Center and Harvard Medical School, has stated:

In our clinic, it is not customary to operate upon newborn infants or those in the first few months of life . . . who exhibit complete sphincter paralysis and total paraplegia. . . . This is true whether or not there is significant hydrocephalus at the time. When examination on the first day of life therefore confirms total absence of neurological function below the upper lumbar levels, custodial care only is recommended. . . . It is the doctor's and the community's responsibility to provide this care and to minimize suffering; but, at the same time, it is also their responsibility not to prolong individual, familial, and community suffering unnecessarily . . . in an infant whose chance for acceptable growth and development is negligible.[6]

Yale University pediatrician Raymond S. Duff and pediatrician A. G. M. Campbell of the University of Aberdeen, Scotland, reported in 1973 that 43 infants were permitted to die during a 30-month-period at Yale–New Haven Hospital in New Haven, Connecticut, because parents and staff members there believed those children had "little or no hope of achieving what theologian and ethicist Dr. Joseph Fletcher terms meaningful 'humanhood.'"[7] The children, who had a variety of profound defects, died because essential medical treatment was withheld from them.

Each of the 43 children was hopelessly ill and had multiple handicaps, but each could have lived at least for some period of time. Not all were newborns. One of the infants, a victim of an incurable lung disease, was kept alive for 5 months in spite of an in-adequate respiratory system and a weak heart. He lived only because of special oxygen treatment. The hopelessness of the situation and the continuous distress of the infant compounded by the severe emotional trauma suffered by the parents and the other children in the family forced the decision to shut off the oxygen. The child died in 3 hours.

"When maximum treatment was viewed as unacceptable by families and physicians in our units," wrote Duff and Campbell, "there was a growing tendency to seek early death."[7] "In lengthy, frank discussions, the anguish of the parents was shared and attempts were made to support fully the reasoned choices, whether for active treatment and rehabilitation or for an early death."

In all 43 cases parents and physicians concurred.

Duff and Campbell acknowledge "the awesome finality" of their decisions and the "potential for error," but they insist these life-or-death matters must be dealt with candidly. Both men charge that medicine has been "hiding" from this issue:

Since major research, teaching and patient care efforts were being made, professionals expected to discover, transmit and apply knowledge and skill; patients and families were supposed to cooperate fully (even) if they were not always grateful. Some physicians recognized that the wishes of families went against their own, but they were resolute. They (the doctors) *commonly agreed* that if they were the parents of very defective children, withholding treatment would be most desireable for them. However, they argued that aggressive treatment should be done for the children of others (italics added).[7]

This arrogant, autocratic approach under the guise of research must be condemned.

Anthony Shaw, pediatric surgeon at the University of Virginia Medical Center in Charlottesville, Virginia, who also believes that quality of life must be balanced against sanctity of life, comments on the same point:

I was called to the newborn nursery to see baby C whose father was a busy surgeon with three teenage children. The diagnosis of imperforate anus and microcephalus were obvious. (The father) called me after being informed of the situation by the pediatrician. I'm not going to sign the op (operation) permit," he said. When I didn't reply, he said, "What would you do, doctor, if he were your baby?" "I wouldn't let him be operated on either," I replied.[8]

The infant was kept comfortable and died 48 hours later.

This pointed question—"What would you do?"—put to the physician by parents of tragic newborns should be heard more often. It would prevent extraordinary and life-long heartache.

For years some physicians have accepted and supported parental decisions that death is the kindest response to the tragically deformed newborn. "This treatment of severely deformed children is a common denominator at every nursery in the country," says Lawrence K. Pickett, chief of staff at Yale–New Haven Hospital. "Other hospitals follow similar practices but are afraid to report them."[9]

This fear is understandable. The world press in 1971 condemned the "inhumanity" of a husband and wife and the staff of a major American medical center. A child with Down's syndrome had been born with an intestinal obstruction at Johns Hopkins Hospital in Baltimore. The parents, who had two normal children, refused to give consent to correct the obstruction. The infant could not be fed and died within 15 days.[10] The parents agonized over the problem. They decided that the impact of a mongoloid infant on their other children, as well as on their own lives, was not acceptable.

The child's death caused a furor in medical and lay circles. It was a major topic at an international symposium concerning medical ethics.[10] Panelists disagreed with the parents. They suggested the child's right to life to the limit of happiness possible was more important than the years of anguish and burden the child would bring on the family. The right to live, they argued, should be the foundation of the decision. The effect of that life on others is secondary. If we agree, however, that the sanctity of life overrides all else, we reach a precipice. We must face the question asked by social critic and writer Michael Harrington: "What if the defect had been much greater?"[10] To answer his question and remain consistent from our hypothetical perspectives, we must agree to preserve the life of the anencephalic child, the newborn without a brain. That life is equally sanctified. But our society comfortably says, "No, that would be going too far." But, if we do not operate to preserve an anencephalic child, we are making a comparative judgment. Comparative judgments deny the sanctity of life over all else. The two are in conflict. We cannot have it both ways.

We must draw the line somewhere. But that line cannot be based on the sanctity of life. That is too narrow a criterion. We must ask the basic question, "What would you or I want if such a child were our infant and should that overrule a parental decision to refuse treatment?" The technical advances of medicine and surgery have been superb. But the question remains, "Does treatment always permit a livable life?" We must not only ask, "Can it be done?" but "Should it be done?"

David Patrick Houle was born on February 9, 1974, in the Maine Medical Center. He had multiple deformities. He did not have a left eye or a left ear. He was physically and mentally defective. His esophagus was not connected properly to his stomach; he was therefore unable to eat.[11] His parents asked that life-sustaining measures be stopped, that surgery to prolong David's life not be performed. But the hospital sought and obtained a court order to allow surgery.

The baby's physician told the court, "We have passed the point where the correction will be of any benefit to the infant. The infant would be physically and mentally retarded and probable brain damage has rendered life not worth preserving.'' In spite of this testimony and the parents' wishes, Justice David G. Roberts of the Cumberland County Superior Court authorized consent for surgery. Justice Roberts' ruling: ''The parents have no right to withhold such treatment and that to do so constitutes neglect in a legal sense. The basic right enjoyed by every human being is the right to life itself.'' The issue, he said, ''is not the prospective quality of the life to be preserved.''

The court order was obeyed. If Justice Roberts were consistent, he would have ordered surgery to be performed to preserve the life of a brainless, armless, legless infant, even if it were his own grandchild.

But would he?

If we accept the concept that certain tragically endowed newborns should not receive medical support, can we devise safeguards to prevent its misuse? There is a danger in trying to establish specific guidelines to evaluate physical or mental deficits accurately. The degree of tragedy varies. There is certainly no sharp line of demarcation. It is one thing to say that the child who is armless, legless, and without a brain of significant size should be allowed to die. But what of the newborn who will be mildly retarded, who with proper training will be totally self-sufficient, able to work at specified jobs, and able to enjoy life? What of the infinite gradations between these extremes?

If specific guidelines cannot be established, are there reasonable safeguards to prevent unwise actions? I believe there are: *the parents*. We should not underestimate the ability of parents to make decisions affecting themselves and the potential of their children. Parents will go to extremes to protect their newborn children. It is the exceedingly rare parent who would allow a newborn to die without an exceptionally good reason. Very rarely, some parents would rather see a newborn not live if the child is not perfectly normal. In these unusual cases, the physician can easily countermand any distorted requests by parents by simply seeking and obtaining a court order to authorize treatment.

The total thrust of medicine is to preserve life. This is the second safeguard. Physicians *will not allow* emotionally distraught parents to prevent treatment when treatment is indicated.

Therefore in spite of a remote possibility for error, I believe that the protective cover of parents and the protective drive of physicians to preserve life are all that are necessary to protect the rights of the tragic newborn.

I would like to suggest what I believe should be the postulates underlying the relationship between the parents of a tragically endowed newborn and their physician:

Parents have the right to understand the medical problems facing their child; only then can they make decisions. It is the obligation of the physician to explain the problems to parents adequately.

If an infant is so damaged that treatment will result in the prolongation of the life of a severely mentally or physically defective child, the parents must be informed of their authority to withhold consent for treatment and their authority to demand that their physician stop treatment if it has been started.

If a physician believes that a child may be able to lead a relatively normal life after treatment—and the parents refuse to authorize treatment—it is his or her obligation to seek a court order to enable treatment to take place.

If the physician's religion demands preservation of life, regardless of quality and contrary to parental demand, he or she should transfer the child's care to another physician and, if necessary, to another institution.

If parents request treatment after full information has been given to them, treatment must be given.

We are dealing with the impact of principles on individual cases. We cannot be absolute, but I do not believe that the inability to be absolute should deter us.

REFERENCES

1. Olmstead v. United States, 277 U.S. 438, 448 Superior Court 564, 572, 72 L.Ed 944, 1928.
2. Erickson v. Dilgard, Vol 252 NYS 2nd 705, 706, Superior Court, Nassau County, 1962.
3. Application of the President and Directors of the Georgetown College, No. 331 F. 2 D 1000 (D.C. cir.) 377 U.S. 978, 1964.
4. Dockett No. 1973-553, Pennsylvania Court of Common Pleas, Northhampton County Orphans Court, 1973.
5. Lecky, W. E.: History of European morals from Augustus to Charlemagne, 1869.
6. Matson, D. D.: Surgical treatment of myelomeningocele, Pediatrics **42(2):**225-227, 1968.
7. Duff, R. S., and Campbell, A. G. M.: Moral and ethical dilemmas in the special-care nursery, N. Engl. J. Med. **289:**890-894, 1973.
8. Shaw, A.: Dilemmas of "informed consent" in children, N. Engl. J. Med. **289:**885-890, 1973.
9. *Associated Press,* Oct. 30, 1973.
10. International Symposium on Human Rights, Retardation and Research, Washington, D.C., October 16, 1971.
11. *New York Times,* February 16 and 24, 1974.

PART IX

Care of the dying patient: emotional survival

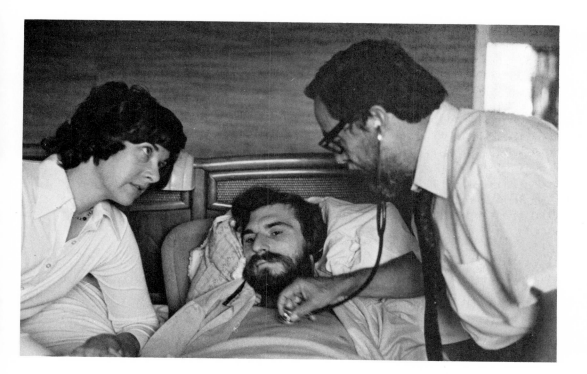

34

The psychology of terminal illness as portrayed in Solzhenitsyn's *The Cancer Ward*

HARRY S. ABRAM

Although Aleksandr Solzhenitsyn's masterful contemporary Russian novel, *The Cancer Ward,*[1] has justly won wide acclaim for its social and political commentary, as well as for its artistic merits, little detailed attention has been given to the vehicle by which he presents his thesis, that is, patients being treated for and dying of cancer. As a psychiatrist working clinically with terminally ill patients, I was particularly impressed with this side of the novel. Solzhenitsyn's insights and vivid descriptions of the cancer patient are so penetrating that they give the reader an unusual opportunity to view the innermost feelings and psychology of the terminally ill patient. In this presentation I shall review these aspects of the novel, particularly as they pertain to psychotherapeutic work with the physically ill and dying patient.

SETTING—AUTOBIOGRAPHICAL ASPECTS

In the publisher's Foreword we are told that:

In February, 1953, just before Stalin's death, he [Solzhenitsyn] was released from a labor camp and entered upon his "permanent" or "eternal"—not merely life—exile. He was confined to a village on the edge of the desert in Kazakhstan, the same region in which Dostoevski had been deported. In this *aul,* or village he taught school.

In the labor camp he had been operated on for a tumor but had not been told the nature of his ailment. During his village exile he suffered extreme pain from a recurrence of the illness. He made his way to the city of Tashkent, where he was treated for cancer and recovered.

Out of this experience came his third novel, his culminating work to date, *The Cancer Ward.*

The story takes place in a hospital, in a city resembling Tashkent, in February and March 1955.

The setting is in a cancer ward ("Ward No. 13"), and various characters in the novel are patients on the ward, who are being treated for and dying of cancer. Solzhenitsyn describes each patient, his reaction to his illness and the treatment, and his interaction with the other patients and his physicians. One of these patients, Oleg Kostoglotov, is a 34-year-old exprisoner in exile who has an abdominal tumor. As the novel unfolds it becomes apparent that Kostoglotov represents Solzhenitsyn. Kostoglotov tells a young woman medical student, Zoya (whose name interestingly in Russian means "life"), with whom he has a transient affair:

The Korean physician who diagnosed my case in the province hospital before I came here . . .

Reprinted from Archives of Internal Medicine **124:**758-760, Dec. 1969. Copyright 1969, American Medical Association.

want to explain things either, but I decided: "Go ahead! I'll be responsible. I'm a
family man and I have to put my affairs in
order," I told him. So he let me have it: "You
have three weeks to live, beyond that I can't
say."

"What right did he have to tell you such a
thing?"

He was a good fellow! A real man! I shook his
hand. I *must* know! I was in agony for six
months, and in the last month I could neither lie
down nor sit nor stand without pain and I slept
only a few minutes a day; I managed to think a
few things out.

DENIAL

Most studies of the physically and terminally ill patient note denial as the major
defense mechanism for handling anxiety
and conflict related to death. This denial
takes many forms and varies from the
patient who postpones medical examination
for an obvious breast mass to a psychotic
denial of death in the terminal phases of
lung cancer. One of the major characters,
Pavel Rusanov, a 45-year-old bureaucrat
with a lymphoma, comments on his initial
physical examination:

But surely I don't have cancer? Doctor? Surely I don't have cancer? Pavel Nicolayevich
asked hopefully as he gently rubbed the right
side of his neck, where the angry swelling
seemed to be growing day by day, stretching the
unoffending white skin.
"No, no, of course not," Doctor Dontsova
reassured him for the tenth time as she continued scribbling the case history in her sprawl-
ing handwriting.

When Pavel enters Ward No. 13, a patient
asks, "Listen, brother, what kind of cancer
have you got? Cancer of the what?" he
asked in a muffled voice. Pavel answers,
"Cancer of the *nothing*. I don't have
cancer."

Later both Rusanov and Dr. Dontsova
continue their joint denial:

"Your trouble is lymphogranulmatosis."
"So it's not cancer!"
"Of course not!" . . . She saw the tumor as big
as a fist under his jaw . . . "But remember," she

hesitated, and then warned in a conciliatory
tone, "it's not only cancer that people die of."

Solzhenitsyn graphically depicts some
patients' use of denial at the time of death:

But here, in this hospital, a man sucking an
oxygen balloon; barely able to move his eyes, he
still used his tongue to prove that "I won't die!
I don't have cancer!"
Like a lot of chickens. A knife at the throat
awaited everyone of them, but they kept cluck-
ing and scratching for feed. When one of them
was carried off to the knife, the others kept
scratching.

DEHUMANIZING ASPECTS OF ILLNESS AND HOSPITALIZATION

Patients in the hospital often lose their
identity, as well as their contact with the
outside world and society. The illness also
becomes all-encompassing, and the libido
turns inward to bodily concern. When
Rusanov enters Ward No. 13, before his
classic statement of denial ("Cancer of the
nothing.") a patient announces, "Here
comes another cancer," as if he had no
other identity save for his illness. This statement is reminiscent of physicians who
speak of "the gall bladder in bed four" or
the "mitral valve on ward two" rather than
identifying the patient as a person first, eg,
"Mrs. Jones who has a diseased gall
bladder."

After Rusanov's hospitalization, Solzhenitsyn writes:

But in a few days this whole close-knit, ideal
Rusanov family . . . had receded until it had
vanished on *the other side* of the tumor . . . the
tumor had divided him from them like a wall, and
he remained alone on this side of it. . . .
The tumor, mute and unfeeling, swelled and
eclipsed the whole world.

Kostoglotov, speaking again for Solzhenitsyn, notes:

Once a patient has entered the hospital, you do
all his further thinking for him. All thinking is
henceforth done for him by your regulations,
your daily consultations, your program, the plan
and reputation of your medical institution. And
I'm just a grain of sand again, as I was in the
camp. Nothing depends on me.

Even Dr. Dontsova (head of the radiology department) is not immune to dehumanization and disintegration. When she realizes she has esophageal carcinoma and becomes fearful of her diagnosis, Solzhenitsyn writes, "Then, suddenly, in a few days, her own body fell out of this harmonious and great system, struck the hard earth, and turned out to be a helpless sack filled with organs, each of which could ail and cry out at any moment."

FEAR OF MUTILATION AND LOSS OF SEXUALITY

Through two young cancer patients who are lovers, Demka, a 16-year-old boy with a bone sarcoma of the lower part of the leg, and Asya, a 17-year-old girl with breast cancer, Solzhenitsyn vividly describes the psychological reaction to mutilative operations, including the sexual symbolism involved in such operations. Asya asks Demka:

"What do you mean, cut your leg off? Are they crazy? Or don't they want to bother curing you? Don't let them do it! Better die than live without a leg. What sort of life is the life of a cripple? Life has to be enjoyed."

Yes, of course, she was right again. What was life with a crutch? Suppose he was sitting next to her, what would he do with his crutches? And what would it be like with a stump? He would never have been able to bring that chair over by himself. She would have to fetch it for him. No. Life without a leg was no life at all.

In a moving scene later in the novel, Asya comes to Demka in tears and in panic,

She was wailing into the pillow.
"Please, Assenka! Tell me what it is. Tell me."
But he had almost guessed.
"They'll am-pu-tate!"
She wept and wept. Then she moaned: "Oo-o-o!"
Demka could not remember ever hearing such a wail of grief as this terrible "O-o-o!" . . .
For the first time Demka saw her wet, red, blotched, pitiful and angered face. "Who wants a woman with one breast? Who? At seventeen!" she screamed at him as though it were all his fault.
"How will I go to the *beach?*" she wailed, as

this fresh thought stabbed her. "The beach! How will I go swimming?" The idea twisted through her like a corkscrew, pierced her and flung her away from Demka and down to the floor, where her body collapsed and she clutched her head in her hands.

Finally she demands that he kiss her cancerous breast and asks,

"Will you remember it? You will remember that I had it, won't you? and what it was like?"
She did not remove it, she did not move away; he returned to the brown nipple, and his lips gently did what her future baby would never be able to do at this breast. No one entered, and he went on kissing the marvel that hung above him.
Today a marvel, tomorrow into the basket.

DEATH AND DYING

Throughout the novel there are multiple references to death, its inevitability, and man's inability to conceive his own death. In describing Rusanov's admission to the hospital, Solzhenitsyn writes, "He walked up the stairs as—how to put it?—a condemned man mounts the scaffold to put his head on the block." And again,

The fact that the time had come for Yefrem [a 50-year-old laborer with tongue cancer] to *croak*. Pronounced like that with evil glee, it seemed easier: Not to die, but to croak.
But these were only words—the mind could not conceive of it, nor the heart accept it.

And again, "He [Rusanov] could not say it. He could not peer into that black abyss. He could not." The stark reality of death is revealed in one remarkably terse sentence, "Now they [the cancer ward patients] had to imagine that he who the day before yesterday trod these boards where they all walked lay in the morgue, cut open along the ventral axis like a split sardine."

CANCER AND TREATMENT

As one can gather Solzhenitsyn's descriptions are so superb that it is difficult if not impossible to give them all. The two which follow are those of a patient, Yefrem Podduyev, with a tongue cancer who is receiving cobalt treatment:

It was Yefrem's tongue that sickened—that flexible, well-knit, imperceptible tongue, hardly ever seen, but so useful in life. He had exercised that tongue much in his fifty years. With that tongue he had talked others into paying him money he had never earned, swore to having done what he never had, paid lip service to what he did not believe, cursed managers, shouted at the workers, intricately piled up his "mother" curses to fall on everything that was dearest and most sacred, and warbled as many tunes as a nightingale. His tongue had also unfolded many a fat joke, though never a political one. It had sung the songs of the Volga, and had lied to countless wenches the world over that he was not married, had no children and would be back in a week to set up house. "Ah, if only your tongue would shrivel!" one of these wenches once cursed him, but Yefrem's tongue failed him only when he was very drunk indeed.

And suddenly it had begun to blow up, to catch on his teeth, and no longer fitted its soft, juicy pharynx.

Through the exposed cells of the skin, through layers and organs whose names their owner did not even know, through that toad of a tumor, through the stomach and the intestines, through the blood flowing in the arteries and veins, through the lymph, the cells, the spine and small bones, more layers, vessels and the skin of the back, through the trestles of the table, through the one-and-a-half-inch planks of the floor, through the foundations and the earth fill and farther and farther, descending to bedrock, poured the harsh Roentgen rays, quivering vectors of electric and magnetic fields inconceivable to the human mind; or, to put it more understandably, quanta missiles, exploding and riddling everything in their path.

THE PATIENT'S RIGHTS AND RECOVERY

A theme, which obviously has political overtones and recurs throughout the book, is that of patient's rights. Kostoglotov angrily and passionately confronts the head of the radiology department, Dr. Dontsova:

. . . and you have drawn the conclusion that I came here to save myself *at any price*. I don't want to do that—at any price! There is nothing in the world I would be willing to pay *any* price for! . . . I came to you *to relieve my suffering!* I said: I'm in great pain, help me! And help me you did,

I'm not in pain any longer. Thank you! Thank you! I am your grateful debtor. But let me go now. Let me return like a dog to his dog house to lick my wounds and rest . . . As for curing me completely—"to the end"—that is something you won't be able to do anyway, because there is *no end* to the cure for cancer.

Yet Kostoglotov accepts further treatment and experiences hope, in place of despair, with the possibility of his recovery:

He stood smoking, filled with enjoyment.
The music came from the park. Oleg stood listening to it, and yet not to it; it was as if he were hearing Tchaikovsky's Fourth Symphony resounding inside himself—the turbulent, difficult opening, one astonishing melody from that opening. This was the melody (Oleg understood it in his own way, though perhaps it should have been interpreted differently) in which the hero, who had either returned to life or been blind and now recovered his sight, seemed to be running his hand over objects or over a beloved face, feeling, and fearing to believe in his own happiness—that these objects really existed and that his eyes were beginning to see.

COMMENT

There are other themes, such as the various ramifications of the doctor-patient relationship with its transference and countertransference problems, and other vivid descriptions, such as that of delirium. However, I fear I belabor my enthusiasm and can only hope this review stimulates some readers who are not familiar with *The Cancer Ward* to read it. What conclusions can be drawn from this presentation? In sum, the book can be read at several levels. I have chosen a medical-psychological one because of my interest and background in the area, as well as its not having been adequately covered previously. Solzhenitsyn's descriptive ability and chartacterization of the cancer patient reveals his deep understanding of human nature. Though he does not use—perhaps the book is enhanced by his not using—psychological jargon or cliches (such as I with the words "denial," "fear of mutilation and loss of sexuality"), he comes up with universal truths and reveals to the reader that life, death, hope, despair, illness, and the basic need for individual freedom are common to all men. The creative writer has much to tell us of the human experience and predicament, more than most of us can comprehend. In such a manner Solzhenitsyn in *The* *Cancer Ward* adds significantly and meaningfully to our understanding of the psychology of the terminally ill patient.

REFERENCE

1. Solzhenitsyn, A.I.: *The Cancer Ward,* R. Frank (trans.), New York: Dell Publishing Co., 1968.

35

The dying patient and the double-bind hypothesis

RICHARD C. ERICKSON and BOBBIE J. HYERSTAY

ABSTRACT—The double-bind hypothesis is applied to the communication patterns surrounding the dying patient. Significant others emit incongruent verbal and nonverbal messages as they attempt to conceal the patient's impending death. Most attempts to conceal are misguided and futile not only because most dying patients suspect and/or want to know the truth, but also because the management of a host of verbal and nonverbal cues is virtually impossible. The potential for psychologically destructive social interactions is documented by drawing parallels with the schizophrenogenic double bind situation. Staff efforts should go into revealing rather than concealing the truth.

Stories come to us from other times and places depicting death as a dramatic moment. Loved ones are gathered at the bedside and the poignant business of settling one's affairs and saying goodbyes is carried out with awesome dignity. A kind of winsome honesty is evident in Kübler-Ross's account of the death of a farmer [1] or the Asian custom of relatives gathering at the bedside of the dying patient two or more days before death is expected, "openly indicating to the patient that they are there to keep him company during his passage out of life" [2]. Granting a measure of romanticizing and a glossing over of unpleasant aspects in these reports, this manner of dying seems infinitely preferable to the impersonal, technological fate we can expect to face.

It is an unpleasant, but probably inevitable, fact of modern times that a majority can expect to die in institutional settings rather than in their own homes and that increasing

numbers can expect to face death at the end of a prolonged decline [2]. It is also inevitable, although not aesthetically pleasing, to expect one's final illness to be invaded by cold hardware—the needles, tubes, wires, and consoles of life-saving, life-supporting, and pain-relieving apparatus. The setting for death could be warmer and more familiar, but in the balance, most would allow that it's a fair trade to increase their chance for survival and physical comfort.

Prevalent in many institutions caring for terminal patients, however, seems to be a consensus bordering on an informal policy that it is desirable and proper to conceal from the patient knowledge of his impending death. Information flows around the patient from doctor to staff to relatives as is deemed necessary, but elaborated precautions are often taken to protect the patient from the fact.

It is the intent of this paper to suggest that most attempts to conceal are not only misguided and futile, but also that they set in motion a brutal set of social interactions

Reprinted from Omega 5:287-298, 1975.

that are psychologically destructive to the patient.

It is probably the case that most patients know their condition whether they are told or not. Avorn [3] cites a study showing that 80% of terminal cancer patients know their diagnosis. Kübler-Ross [1] notes that the outstanding fact of her work with over 200 dying patients was that they all had an awareness of the seriousness of their condition whether they were told or not. Reeves [4] concluded on the basis of his experience that the terminal patient is rare who does not know "regardless of the protective fictions spun by staff and family." Feifel [5] reports that 82% of sample of patients wanted to know about their condition. Kelly and Friesen [6] questioned three groups of people. Eighty-nine per cent of a group of 100 cancer patients who had been told their diagnosis reported they would have preferred to be told. Eighty-two per cent of a group of 100 non-cancer patients reported they would want to know the truth if they had cancer. 98.5% of a group of 740 patients who were undergoing diagnostic tests at a cancer detection center indicated they wanted to be told the truth if they had cancer. Feifel [5] compared studies concerning whether or not to tell patients about their diagnosis. Depending upon the specific study, 69-90% of the physicians studied favored not telling. In an opposing vein, 77-89% of patients wanted to know.

Thus, it seems, an abundance of time and effort goes into producing an elaborate deception for an audience that 1) doesn't want to be deceived and 2) already suspects the grim denouement of the drama.

But setting aside for the moment whether the patient knows or wants to know, what in fact takes place when deception is undertaken? Briefly, an attempt is made to invest a terminal patient with a "fictional future biography" and control his assessment of cues and events that might lead him to suspect the truth [2, 7]. Staff, family, and even other patients may be directly or indirectly informed and enlisted so the

proper behaviors are elicited. The deception presumes to encompass verbal and nonverbal levels.

Controlling verbal behavior would appear to be relatively easy, but, in point of fact, an elaborate system of evasions, double talk and falsehoods is necessary. Glaser and Strauss [2], among others, describe the intricate footwork attempted by staff: misleading explanations for medical decisions, hints and fabrications to suggest favorable progress, discounting symptoms, encouraging the patient to make optimistic interpretations, undue attention to irrelevant statements or events, reducing the range of expression and conversational topics, and focusing talk on the present. The task of keeping a number of staff cued in seems monumental. Inconsistencies will destroy the fiction unless specific measures are taken to transmit information to staff on another shift or to new staff. The sheer complexity of maintaining a consistent verbal facade on the part of the staff, let alone family and other patients, guarantees the eventual collapse of the enterprise if the patient lingers.

The futility of attempting deception is evident when one recognizes that every person also understands and responds to a concurrent set of nonverbal cues. In interpreting a message, a person also attends to the other's gestures, voice pitch and inflection, facial expression, nonresponses, etc. The grammar of body language has been closely studied by Birdwhistell [8] among others. Body language may serve as an indicator of attitudes, status of relationships, degrees of anxiety being experienced, and may accentuate or contradict a verbal statement. For example, Dittman [9] found patterns of body movements indicative of a person's mood. As fleeting as nonverbal signals may be, they likely play a key role in making deception nearly impossible and conveying powerful expectancies affecting performance.

People receive and respond to nonverbal cues even though they may not be able to label or "put their finger on" what they are responding to. It is reasonable to say that people place at least as much, if not more, reliance on subtle, nonverbal cues as verbal cues. In fact, Mehrabrian [10] contends that 93% of the total communicative message is nonverbal.

Several investigators have observed and reported on an abundance of revealing nonverbal cues in the institutional setting [2, 7, 11-13]. The dying patient may be moved to a separate room, a room with a comatose patient, or a room at the end of the hall. There is a tendency to withdraw and have fewer direct communications with him. Staff and visitors behave in tight, constricted ways. Interactions are marked by shallow, brittle cheerfulness. Topics like death and the future are evaded. Visits may become shorter, more perfunctory, or may stop altogether. Extra doctors may appear and tests and procedures are carried out with little explanation given as to their specific purpose. There are tell-tale pauses, eyes that don't meet or drop, unexplained solicitude or privileges. Staff may tend to avoid the room or may look in and leave without coming in. Nurses take longer to respond to call lights from terminal patients. A quite marked pattern known as the "death watch" may be carried out by the nurse if she suspects the end is near. Strauss and Glaser have observed that staff and family organize themselves firmly around an assumed "dying trajectory" and they experience problems if the patient does not follow this pattern.

The sequence of nonverbal cues tells its own story. Unless we are willing to assume that the patient has forgotten what lifelong experience has taught him, we must conclude that he is more or less explicity aware of this deception, or consuming a considerable amount of psychological energy to ignore it. A pathetic note is struck when the patient, aware of the deception, engages in mutual pretense with those attending him [7].

In short, we submit that it is untenable to assume that the truth can be withheld from a patient, i.e., that an elaborate fiction can be carried out for any length of time by a large company of people, none of whom has had a lesson in acting. Whether the patient will suspend his disbelief in response to a good act is questionable. If he does, it will cost him psychological energy to do so. Reality has a habit of continually insinuating itself.

Doctors and other medical staff are invested in trying to alleviate suffering, but often little emphasis is placed in their years of training on how to deal with the enormous crisis an awareness of impending death precipitates nor are they adequately prepared to operate in a context of accountability regarding the psycho-social aspects of death [2, 7]. Their intent is to provide an orderly, tranquil and hopeful setting for the dying patient and for other patients in the setting and they must attempt this in the face of the most disturbing and disrupting event of all. Society expects them to deal with a reality it takes great pains to ignore. Granting their good intentions, it is tempting to conclude that they are making the best of an extremely difficult situation. Perhaps, in the final analysis, they cannot withhold the truth, but at least they have alleviated suffering in the attempt.

Unfortunately, a case can be made that attempts by the staff and family to protect the patient from his diagnosis and prognosis may, in fact, set in motion a set of social interactions that are psychologically destructive to the patient. To explain this, we will need to introduce the reader to the "double bind hypothesis" and its psychiatric consequences.

Briefly defined, the double bind is a situation "1) in which a person is faced with contradictory messages, 2) which is not readily visible as such because of concealment or denial or because messages are on different levels and 3) in which he can neither escape or notice and effectively comment on the contradictions" [14]. The inability to escape to the result of dependence on those giving the contradictory messages, a dependency inherent in childhood or illness.

A simple illustration of a double bind would be a mother saying "Come here, dear" to her child in a slighty hostile tone accompanied by slight bodily withdrawal. Nonverbal and verbal cues don't match, but attempts by the child to clarify meaning by calling attention to the incongruity are met with guilty denial or protests of benevolent concern on the part of the mother. Her attempts to cover up the first incongruity comprise another pair of incongruent messages and so on in a progressive and cumulative manner.

Double bind messages are common enough that most of us recognize them and deal with them using confrontation or humor. We seldom find ourselves sufficiently dependent or subjected to double binds as a recurrent theme. We probably experience them as a transient disruption in the flow of a relationship.

Bateson, Jackson, Haley, and Weakland [15], suggest that when a normal person is caught in a double bind situation he will respond in a defensive manner similar to that of the schizophrenic. Given the double bind as a recurrent theme in a person's experience so that the double bind structure comes to be a habitual expectation, more serious effects may follow. The person may experience increasing difficulty in discriminating communication modes in the messages he receives from others, the messages he emits, or even within his own internal experience. The victim of the recurrent double bind may find himself unable to judge what others mean and resort to continually searching for hidden meanings detrimental to his welfare (paranoid), treating all messages as unimportant or to be laughed at (hebephrenic), or cutting off more and more interaction with the outside world (catatonic). Without help, the person cannot discover what people mean and is subject to a vicious cycle of distortions.

The classic double bind involves the ambivalent mother who emits hostile, withdrawing behavior when the child approaches and simulated loving or approaching behavior as a way of denying that she is withdrawing when the child responds accurately to her behavior. The mother needs to control her anxiety by controlling her distance from the child. "To put this another way, if the mother begins to feel affectionate and close to her child, she begins to feel endangered and must withdraw from him; but she cannot accept this hostile act and to deny it must simulate affection and closeness with her child" [15]. To discriminate, the child must see that the mother doesn't want him and is deceiving him by her loving behavior. All the while, the mother is "benevolently" defining for the child what is going on. The child is punished for correct and incorrect discriminations. And support from others is lacking or cut off.

Little wonder that the victim of a double bind situation experiences helplessness, fear, and rage and may respond with misinterpretations and distortions of reality, constricted and inappropriate emotional responsiveness, loss of empathy with others, and withdrawing or bizarre behavior (the diagnostic description for schizophrenia).

How all this applies to the terminal patient is perhaps becoming evident to the reader. A rereading of the preceding paragraphs substituting staff and /or family for mother and the terminal patient for child is disturbing in its appositeness. We hasten to underline the fact that this material is being presented as a hypothesis, not a demonstrated finding. Reports of interactions between staff and patient and family and patient are too sketchy and anecdotal to offer convincing support at this time. On the other hand, on the basis of published observations and the logic inherent in the situation, it is hard to see how any other interaction can prevail if the patient is not informed of his condition. The reader is invited to test his own experience.

The patient enters the hospital quite literally full of hopes and fears. The very act of entering expresses his willingness to place his life and well being in the hands of an institution and its personnel and his declaration that he sees this place and these people as noble, trustworthy, benevolent and full of life-saving powers. In submitting to treatment he is ascribing almost superhuman powers and rectitude to doctors and staff. At the same time, the act of entering constitutes an admission that he is facing a serious threat which he cannot handle by himself. He is at least apprehensive about how serious the threat is and may entertain the possibility that his life is in danger. Hospitals are not for run-of-the-mill diseases. In short, the patient is more dependent, less self sufficient, more vulnerable and more apt to ascribe magical powers to powerful others than at any other time in his life save childhood. The mode of his interaction is childlike: "I'll do what you say. You must take care of me."

Medical staff are defined by themselves and society as those who are able to take care of sick people. Their task is to save lives, to prevent pain and anguish, to make people comfortable. They are expected to know how to handle things. Never mind their training or temperament. They always do what's best for the patient. "I will take care of you if you do what I say." So death signals a failure and manifest anguish arouses anxiety.

The doctor, most pressed for time, most responsible for the life or death of the patient, is alone granted the authority to withhold or permit revelation of the fact that the patient is about to die. Family and staff can be expected to defer to his spoken or implied wishes. They are unlikely to reveal the truth except with his expressed permission.

The scene is set. Doctor, staff, and family know. The patient does not. All are defining their role vis a vis patient in terms of benevolent concern. All approach the patient with anxiety and a host of ambivalent feelings. The patient is extraordinarily dependent and vulnerable and the messages he receives are of the gravest significance.

The patient begins to pick up nonverbal cues that all is not well. But people keep talking reassuringly. He may be receiving alarming signals from his own body, but these are discounted. Something's wrong, but the evidence for it is so elusive. He can't quite put his finger on the discrepancies. Are visits really shorter, or does it merely seem that way? Is the atmosphere more ominous? Really? Why did the doctor pause that way? Why won't the nurse look me in the eyes? Surely they would say if something was wrong, or would they? The inconsistencies and incongruities pile up and the patient's apprehensions and suspicions increase.

Under the pressure of anxiety, the patient begins to formulate information-seeking questions, probably tactful and approximate. How will he gather evidence for the question, "Are things more serious than I've been told? Am I going to die?" He asks his tentative question of the nurse, or the nursing aide, seemingly innocent but loaded with importance. And the nurse refers him to the doctor, and/or comments with ritual, professional cheerfulness, "Don't you worry about a thing, you're doing just fine." If he tries to pursue it, he may notice subtle signs that the nurse is becoming anxious and she may excuse herself prematurely and tend to avoid the room. If he comments on that, she will deny it and may appear confused or hurt. Yet, if he tries to go along with her verbal reassurance in any serious way, he again notices her discomfort or desire to withdraw from any but the most ritual interactions. Or the family. It's harder to raise the issue with them. It could cause them pain. But how forced and brittle with cheerfulness the visits are getting. If the patient hints of his apprehension, others, with a glance at one another, rush in with reassurance: "You'll be up in no time." But if he tries to approach them as if they had a future together, he notices that he arouses discomfort and precipitates withdrawal. If he tries to comment on that, he gets the message "You are to treat me like I want to be approached."

Reality continues to insinuate itself thru repeated exposure. The patient's suspicions grow and apprehension gnaws at him. Yet no one will settle the issue. The patient begins to doubt himself, feeling he must be missing something. Others act as if the situation were quite logical and consistent. Every comment he makes on the situation seems in some way inappropriate. Something must be wrong with the way he's looking at things.

Should he ask the doctor? He has the authority to say. But consider the doctor's problem. He is most pressed for time. Who can and will deal with the patient's response to the revelation? He has his own anxieties about death. He was supposed to save this man's life—he has failed. On top of his own professional concerns and personal anxieties, he is expected by the family, staff, and perhaps the patient himself to manage so that the situation remains calm, orderly, and hopeful. More than any other person, the doctor is under pressure to evade and postpone revealing the truth. But because of his position, the incongruity in his messages arouse the greatest anxiety. The patient is ill and uncertain. "If the doctor knew, wouldn't he tell me? If he won't tell me, he must be afraid of how I would take it. Perhaps he knows I am dying and has reasons to feel I can't handle the truth. Maybe I couldn't."

In order to get out of the bind, the patient is asked to take on an unbelievable task. He must, on his own, accept the fact he is dying and take the risk of expressing the metacommunicative message: "It is obvious to me you are uncomfortable and evasive around me because I am dying and you are having difficulty dealing with me as a dying person." Such a courageous act may be rewarded with the revelation of the truth and relief on everyone's part. But there is also a great risk that it will set in motion more spirited denial and concealment. The patient faces here the greatest threat that he will experience punishment in the form of anger, withdrawn love, avoidance, and abandonment. How will the doctor, staff and family deal with him when he violates the communication pattern so essential to their security? In fact, he is asking a great deal. Others must admit their own vulnerability and misguided efforts and rely on the dying patient to show strength and concern for them. They must be able to let the patient comfort them in their anxiety and grief.

In summary, then, while the patient may give out his own incongruent messages, this is of secondary importance since the family and staff are not so dependent and can escape the situation and find allies. The patient is deeply dependent on staff and family who may systematically convey the following incongruities: 1) on the verbal level and all controllable nonverbal levels, others attempt to propagate the fiction "You will live." The patient is enjoined (cf, the command aspect of the message [16]) to act confidently and hopefully, to make plans for the future, and to behave as if the present situation were a passing unpleasantry. 2) A pattern of nonverbal cues declare "You will die." The patient is enjoined to come to terms with this reality and to help others—staff and family—to be reconciled to the loss. An undercurrent is the emotional ambivalence on the part of the staff and family similar to that discussed above: they can neither approach or avoid comfortably.

A patient's attempt to respond to the verbal message, i.e., to decrease interpersonal distance by acting on the hypothesis that he will live, not only makes the nonverbal cues more evident, but compounds them as the other person's anxiety increases and he attempts to maintain and embellish the fiction. An attempt to respond to the nonverbal cues is met with denial and protests of benevolent concern. The terminal patient is called upon to distort his perception of reality in order to protect the feelings of the other person and incongruity is piled on incongruity in a progressive and accumulative manner.

When the patient lingers, the theme is recurrent and is played out with ever increasing elaborateness. The institution may programatically deprive the patient of honest informants among staff, family or other patients [2] and he literally cannot leave the field.

At this point, we can anticipate the results observers will report. The patient approaches the time of death with an increasing sense that he has no one he can trust. He feels dishonored and abandoned, anxious and worried [3, 4]. ''At a time when closeness is one of the only remaining sources of joy, it is undermined by an unacknowledged system of deceptions whose intricacy can reach Laingian dimensions'' [3]. ''A patient who is in a life and death crisis may also be caught in an antitherapeutic atmosphere, in which salient facts and perceptions are avoided and distorted. Consequently, he may slant his own communications and thoughts. Then, because people surrounding him mouth platitudes and truisms, the double edged effect may be for everyone involved to repudiate each other, while remaining physically present and officially concerned. For example, if a dying person finds himself treated like a hopeless case or like a child who cannot understand, he may become hopeless about himself, plead that he does not understand, and be convinced that he is worthless as well'' [17]. Strauss and Glaser [7] have noted that withdrawal and apathy may follow the unprogrammed revelation that death is imminent and the trusted family members have been part of the deception. Glaser and Strauss [2] and Reeves [4] have noted that in the end, the patient may need to be stupefied by drugs to manage his behavior or to keep the truth from coming out.

A penultimate experience of abandonment and confusion: a terrible finale. And largely because some scarcely tenable assumptions are made. 1) That a large number of people can effectively carry out an elaborate deception for an extended period of time in the face of a suspecting audience. 2) That revelation of the truth is the only painful or most painful course of action others can carry out. Glaser and Strauss [2] comment on how these assumptions are perpetuated by medical folklore.

An attempt to maintain tranquility in the face of death is similar to the attempt by an estranged couple to smooth over the rift. It only exacerbates the problem. It is certainly true that the truth will precipitate an emotional crisis, but as any psychotherapist will

testify, the pain of expressing pent up feelings is far preferable to bottling them up in an insidious context of deception and distortion. In the balance, it must be acknowledged that the crisis is disturbing and time consuming. Family and staff must be prepared to invest time and emotional energy.

But patients do work thru the crisis [1] and the possibility opens up for loved ones to share honest last few days together [3] and patients can even give support to one another and to the staff [7].

We are not suggesting that the terminal patient is to be told the truth with all due haste and bluntness. There are weighty issues to take into account which have been sensitively discussed at length elsewhere [18]. We are suggesting that deception is usually a futile and destructive strategy. The task facing the staff is how to present to the patient tactfully and with sensitivity that he is probably going to die at the juncture where staff usually begins to implement their deceptions. All the elaborate effort and good will which go into withholding the truth should rather go into revealing the truth. The skill required is similar to that of the psychotherapist who neither bluntly confronts his patient with the truth from the first moment he, the therapist, apprehends it, but neither does he establish or participate in the patient's self deceptions. Rather the therapist bends his efforts to lead the patient to the discovery of the truth about himself.

How might our hospitals be modified and their staff be encouraged to respond more personally, more individually, more humanly to the dying person and his family? How might they be designed to help alleviate the double-binding ''no exit'' situation in which the dying patient may find himself?

Changes might be made within the design of the physical structure itself. Places which provide opportunities for patients and/or their families to engage in either private conversations or more intimate caring relationships would be significant beginning. How can a person share his very most inner, intimate thoughts and feelings of impotence, anger, grief, and helplessness in a two or four bed ward? Difficult, at best! There is isolation in hospitals, but little privacy. Day rooms that invite conversation with others could also be a place where patients and their families could gain support and understanding from each other.

Allowances could be made for live-in situations which are now only accorded the rich. Arrangements could be made for spouses to stay with the patient through those particularly stressful periods when it would be comforting to have the hand of someone close to you to touch for reassurance. This could significantly help the patient deal with his fears of being rejected and abandoned.

Every patient who enters a hospital is expected to unlearn many of the roles which have become so familiar to him and go into making up his identity as a person. He is expected to assume the role of the patient. As institutions are unlikely to change greatly, counselors could assist in interpreting and clarifying with the patient and his family what is going on, what is expected of him, by talking to and with him rather than around and about him. Nothing is more devastating to one's individuality and identity than to be referred to as the "colostomy in Rm. 8."

Being able to bring familiar items from home may also help to take some of the strangeness and unfamiliarity out of the hospital situation. Merely wearing one's own pajamas or laying one's head down on a familiar pillowcase can make a difference when everything else about one is foreign and threatening. Some familiar items are important because they give one a known base from which to begin to tentatively explore new awarenesses and realities.

Rules which prohibit children from visiting their parents may be appropriate to the physical needs of the patient; but are often devastating to the psychological relationship and needs of both child and parent.

It is important that the patient be involved in the planning and decision making processes of his treatment . Having the ability to make input and decisions is an essential part of gaining and maintaining one's individual identity. Explaining what medical procedures, tests, medication and medical terms mean to the patient can begin to reduce some of the ambiguity of the situation. Involving the patient as an active agent in his own treatment can enable him to trust those around him. He can get a better grasp on the reality of his situation rather than having to fabricate his own reality or psychologically withdraw. Forming trusting relationships is one of the most effective ways to encourage open communication.

In addition to the attending physician, an interdisciplinary team including a counselor or psychologist, a social worker, a minister, a recreational therapist and a nurse could be specifically designated to respond to the various needs of the dying patient and his family. As non-medical personnel, they are not conflicted over their "failure" to save the patient's life. The team could focus on the "whole person." The psychologist could meet with dying patients as individuals and in groups and with their families to help them work thru their emotions about the impending death. The social worker could help the patient and his family work out the concrete financial and social problems posed by this drastic change of circumstance. He could also serve as a liaison and an advocate for the patient with other staff and services in the hospital. The social worker would be a key component in helping the patient to understand and adjust to the complex hospital community.

A recreational therapist may seem a strange component on such a team; but pleasure needs of the dying person and his family are sadly neglected. Attendance to individually declared needs may help the patient gain some perspective on his situation and enable him to cope with the long hours in the hospital. A minister would be helpful to responding to the spiritual needs of the individual. A nurse could interpret the "unintelligible" medical terms, tests and procedures to the dying patient as well as providing a liaison with the attending physician. Even patients who are quite ill can benefit from group interaction with the assurance that a nurse is close by if they need her.

Such a team could provide the supportive *core* to which a patient and his family could turn as they try to clarify, understand, and integrate the complexities of the entire situation. It would be the goal of the team to help the patient and his family to live as fully and meaningfully as possible while at the same time assisting them in coping with the many tasks of an individual's dying.

Many have spoken of the need for specialized training for medical personnel in how to respond to the psychosocial needs of the dying patient. The point will not be belabored here. But few have addressed the equally important needs of medical staff, from the physician to the nursing aide. They need an outlet for the feelings of frustration, anger, helplessness and grief that they may experience in caring for the dying person. Counseling services should be provided for staff members who are constantly charged with the task of saving lives, an ultimately impossible task. Medical staff members should have an opportunity to share their thoughts and feelings in a supportive atmosphere, so they can in turn be responsive and supportive to the patient and his family.

Essentially, we are speaking of designing an institution and forming a staff that are person-centered. With a more humanistically oriented institution and staff, it is hoped that the patient might look forward to receiving support and acceptance in his sharings and an "exit" to a double-binding situation. The patient is given an ample opportunity to test with a *core* of others (an interdisciplinary team) what he perceives as reality in an open, honest, supportive way, making it unnecessary for him to resort to a defensive schizophrenic-like reaction to cope with the situation.

REFERENCES

1. Kübler-Ross, Elisabeth, *On Death and Dying,* New York: Macmillan, 1969.
2. Glaser, B. G. and Strauss, A. L., *Awareness of Dying,* Chicago: Aldine, 1965, 3-46.
3. Avorn, Jerry "Beyond Dying," *Harper's,* March 1973, 246(1474): 56-64.
4. Reeves, R., "To tell or Not to Tell the Patient," in A. H. Kutscher, (ed.), *Death and Bereavement,* Springfield Ill.: Chas. C. Thomas, 1964.
5. Feifel, Herman, "Death," in N. L. Faberow, (ed.), *Taboo Topics,* New York: Atherton, 1963, 8-21.
6. Kelly, W. D. and Friesen, J., "Do Cancer Patients Want to be Told?" *Surgery,* 1950, 27, 822-826.
7. Strauss, A. L. and Glaser, B. G., "Patterns of Dying" in O. Brim, et al, (ed.), *The Dying Patient,* New York: Russell Sage Foundation, 1970, 129-155.
8. Birdwhistell, R. L., *Kinesics and Context,* Philadelphia: University of Pennsylvania Press, 1970.
9. Dittman, A. T., "The Relationship Between Body Movement and Moods in Interviews," *Journal of Consultive Psychiatry,* 1962, 26(5): 480.
10. Mehrabian, A., "Communication Without Words," *Psychology Today,* September 1968, 2(4): 52.
11. Sundow, D., "Dying in a Public Hospital," in O. Brim, et al., (eds.), *The Dying Patient,* New York: Russell Sage Foundation, 1970, 191-208.
12. LeShan, L., cited in Bowers, M., Jackson, E. N., Knight, J. A., and LeShan, L., *Counseling the Dying,* New York: Thomas Nelson, 1964, 6-7.
13. Kalish, R. A., "Social Distance and the Dying," *Community Mental Health Journal,* 1966, 2: 152ff.
14. Weakland, J. H., "The Double Bind Hypothesis of Scihzophrenia and Three Party Interaction," in D. D. Jackson, (ed.), *The Etiology of Schizophrenia,* New York: Basic Books, 1960, 373-388.
15. Bateson, G., Jackson, D. D., Haley, J., and Weakland, J., "Toward a Theory of Schizophrenia," in G. D. Shean, (ed.), *Studies in Abnormal Behavior,* Chicago: Rand McNally, 1971, 252-271.
16. Haley, J., *Strategies of Psychotherapy,* New York: Grune and Stratton, 1963.
17. Weisman, A. D., *On Death and Denying,* New York: Behavioral Publications, Inc., 1972.
18. Pemberton, L. B., "Diagnosis: Ca—Should We Tell the Truth," *Bulletin of the American College of Surgeons,* 1971, 56, 7-13.

36

Easing the inevitable

CHAUNCEY D. LEAKE

Neither the sun nor death can be looked at with a steady eye.

La Rochefoucald, 1613-1680

Suddenly, as with so many other skeletons, death has come out of the closet. It is quite socially acceptable to talk seriously about death, which is currently the subject not only of operas, but also of organizations, academic course work, and conferences (both professional and lay). There is little professional psychologic technology or in-group jargon associated with death, so that lay people can often contribute as much as health professionals to an understanding of death.

Health professionals, however, have an increasing obligation to handle dying patients and their friends and relatives. In this work they are wise to deal with death in a dignified, comforting, gently effective way, with genuine empathy, human tenderness, and understanding.

There are so many of us, however, and so many of us who die that it is very difficult to get around the often callous, institutionalized, or bureaucratic routine of dealing with death in a crowded anonymous urban area. This is a disgrace to our vaunted humanity, as Jessica Mitford has emphasized.[1]

Often the disgrace is compounded by venal commercialization of the necessary disposal of the dead. There are signs, however, that this situation is improving, thanks to books and other publicity exposing the unctuous hypocrisy and fraud sometimes associated with the business of disposing of the dead. We should now work on spon-soring some publicly supported dignified places for holding services for the dead—free from bureaucratic callousness—to ease the burden of the inevitable for poor people.

Rural areas have a much better way of dealing with their dead. With fewer people nearly everyone knows everyone else, and there is thus a greater sharing of our common humanity in births, marriages, and deaths than is possible in crowded cities and slums. In rural areas sham and fraud are quickly detected, and false emotionalism is rarely tolerated. Wise grandmothers deal with death openly and honestly, comforting the dying and those near and dear with tenderness and understanding. They know from long experience how to ease the inevitable.

Women are generally better than men in dealing with death and other inevitable crises. Their emotions are more open and thus more real. Men feel that it is a part of their manliness to suppress their natural emotions, especially in the face of death. This seems to be the case in all cultures.

Ethnic groups handle death and dying patients with the dignity and decency of long tradition. The Chinese, the various Latin groups, the Irish, the Germans, the Poles, the Scandinavians, and the English all have established customs for dealing with death in a dignified way, as do Greeks, Muslims, Hindus, Japanese, Africans, American Indians, and Slavs. It would be wise for us to foster these aspects of ethnic culture to preserve the social benefits of a variety of traditions that have so far managed to survive even the pressures of urban and slum life. A sympathetic understanding of how other cultures deal with death might benefit all of us.

We all go through the cycle of birth, life, death, and rebirth through the next generation. In the Stone Age culture that instructed people to worship the Great Mother, the initiation of teenagers into adult life included the ritual of portraying how our species continues to exist through individual birth, death, and then rebirth. As Robert Graves the great English poet emphasized, there was much wisdom among people in antiquity. It would aid us to become familiar with it again.

PUBLICITY ON DEATH AND DYING

Many publications, popular and professional, have appeared on various aspects of death and dying. Publicity in the matter was well under way a decade ago. My colleagues Barney Glaser and Anselm Strauss, sociologists in the University of California School of Nursing, offered a helpful volume, *Awareness of Dying,*[2] many years ago. Its dust jacket depicts the usual reaction to death on the part of health professionals: seeing nothing, hearing nothing, and saying nothing.

The wisdom of these same sociologists was again shown in *Time for Dying,*[3] in which health professionals are advised about their conduct, their demeanor, and their attitude when handling dying patients.*

---

*A compassionate article for physicians was that by William Easson: Care of the young patient who is dying, (J.A.M.A. **205**:203-207, July 22, 1968). The American Association for the Advancement of Science held an important symposium, "Problems in the Meaning of Death" at its Chicago meeting, December 29, 1970. This symposium was sponsored by the Institute of Society, Ethics and the Life Sciences, Hastings, New York. One of the more philosophical of the discussions at this symposium was given by sociologist Robert S. Morison of Cornell on "Death: Process or Event" (*Science,* **173**:694-703, August 20, 1971).

Meanwhile the late distinguished anesthesia expert at Harvard, Henry K. Beecher, chaired a committee that tried to set specific guidelines for determining the time of death,[4] for years commonly held to be 5 minutes after the last detectable heartbeat. Beecher's criterion of death was cessation of electrical activity of the brain as shown by electric encephalogram. Beecher sought "agreement that brain death is death indeed even though the heart continues to beat." His reasoning was physiologically sound, and general agreement with it is slowly emerging.

Austin Kutscher of New York organized The Foundation of Thanatology, which has for a decade sponsored symposia on death and dying. The tenth anniversary symposium in 1977 dealt with the education of medical students in thanatology, a helpful addition to the sterotyped medical curriculum.

At its Denver meeting in February, 1977, the American Association for the Advancement of Science held a symposium "The Right to Die." Mansell Pattison of the University of California, Irvine, discussed psychosocial factors in coping with dying. He emphasized that dying is a process. Seldom do we face dying rationally. Seldom is our comprehension of and meeting with death the same in every instance; we face death at different times in our life cycle. An appropriate death means different things to different people. Decisions made by health professionals about a dying patient make sense only within the context of the quality of life of the dying person. People are rarely left to fend for themselves when faced with dying. We help each other as we can often by projecting ourselves into the other's thoughts. This may even apply when the useless aged among the Eskimos finally of their own accord go out alone in the cold snow to die.

The English view of death is well expressed by John Hinton, Professor of Psychiatry at Middlesex Hospital Medical School in London.[5] He discusses attitudes toward death, from fear to acceptance;

physical and emotional distress in terminal illness, including the patient's awareness and denial, struggle, and acceptance; care of the dying, from treatment through speaking of death, to the question of whether to prolong life or hasten death; and finally mourning, including reactions to bereavement and the eventual reestablishment of equanimity. Professional health personnel could learn much from this approach.

DEALING WITH DYING PATIENTS

Fortunately there are many tools available to help professionals improve their care of dying patients. Drugs in abundance can alleviate pain, induce sleep, and effect euphoria. For the comfort of the dying, health workers would be wise to use such drugs in large enough amounts to give the desired effect. There is no point in worrying about an excessive use or possible addiction. Certainly, if pain is present, morphine should be administered in appropriate amounts to give relief. Morphine, with its relaxing power, induces some euphoria as well as provides relief from pain. None of the recent commercialized substitutes for morphine is as satisfactory as morphine itself.

The gentlest and kindest way of easing the inevitable in a dying patient is to give the blessed comfort of sleep. Death can come mercifully when one is asleep. Barbital and phenobarbital are approximately as satisfactory as any chemical agent for bringing on sleep.

The psychologic approach to easing the physical and mental pain of dying is much more difficult. It is usually overdone. Dying people are embarrassed if people make too much of an effort to be helpful. Such an effort is apt to be hypocritical anyway. It is better to hold the hand of a dying person and to hold one's tongue. It is better to be honestly empathic than to be fussily solicitous.

Dying people can often be made comfortable, euphoric, and tranquil with what is quite readily available. It is not always necessary to have all the facilities and expensive surroundings of a hospital. fessionals may not be needed if t sensible older person around. A full of whiskey diluted a bit can be pain-d pressing, euphoric, and comforting. It is usually easy to obtain and may be the most satisfactory first aid in an emergency when death seems imminent.

Also in the slow anguishing dying caused by terminal cancer, the usual drugs, such as morphine to relieve pain or phenobarbital to induce sleep, may well be supplemented by alcoholic beverages. Sipping wine or beer at mealtime, whether at home or in a hospital, may make more agreeable the difficult task of eating.

Professional health personnel would wisely strive for empathic gentle ministration during the terminal illness of their patients. It is unwise to engage in frivolous conversation, but it is humane to be understandingly empathic. Professional health workers see death in many forms. Team work with advance planning is essential for effective care no matter what the eventuality. Although physicians will lead the team, the nurses, who spend more time with the dying, will be called on most to bring comfort to the patient.

Professional health personnel should be familiar with the religious and legal formalities associated with death. If religious aid seems to be indicated, it should be promptly obtained. The same goes for legal advice. In easing the inevitable for the terminally ill, it is essential to attend to the welfare of the patient, even at individual self-sacrifice.

There is frequently the temptation in caring for the terminally ill to do everything possible to keep the patient alive. This may be very cruel, and it sometimes becomes a game, unconscious though it may seem to be, to see how long a health team can keep a terminally ill person alive. We must not play games with death.

Modern technology makes it possible to keep people alive long after they might otherwise have died. But is the lengthened life worth living? It might be distressful and ned, but again it

87, he fell on the
ig our car and frac-
ad a complete heart
ere unaware, but his
skillful neurosurgeon
ine, and my father had
When he had regained
cons~ er a couple of weeks, he
said to me, .. didn't you let me die: that was my time to go. Now I'll be a burden to myself and to you, and I do not like it." He lived quietly and happily for 7 more years, dying at 94 of pneumonia, the merciful friend of the aged. This was a fortunate case. Not all attempts to prolong life come out so well. When one's father asks why he wasn't permitted to die, one may well begin to think about death and what it means.

An ancient tradition in the medical profession calls on physicians to do everything possible to save a life. On occasion, however, they may go beyond reason. Governmental agencies, in particular, are prone to go to great extremes to prolong life. A distressing case concerns the Veterans Administration. A distinguished scientist was in an automobile accident in which his brain was severely injured. He was comatose with no electric activity in the brain except in the medullary areas. His heart and circulation functioned well, but he had to be maintained in a respirator. He was kept alive in this way, although completely comatose, with intravenous feeding for 8 long years. Meanwhile his wife, in her thirties, had to wait it out. Finally the respirator went off, accidentally or deliberately—who can say? We may well ask whether any useful, kindly, sensible good was accomplished by this expensive long effort to keep a body alive without a functioning brain. Karen Quinlan is another case in point. With my long time friend, Irvine Page, I question the wisdom of supplying elaborate life-prolonging techniques to every patient.

It takes long experience and much wisdom to make sound judgments in medical practice, especially when death ap-

proaches. The ancient Hippocratic wisdom of the Aesclepiads of old Greece is still applicable. Their first aphorism cautions: "Life is short, and the Art long, the occasion fleeting; experience fallacious, and judgment difficult." The harmony ethic of the Chinese sages, the Buddha, and Aristotle is also still appropriate for medical practice. It advises moderation in all things and living in harmony with oneself and one's environment. It suggests calm effectiveness, gentleness, kindness, and understanding in dealing with death and the dying. Such an attitude can ease the inevitable for professional personnel as well as patients.

DEALING WITH RELATIVES AND FRIENDS OF DYING PATIENTS

Sometimes it is more difficult for health workers to deal effectively with the relatives and friends of dying patients than with the patients themselves. The relatives and friends are usually anxious, apprehensive, nervous, and critical. They often seem to blame the professional health personnel for the death of their relative or friend. This emotional response is behind many malpractice suits involving the care of dying patients.

The difficulty in handling the relatives and friends of dying patients seems to be chiefly because of their preoccupation with feelings of guilt, which greatly confuse their emotional reactions. Their grief is often guilt at something they did or failed to do for the dying person. Professional health personnel may find it helpful to get some training in psychosocial approaches to grief and bereavement.

Again, health care professionals should exhibit kindness, gentleness, calm efficiency, and empathic understanding. Conversation may aid. Guilt feelings are often relieved by talking about the misdeeds: confessing, feeling sorry, and then receiving assurance that the dead person has long ago forgiven or forgotten.

To open the way for conversation, members of the professional health group can pleasantly ask about some of the things the dead person might have done or been interested in. They might also take the opportunity to help the bereaved ones recall some of the happy moments they shared with the dead one. The example of the dead or dying patient can be presented as an inspiration to carry on for those left behind.

Health care professionals can also help the bereaved family by assisting them in attending to the various legal matters associated with the dying patient. Obtaining a postmortem examination is not always easy. The legal permission for one may sometimes be obtained by expressing doubt about the real cause of death or by showing that the examination will add to the overall knowledge of pathologic processes and aid in the diagnoses and treatment of people in the future. It is helpful to give aid in the selection of an appropriate undertaker and in arrangements for a funeral or memorial service. It is also important to help the family take prompt care of Medicare or Blue Cross red tape.

The bereaved in the immediate family of the dying will gain much comfort from knowing that the health workers who are caring for their terminally ill relative are functioning smoothly, efficiently, with kindness, good will, gentleness, and calm unhurried good sense. This eases the inevitable in the most satisfying way to all concerned.

A FEW PERSONAL NOTES

We cannot come into old age without having many encounters with death. Each situation is different. Each experience is humbling. Each time we may learn more about our common humanity and thereby come to deal more humanely with friends, neighbors, and relatives. Gradually we learn not to do those things we ought not to do and to do more graciously those we ought to do, and thus there may be more health in us.

When I was a boy approximately 11 years old, my maternal grandfather and grandmother lived with us in a rather pleasant old home. My grandfather apparently died suddenly from a stroke when he was out in the garden. I remember how hushed and solemn were my usually cheerful mother and grandmother as they carried him limp and ashen into the library and laid him on a couch. He did not respond at all to my greeting, and my mother hushed me and took me upstairs without comment. I was puzzled and hurt. Only at the solemn funeral did I begin to realize that he was no more, that he was dead. Long did I ponder over where he might be. We never discussed his death, and only rarely did we recall episodes from his life. It was a devastating experience, for we had so often played happily together in the garden. Slowly as life so busily rolled on I realized that it was up to me to carry on and do what was to be done day by day. So I got a healthy respect for death, but somehow the thought lingered that we had not been able to meet death appropriately. That doubt persists.

My paternal grandparents had long been gone, and I knew of them only by occasional comments usually given with a respect that I learned to appreciate. I was away when my wife's father died, but the memory of the grief at his passing remains with me. My wife's mother died in my arms.

She had come from her longtime home to be with us, as she seemed to know her time was near. She was 87. We often talked after dinner of her long life with her friends and relatives, learning of the background of both her family and that of her husband. She seemed happy in giving us family history. One evening she was lying on a couch in her room, and she asked me to come sit by her. My wife came too. We held her hands, as she took longer and longer breaths, and then, asking me to hold her, she smiled and sank back dead. This was a shattering experience.

She was very much a churchwoman, believing ardently in the future happiness of her soul. These beliefs are powerful supports to the dying and should be strongly respected, as William James has emphasized. In his famed essay *The Will to Believe* (1897) he insisted that everyone had the *right* to believe as he or she wished. It is wise to remember this bit of philosophy.

I am a scientist, accustomed to look for solid evidence on which to base belief. There is no such evidence regarding the concept of soul, which has, however, a long history of psychologic and anthropologic justification. So it is with that equally baffling concept of mind. My wife and I often talked about these matters and gradually evolved a satisfying way of thinking, that has long been a comfort for us. It is expressed as "humanism" and has been brilliantly expounded in *Dragons in Eden* by Carl Sagan. I have always been careful to show respect for other people's beliefs and indicate that I expect them to show respect for mine.

It is distressing to watch the slow torture of death by inoperable cancer. We had such an experience with our sister-in-law, a keen scientist in her own right. She was game to the end, holding her own in conversation even when in much pain and distress. She died in the University of California Hospital with my wife, my brother (her husband), and me holding her hands. My brother went out suddenly with a bad heart while bowling. He knew it was coming from his anginal attacks, but he was cheerfully ready for it. He even laughed over the way nitroglycerine would relieve his angina.

My colleague at the University of Texas Medical Branch, the distinguished tissue-culture expert, Charles Pomerat, developed cancer of the bowel. It became inoperable, but he maintained his good humor, joking about the misbehavior of his colostomy until the pain was no longer containable. He then did what we had often talked about: He gave himself a fatal dose of morphine, writing out his feelings until coma came on. It was a dignified death in the privacy of his bachelor apartment.

Only a generation or so ago it was impossible to talk openly about death. Children in their natural curiosity might ask, but their elders would quickly shush them with,

"That's something we don't talk about," as though it were something evil. Now it has become quite socially acceptable to talk and ask questions about death and dying: how to accept it, how to prepare for it, how to meet it. This helps to ease the inevitable.

In October of 1976, my wife Elizabeth and I celebrated our eightieth birthdays and our fifty-fifth wedding anniversary. We were given a gala dinner with more than 200 guests. It was a touching affair. When we were alone with our two sons and daughter-in-law, we talked about our happy life and wondered laughingly how long it might last.

In March 1977, we had a blow. Our cousin, Virginia Williams of Novato, beautiful at 16 and a splendid horsewoman who had won some 50 blue ribbons, was killed in an automobile accident. When we joined the despondent family I read to them something that occurred to me on the spur of the moment:

> Ask not of Death, why?
> For Death cannot answer, being dumb.
> Nor can we answer, either,
> For we are stricken, paralyzed and numb.
> But let's recall her life:
> It was a triumph, full of joy and verve;
> It was sheer delight!
> For us, it is a memory to preserve.

This seemed to comfort all especially at the memorial service when the rector read it. It has since seemed to comfort others also. What more can we say?

In April of 1977, the San Francisco Spring Opera put on a triple bill of one-act operas: A Monteverde number, one with a Hindu theme, and one composed by two men in a Nazi prison camp who knew they would probably be killed. All three dealt with death, but with death as a kindly merciful character who is always with us, as the medieval Europeans realized and pictured. Afterward Elizabeth and I were talking, and she said, "If you go before I do, I intend to carry on; If I go before you, I'll expect you to carry on."

For Mother's Day, our elder son planned a happy outing. We had a noble dinner such as Elizabeth loved to prepare and serve, and we had fun deciding where to go. But that night Elizabeth did not feel well. Next morning she had pains in her chest and was nauseated. So we called her physician, and he said to get her to the hospital promptly. She dressed neatly as usual, and we soon had her comfortable in bed with most efficient and gentle care. She was cheerful when we were with her and laughed about how we'd be on our way in a few hours. She went to sleep and never woke up.

We've been swamped with letters from all over, each one a comfort in itself and all testifying to the real affection people had for Elizabeth. I had already committed myself to writing this paper on death and dying, and indeed it was Elizabeth's idea for me to talk about "easing the inevitable." So we are carrying on.

AVE ATQUE VALE

Life is continually "hail and farewell": Hail the newborn; farewell to the dying. Professional health personnel are closer to these realities than any other group of people. They have an almost sacred obligation to ease the inevitable. Increasingly they are doing it well with compassion, with gentleness, with efficiency, with tenderness, and with understanding. Realizing these ideals may bring them deep satisfaction.

REFERENCES

1. Mitford, J.: The American way of death, New York, 1975, Fawcett World Library: Crest, Gold Medal & Premier Books.
2. Glaser, B., and Strauss, A.: Awareness of dying, Chicago, 1965, Aldine Publishing Co.
3. Glaser, B., and Strauss, A.: Time for Dying, Chicago, 1968, Aldine Publishing Co.
4. Beecher, A. K.: J.A.M.A. **205**:337, 1968.
5. Hinton, J.: Dying, Baltimore, 1967, Penguin Books, Inc.

37

A child dies

CHARLES A. GARFIELD

"My child should be protected from it as long as possible. . . Susan is still too young to think about death. It just isn't normal for her to concern herself yet. Besides, she wouldn't understand." Parents of healthy children often believe and act upon these notions.

As adults we assume that we have the power either to tell children about mortality or to keep them protected in insulated ignorance. Believing that the child's awareness of death is unnatural or may be harmful, we discuss death with the child in such a way that the goal is usually one of deft "management" of the issue—so that death can go away again. But can we actually stave off all these intrusions of death awareness? Can children then resume their supposedly sheltered existence? More important, what should we tell the child who is dying, for whom death is least likely to go away?

The view that young children are not or should not be aware of death remains with us, not because it is true, but because it serves to protect adults at certain vulnerable points. Although the dying child may never have been told in explicit terms of the severity of his condition, he has received other communications. He has seen and heard the normal, understandable adult response to watching a child die—the voice that trembles, the eyes that look away, and the shoulders that sag, belying the forced smile. Between 70 and 90 percent of the communication between adults is non-verbal. Less attached to words than most adults, children may rely even more heavily on nonverbal information. Verbal attempts at massively sugarcoating the real situation of the dying child are most often contradicted by the obvious stress and anxiety of parents and hospital staff. What results is an ambiguity and confusion far more likely to torment the child than the truth.

"Sarah knows each time there is something seriously wrong," a mother whose 8-year-old daughter was dying said. "She imagines that terrible things will be happening and has terrible fears. As soon as we label the problem and give it a name, there's only one thing she has to be scared of. She doesn't have to worry about turning into a yellow monster tomorrow."

Judith Viorst, in her article "The Hospital That Has Patience for Its Patients," (Redbook, February, 1977) quotes a 9-year-old boy: "The baddest thing is to lie to a kid. It's much badder to lie to me than to scare me by telling me the truth. To lie to a kid is the baddest thing of all."

A nurse in pediatrics told me recently that Ben, a 10-year-old boy, was admitted to the hospital to be treated for leukemia. Although obviously frightened, Ben was proud of the fact that he had deciphered the nature of his illness "before anyone told me a thing." He remembered riding up in the elevator to the appropriate floor, exiting, and immediately seeing a sign that said "Comprehensive Cancer Center." Ben asked several people if he had cancer. He could not help noticing the obvious distress of the adults he asked, the tears in his mother's eyes, the stress of his doctor and nurse, and their reluctance to answer his questions. Undaunted, he decided that what he needed was a dictionary. From it, Ben learned that cancer is "a very harmful growth in the body, a malignant tumor" and that it "destroys the healthy tissues and organs of the body." He also discovered that it is an "evil or harmful thing that tends to spread." As a painful bonus he found that malignant means "very evil; very hateful; very harmful; very dangerous; causing death."

When Ben watched Dr. Marcus Welby on television fail to cure a patient with cancer, the situation became even worse. When Ben noticed wall plaques in memory of patients who had died, that was the last straw. Once gregarious, he now became withdrawn and depressed.

Fortunately Ben's nurse was supportive. She understood that fear, depression, and anger are normal responses for children (and adults) facing life-threatening illnesses. Deeply caring, she realized that being emotionally involved with Ben was good for both of them. She spent extra time with him talking, drawing, and examining baseball cards. Ben learned that when his nurse was 9 years old she had sometimes been very frightened and sad. What she needed most then, she told him, was a close friend with whom she could talk, cry, and even laugh when things were funny. Ben and his nurse exchanged stories about their favorite pets. Each had had a dog who had grown old and died. How wonderful to have a dedicated friend—how sad when he died! Together they mourned the loss of their childhood companions, an ageless grief uniting the two of them.

"The saddest thing of all," cried Ben, "is that I won't even live as many years as Kip. He died when he was 12 and I'll never be 12." It was then that he told the nurse how he'd learned of his illness. She assured him that although his illness was a serious one he was not likely to die very soon and that

he had not done anything "evil" or "hateful." In fact, she assured him that he was a wonderful boy to have as a friend.

Gradually things began to change for Ben. (Later the hospital staff recalled that things began changing for them then too.) His nurse played a big role in this. The staff encouraged Ben to ask questions and answered them honestly and kindly. It became a staff policy to keep Ben regularly informed (even if he did not ask) about what would happen next and why and about whether or not it would hurt and, if so, how much. This gave Ben some preparation time for each trauma, time to muster the strength necessary for coping with the emotional and physical jolts.

For most people—and especially for children—hospital experiences are strange indeed. The pain of illness or treatment, the absence of their parents, the fear that illness is some sort of punishment, and the fears of separation, mutilation, and helplessness can be powerfully disorienting. To assume that children will quickly recover from the emotional assault of hospitalization is to underestimate children's intelligence and sensitivity.

In her article, Judith Viorst discusses some fascinating (albeit painful) misconceptions concocted by hospitalized children fearful that illness and pain were punishment for sin.

"God makes you sick because you're bad," one child said.

Imagine the anxiety of a young boy who knew that touching his penis would make him ill. Proving the point, he cited the example of a friend of his having fallen ill in just this way, who was cured by "peni(s)cillin"!

Hospital terminology is far more unfamiliar than we realize and can often be translated by a child into something more understandable and terrifying. As Viorst observes, a "bone marrow test" becomes—with all its ghastly implications—a "bow and arrow test." A blood test may mean "they'll drain out all of my blood." One terror-stricken child whose doctor planned to inject her with dye collapsed in tears believing that what he was administering was spelled d-i-e and was surely fatal.

Like most children, Ben knew little of how a hospital operates. Everything seemed unfamiliar: the endless pieces of equipment and instruments, the food that tasted strange, and the new children he met in the playroom. Accordingly Ben appreciated the tour of the hospital arranged by his nurse. Discussions with such resident luminaries as playful puppets and erudite clowns (as well as the staff behind them) did much to reduce his anxiety and confusion. His doctor explained patiently and accurately about Ben's particular form of leukemia, the benefits and side-effects of each drug he recommended, and his intention to help Ben spend as much time at home as possible.

One day following such a discussion, Ben proudly announced, "Now that I know all about leukemia, I really wish I could grow up and be a doctor."

"You'd make a fine doctor, Ben," his father agreed. "We'd love to have you teach us all about your illness right now."

So "Dr. Ben," after preparation, gave several careful talks to his parents, sister, and nurse about pediatric leukemia and its treatment. After each lesson, Ben and his family discussed their feelings about his illness and about each other. Ben's 12-year-old sister Sandy shared her fear and sadness and the annoying fact that everyone paid much less attention to her than before. Sandy's emotional needs, like those of many siblings of seriously ill children, had been virtually forgotten. Ben's parents decided to include her in more family discussions and to encourage her to express her feelings more freely.

Sandy, having begun to grieve the loss of her brother, was frightened and confused. Her parents, who were grieving too, were emotionally drained. They wondered where they could get the strength to help Ben and at the same time cope with such a sad, painful loss. Sandy and Ben agreed to have a private meeting each day to discuss how they could best "take care of their parents."

It is to parents of a dying child that fate delivers the severest blow. We fear for our children as we fear for ourselves. Never have we lived or loved enough. Death always comes too soon.

It was all too obvious to Ben's parents that he had not lived enough. They agreed that what he needed most was the feeling of being loved enough. Through the remainder of Ben's illness, the family grew closer, spending more time together and sharing more personal feelings and experiences. Ben, Sandy, and their parents found that this new family closeness was their single most important form of emotional support.

At first Ben responded well to treatment and was able to return to school. Later as his illness progressed, he came to the hospital weekly for massive doses of powerful drugs. The drugs made him vomit and lose his hair and left him pale, exhausted, and at times embarrassed. As the disease began to spread through his bones, Ben was in constant pain and very vulnerable to infection. "We have a problem," Ben announced one day after his daily conversation with Sandy. "I think I'm getting worse."

Ben revealed his fears about dying and pain, leaving his parents and sister, and the awful thought that he might have to be "put to sleep like Kip." Reaching for their son, Ben's parents assured him that they would be with him no matter what happened. They reminded Ben that his doctor promised to do everything possible to control the pain if it got worse. Although there might come a time when he felt like sleeping more often, never would anyone "put you to sleep like Kip."

After consulting with his physician, Ben and his parents decided to concentrate their efforts on keeping the boy comfortable. During his last months of life, Ben often played alone as if quietly contemplating the task ahead. Most of this period Ben spent at home. His favorite nurse visited often. Sitting on the living room floor they talked, drew with crayons, and played with finger paints or clay. The nurse understood that children often communicate a great deal of their emotional reality through pictures and stories. Huge doctors with tiny patients, hungry lions and helpless children, towering mountains and struggling cable cars, all revealed Ben's unspoken fears.

These long hours of caring for Ben were understandably difficult for his parents, but through it all—the pain, their son's agonizing physical changes, their own fear—they remained at Ben's side, often barely coping with their own terror. Frequently consulting each other about Ben's status—and their own—was a way of expressing mutual appreciation and taking care of each other. By preserving a sense of humor and consoling each other during midnight outpourings of grief, they maintained the emotional strength necessary to continue. Alternating shifts and taking breaks—sometimes short ones, occasionally for an entire day— helped, too.

During it all Sandy played an active role in caring for her brother, even managing to allow her parents an infrequent evening's respite together. Although these breaks were necessary to stay sane and replenish their energy, Ben's parents often found that being away from their son was actually more stressful than being with him. But the biggest stress of all, they acknowledged, would be to feel later that they had not given Ben every ounce of love and caring of which they were capable.

Although Ben himself had long since been resigned to death, he still spoke occasionally of "fighting the leukemia with all my might, because I don't want to die." Progressively, though, he grew weaker. A massive infection had invaded Ben's body, causing him to drift in and out of waking consciousness. Still, although he was occasionally restless, Ben seemed in less pain than before. Early one evening Ben's breathing became gradually more shallow. With his parents and sister gently holding him, Ben died. Still holding her brother's hand and through a torrent of tears, Sandy broke the eerie silence that followed.

"I can't believe Ben's gone, that he's not here. Why did he have to die? It's not fair!"

"It isn't fair, Sandy," replied her mother. "It's not fair at all. Go ahead and cry for Ben because you love him and because it's the only thing that makes any sense."

For several minutes they sat with Ben's body, all saying their silent goodbyes. A huge part of their world had come to an end. Things would never be the same again.

38

Dying in a system of "good care"; case report and analysis

MARTIN G. NETSKY

The ·circumstances of the case to be presented are factual, but a particular institution is not implied. The report is intended to reveal what may commonly occur, as a basis for the analysis and conclusions.

An 80-year old woman, my mother, became unable to manage her daily needs and was unwilling to be attended by those closest to her. She therefore decided to go to a nursing home. Mother's mind began to wander in those last months, but at lucid times she would ask, "Why does God let me live so long?" I usually turned away from the question; I simply did not know the answer. She made me promise she would not be allowed to linger under the devices of modern medicine. I agreed, but in the end I was unable to fulfill her wish.

In the nursing home my mother felt that she had lost her usefulness, was a burden to her children, and was not her "old self." Repeated episodes of involuntary urination and defecation were extremely distressing to her, as well as to the staff of the nursing home, especially when the cleaning was delayed. A sudden alteration in her physical condition led to transfer to a hospital. There, she was at first partially conscious, but soon lapsed into coma. Extensive investigation and treatment failed to alter the

coma, which persisted except for occasional lucid moments.

Upon arrival in the hospital emergency room, my mother entered into a course of diagnostic evaluation and treatment in an institution priding itself on good care. A course in medical ethics was offered at the associated medical school. At no time, however, could I determine who was responsible for her management. Many physicians entered and left the emergency room, but I was unable to identify which one decided to move her from the emergency room and to admit her to the hospital as an inpatient. Residents, interns, medical students, nurses, and aides moved around her in a swivel. Despite the fact that she was a "private" patient, she was assigned to an attending physician without anyone inquiring about my wishes or even informing me of the assignment. After the initial shock of the events disappeared, I was annoyed that I had not been asked what I wanted done, or whether I would approve of the physician selected. In the light of later events, it probably did not matter. Most doctors in the institution were trapped by the system.

What happened was a nightmare of depersonalized institutionalization, of rote management presumably related to science, and based on the team approach of subdivision of work. The nurses gave by far the best care. My mother's unconscious body

Reprinted from *The Pharos of Alpha Omega Alpha,* **39**:57-61, 1976, with the permission of the Editor.

was cleaned and bathed regularly, but no regularly indentifiable person performed these functions. Different nurses wandered in and out of my mother's room each hour, each shift, each day, calling for additional help from nameless others over a two-way radio. They rarely introduced themselves to me. They were trained as part of a team "covering the floor" rather than aiding a sick human being.

A few months before, when undergoing minor surgery in the same hospital, I had noted similar nameless packs wandering into my room—residents, interns, registered nurses, licensed practical nurses, student nurses, nurses' aides, takers of blood pressures, takers of temperatures, cleaners of the floor, cleaners of the woodwork above the floor, orderlies, technicians, and indeed almost everyone but the surgeon. Most elements of this impersonal horde never identified themselves. It was as if each was obligated to perform a set task in relation to tended bodies in various rooms. The teamwork and subdivision of labor presumably made each person more efficient at his work, but the depersonalization chilled me.

The physicians began the routine ministrations to the patient, my mother. The resident told the intern and the medical student what tests to order, initiated the giving of fluids, oxygen, antibiotics, set the frequency of recordings of blood pressure, pulse, respiration, temperature, and the insertion of tubes. From my knowledge of the system I supposed that the resident was consulting with the attending physician, but my assumption was never verified. My inquiries resulted in vague reassurances, and I was reluctant to press the issue.

Occasionally, the initials of the attending physician appeared on the progress notes, which I was privy to read, but there was no progress. I was a regular visitor, but I did not see this doctor for many days. He was "on rounds," in conference, lecturing, out-of-town, or simply not available. The resident came to his "end of service" and a fresh, unversed man became visible. I tried

again to see the attending physician and asked the new resident for assistance. He had no knowledge of how to locate the attending physician, nor the method of obtaining an audience. I called the medical secretary, saying that I wished to talk to the physician-in-charge. The peremptory answer was, "Is this an emergency?" Possibly she was shocked when I replied, "Yes, my mother is dying." Clearly, the secretary saw her function as a shield against anxious relatives.

When the meeting between me and the attending physician was finally achieved, I explained what my mother had said when lucid: she and her closest relatives, including my brother, did not want unnecessary prolongation of the agony of dying. We would prefer, for example, that oxygen and antibiotics not be given. The attending physician listened sympathetically, understood fully, and agreed completely; but *nothing changed*. He who should have been in control of the system was dominated by it! Laboratory studies of blood and urine continued to be performed, fluids were given, oxygen was bubbled in, antibiotics were administered; and days went by but seemed to be years. The patient was seen occasionally by large groups of physicians making rounds, presumably learning the art of practicing medicine properly.

I began wondering who looked at the accumulating mass of data. The nurses recorded their detailed observations of vital functions and behaviors, but did anyone except the nurses see the comments? The chart was enlarged regularly with the "progress notes." These hastily scrawled writings always dealt with laboratory data, never about the feelings of the patient or her family, and certainly never with the question, is this effort necessary or wanted? Yellow slips of laboratory data and reports of special procedures continuously added to the thickness of the chart. My mother's inert body was regularly weighed, but for what purpose I did not know, except that it was part of standard management for medical patients, and gave a member of the team another routine duty to perform. Life was being preserved, but little thought given to the means or the purpose.

One report stated that occult blood had been found in the stool. Someone responded by writing in the chart that, in view of this finding, sigmoidoscopic examination and a barium enema were indicated. I suggested to the author that his conditioned reflexive act was not warranted in the care of an unconscious 80-year-old woman who wanted to die gracefully. If a cancer of the bowel were found, would he subject her to major surgery? He admitted that he would not. Then why make the suggestion? "That's what I have been taught," was his answer. The laboratory studies continued to grow, and the records now were massive.

I managed another conference with the attending physician. His response was to ask for a consultant to see the patient. The new person stated on the chart, but not to me, that the care being given was the best and the "regimen" should continue. The residents reacted similarly, regularly calling for other physicians—"consultants." The usual function of the consultant is to offer ideas of diagnosis or treatment not previously considered, not in the domain of expertness of the attending physician. Most consultants suggested additional studies in the sphere of their own competence. I did not want more studies, preferring compassionate care, and I refused the services of one consultant. Another offered *me* the opportunity to be the physician for my mother by *my* deciding whether she should have burr holes placed to look for subdural hemorrhage. I decided he was treating me rather than her, and that he should make the decision, allowing me to approve or disapprove.

At this juncture, I considered removing Mother from the hospital. The nursing home would not take her. What about another hospital in town—would they offer more humane and individually responsible treatment? Being uncertain, I decided to wait until further inquiry revealed whether the present treatment would be repeated

elsewhere. I even contemplated bringing her home, but decided, perhaps foolishly, that a hospital was more appropriate and that the end might soon come.

Agonizing time went by. We waited for the merciful end, but experienced no mercy from the physicians treating her. Each did his routine job of saving life when it was almost not present. A formerly vivacious and attractive person now existed only as a human body with a beating heart but little other evidence of humanness. Suddenly, the action of the heart became irregular, clots were formed, some entering the lungs, and then even the mechanics of life ceased.

The enormous monetary cost of this case was paid fully by various agencies. The time, energy, and personnel expended were incalculable, the prolonged anguish of the family inexpressible. Lives of starving children or of socially deprived people could have been saved with less expenditure, but the system, confronted by the body within its halls, was put inexorably in motion. The people trapped by this routine performed their actions because they had been taught that life must be saved at all costs and at all times. They sincerely acted as if they offered good care. They paid no heed, however, to the wishes of the living, nor of the almost dead, but only their own presumptions. It struck me that similar events were occuring in almost any "teaching" hospital in the United States.

After my mother's death persistent questions arose in my mind about saving life, and about what constitutes proper care of those patients who are not salvable. If the care offered by a "teaching" hospital produces undesirable results, what is it that is wrong? Legalities and religiosities aside, can both compassion and clear assessment of the particular case be applied? Why do those dedicated to giving so-called good care not accept differences in effort made to prolong life? Some physicians clearly do pay attention, but why do so many not consider the differences, and the desires of each individual? Why is there no presently acceptable way of saying, "This person is very old and has had a long full life, and now it is impossible to make her well again. I will therefore do nothing to discomfort, demean, depersonalize, deform, or deter the natural process of dying serenely"? The treatment given my mother would have been appropriate for a young person with years ahead of potential value to self, family and society, but the system did not alter its methods, nor recognize the difference.

If a life is to be saved at all costs, should we not be certain that the life is worth saving? If an inert body has cardiac and respiratory action, can that body always be said to be alive? What about prolonging the suffering of family and friends as they face the certain death of a loved person—who calculates or even thinks of that? What of the known wishes of that person? Do those offering "good care" contend that a person has no right to express a preference as to how he or she will die? Why do they ignore the wishes of the family and fail to communicate? Does the system devote itself undeviatingly to its routine? Can it learn to adjust to different needs? Must all human beings admitted to an institution surrender to the conditioned reflexes of scientific teamwork? Where is love and compassion? Why prolong life when it exists only as a remnant, without hope, and is undesired by the person and the family? Who made the rule that life must always be saved, and at any cost? Is death a disgrace? Is it not the expected end of life?

The medical personnel gave what they were capable of giving impersonally: brain scans, antibiotics, oxygen, fluid by vein, measurement of blood, urinary constituents, blood pressure. The specialists and consultants supported these activities, not to save a life, but to give the outward appearance of "good care." The system of specialization allows a superior knowledge of one subject, but usually limits the specialist to the performance of what he knows well. Calling multiple specialists increases the risk of this type of care. Who looked at the patient and the problem as a whole? What was lacking was good judgment.

The system expropriated the right of this patient to make her own decisions about her

life or death. To have fulfilled her wishes would not have required illegal methods. She was not in a respirator: the question of "pulling the plug" was not an issue. If antibiotics had not been given, she might have acquired a merciful pneumonia. Without oxygen, she might have stopped breathing sooner—an outcome she had requested when her mind was clear. Much of the recorded data was useless. The team worked valiantly, but had they been successful, the patient would have gone back to the nursing home, where her days were without meaning. My mother did not fear death; had she known beforehand the circumstances of her prolonged treatment, she would have preferred her wishes to be honored.

Later, at a time of less emotion, a different question arose. How had this senseless fight against the process of dying developed? As a medical educator, first as a clinician, and then as a pathologist, I tried to inculcate in my students a respect for the living, the dying, and the dead. Concern for the healable patient is not the issue here. An ethical concern for the preservation of life at all costs has been inculcated in us. Even when death was certain, we would vigorously treat persons with severe burns covering 95 percent of the body surface. For the patient in our institution no effort, no cost was too great. The concept was that life must always be preserved. Death, then, was an affront to the physician, a challenge to his wish for omnipotence. We paid lip service to "public health and preventive medicine" but few medical schools, hospitals, or physicians made efforts to help the millions of people outside their halls who died for lack of food or love.

Some factors now run counter to our concept of "save life at all costs." Slowly, we have begun to realize that resources are limited—what is given to one may be taken from another. The idea that costs must enter the consciousness of the physician still is reprehensible to many. In addition, medical ethicists have raised, but usually not answered, difficult questions concerning the quality of life. Is a person in a vegetative state living? When the brain is without function, can the body be called human and alive? Is it a proper concern of relatives to avoid prolonging the agony of death; how should physicians respond and under what conditions?

It would be simplistic to say that enforcement of an ethical principle is the entire answer. Medical education is a dehumanizing process, not intentionally, but effectively nonetheless. Anatomy often begins with dissection of a dead body. Western culture promotes fear or dislike of death. Some students must harden their feelings to deal with the cadaver, and to overcome this cultural bias. The remainder of basic science largely has become "molecular biology," so that students know much about mitochondria, and the effects of cyclic AMP, but receive little information about the personal problems of human beings. Courses in medical ethics are given, but students recognize that the intellectual excitement lies elsewhere in the minds of most members of the faculty. They meet few physicians who model primary concern for the overall care and well-being of the patient, but daily see those with an overriding concern for knowledge in fragments of differing importance.

Pathology, a field not related directly to the patient, makes its contribution to the dehumanizing process. Disease is the primary interest rather than the reaction of a person to illness. Indeed, the definition of *disease* cited in American medical dictionaries emphasizes the impersonal or mechanical aspects: "A definite morbid process having a characteristic train of symptoms, it may affect the whole body or any of its parts, and its etiology, pathology and prognosis may be known or unknown" (Dorland's Illustrated Medical Dictionary, 24th Edition).

By contrast, in Butterworth's Medical Dictionary (formerly the British Medical Dictionary) *disease* is defined in terms of a person: "In general, a departure from the normal state of health. More specifically, a disease is the sum total of the reactions, physical and *mental*, made by a *person* to a noxious agent . . . a metabolic disorder . . .

a food deficiency . . . Since a particular agent tends to produce a pathologic and clinical picture peculiar to itself, although modified by individual variations in different *patients*, a mental concept of the average reactions or a composite picture can be formed which, for the convenience of description, is called a particular disease or clinical entity. *But a disease has no separate existence apart from a patient, and the only entity is the patient.*" (The emphasis is mine.)

In a course in anatomic pathology a case of cancer may be described as a "beautiful example." Organs are less personal than the human body. Slides of tissues are numbered, but usually lack the name of the patient. Living persons become cases, and those with "interesting" diseases are important. The clinocopathologic conference (CPC), an exercise in achieving the correct diagnosis, does not ordinarily include consideration of the social or psychologic problems of the patient, or their impact on the family. The CPC may become an aggressive attempt to reveal shortcomings in the clinician, causing him defensively to request every conceivable examination lest he be criticized for lack of effort and data.

Another aspect of pathologic teaching is designated "laboratory medicine." Technologic advances have resulted in enormous increments in numbers of tests. With this increase, attention becomes directed more to the data and less to the patient. Still more recently, the automatic determination of many tests as a unit superposes another distraction from concern for the patient as a person.

Even the teaching of clinical medicine is too often similarly dehumanizing. The "good case" is more important than the "crock," a derogatory term for a person whose problems are not solved by a scientifically trained physician. Clinical rounds commonly are exercises characterized by large groups of doctors, nurses, social workers, and dietitians gathering around the bed of the patient. The discussions concern laboratory data and making the diagnosis, rather than the patient himself. Demonstrations reveal physical signs or operative incisions, not the hopes and fears of the ill person.

The training of the physician minimizes emotional involvement with the patient and his family, in part to prevent these considerations from interfering with decisions, and in part because too great an emotional concern may be self-destructive. As a result, conversation with other physicians is likely to be about the disease rather than the patient: "The ulcer in the second bed is getting better." The student reads textbooks describing symptoms and signs as if they occured in a disease, not in a sick person: "weakness, atrophy, and Babinski signs occur in amyotrophic lateral sclerosis" rather than in a human being ill with this disease. Dictionary definitions, conferences, recording of notes, discussions, and use of language all serve to enlarge interest in the process of disease, and to decrease concern for the person who is ill. None of these features alone is bad, but their cumulative effect lessens the importance of the sick human being.

Mechanical procedures for dealing with the patient add to the problem. The student in the intensive care unit and postoperative recovery room sees physicians and nurses scanning the cardiogram, encephalogram, and recorded blood pressure rather than the patient. He enters the out-patient clinic where the flood of sick people creates a bureaucracy with predominant interest in schedules, correct forms, and insurance coverage. Patients may drive a hundred miles to be present in the clinic at 8:00 a.m., and be required to sit until 4:00 p.m. before being seen by the physician. The hospital routine, too, is determined by rule rather than for the benefit of the ill person. Anyone whose sleeping habits are different must surely be annoyed at being roused at 6:30 a.m. to have a temperature taken by the last of the "night shift" leaving at 7:00 a.m.; or by meals served at 8:00 a.m., noon, and 4 p.m., so that workers in the kitchen can go home at a time proper for them. Few of the laity know the problems they create by requiring medical attention late in the evening or on weekends!

The practicing physician faces many other difficulties in dealing with death. Often he has not participated with his teachers in the consideration of dying patients. He may fear or resent the death of a patient, finding it an affront to his strenuous efforts. He may salve his conscience by escalating orders for diagnostic procedures or treatment. At the same time, doctors and nurses tend to visit a dying patient less often, although the person facing death may need human contact even more. Dying patients undergo "social death"[1]; relatives, friends, and medical personnel view the patient as not existing. The physician has limited time. He enjoys visits to patients who can be cured, and allots shorter periods to the dying person.

To these factors has been added the impact of courts of law and the legal profession, as well as the personal and financial burden of suits for malpractice. In practicing medicine in such a way as to avoid lawsuits, the physician may damage the patient, feeling compelled to request excessive numbers of tests, many not innocuous, and to order procedures to maintain life beyond any usefulness. Humane medicine deals with *this* patient and *his* problems. The law works by rule. For a physician, every patient should be exceptional; past experience offers a guide to action but is not necessarily a determinant. A lawyer views all cases by the same standards, and precedent is important. But should the practice of medicine be conducted for the patient, or for the lawyer? Laws can be changed. Unnecessary suffering or harmful drastic measures should not be legal; excesses of this sort should be exposed, fought and eliminated.

What is needed is the rare quality of good judgment. Benefits and risks should be weighed for each person, and decisions made by careful reasoning within the framework of enlightened law rather than by rote or system. The feelings of the family should be carefully weighed, and the opinions of other physicians or non-physicians sought, but in the end, a decision should be made through the merciful judgment of one properly trained human being who has full responsibility.

The teaching of compassion to a medical student is more effective by precept than by word. Some physicians never lose sight of the importance of the patient as a person, but much of present-day education tells the medical student that the science of medicine, as well as the existing system of patient care, is good and that advances come only from research. Few voices are heard to say that the practice of medicine is an art as well as a science. The best method is not necessarily the most relentless and vigorous, without regard for the particular and special needs of the patient. Compassionate concern for human beings *as persons* is part of good medical care, and is needed as much as the brilliant application of medical science.

These paragraphs were written long after the actual events. When in the midst of the incident, I was disturbed but, in general, accepted what was done. I was as much a part of the system as the physicians who treated my mother. Recently a personal memoir by Lois Wheeler Snow[2] concerning the death of her husband revealed further evidence that insensitivity to the personal needs of the patient and the family is related to our training. A private Swiss clinic treated Edgar Snow and his wife; their major concern was with the disease. Open discussion with the family was actively resisted. The medical team of another culture managed the individual problems of the patient and the family far better. When the Chinese came, they shared all information: doctors, nurses, the patient, and the family discussed problems openly. Medical personnel were freely available to the family. The patient received companionship whenever he wanted it. Emphasis was on the person, and the family, as well as on the incurable illness. "There is yet a limit to technology; there is none to humanity, beyond our own making."[2]

REFERENCES

1. Kastenbaum, R., and Aisenberg, R.: The Psychology of Death. New York, Springer, 1972.
2. Snow, L. W.: A Death With Dignity: When the Chinese Came. New York, Random House, 1974.

39

Hospice care in terminal illness

ROBERT WOODSON

WHAT IS HOSPICE?

Hospice is a concept whose time has come.[1] It involves the skilled and compassionate care of dying patients and their families. Pioneered successfully throughout England and Europe for centuries as a place of rest for travelers on their way, the hospice is becoming a major medical innovation throughout America and Canada in the treatment of the terminally ill. It is an innovation in the sense that until only recently the specialized palliative care of the dying patient was left largely to chance or to the charge nurse. Consciousness raising efforts by Elisabeth Kübler-Ross[2] and others to sensitize American medical practitioners to the denial of death syndrome and the death with dignity notion did much to alleviate any further need for placing dying patients in rooms at the ends of hospital corridors where they could die in peace, alone.

Today there are some three dozen programs throughout America and Canada where the dying patient may receive this highly specialized palliative care. They are called hospices. Patterned largely after England's world famous St. Christopher's Hospice in Sydenham, these hospices all have the same common goal: to keep the patient pain-free, comfortable, and fully alert during the final phases of his illness and his life. This goal is achieved through a highly sophisticated—although basic—scientific and artistic system of palliative care developed over the years largely by Cicely Saunders and her hospice staff. The system includes the following major components.

A FOURFOLD APPROACH TO PAIN CONTROL

In terms of the hospice concept pain may be either physical, psychological, social, spiritual, or any combination of these four. The task of the skilled clinician in alleviating pain is to tease out through careful observation and examination of the patient specifically which of the four components of pain are present, active, in what combination, and to what degree. Once the combination has been determined, then the *appropriate* combination of intervention strategies can be initiated.[3] Since pain control measures must be adjusted to each individual patient's needs, his own particular social-cultural response to pain, including his own unique autoplastic pain process, must also be considered in any initial assessment. Pain control then, in terms of the hospice approach, becomes one of pain management involving several forms of intervention all aimed at keeping the patient

Reprinted from Psychosocial care of the dying patient by Charles A. Garfield. Copyright © 1978 McGraw-Hill Book Co. Used with permission of McGraw-Hill Book Co.

[1]Alice Heath, Founder, Santa Barbara Hospice, Inc.
[2]Elisabeth Kübler-Ross, *On Death and Dying,* Macmillan, New York, 1969, pp. 1-37.

[3]Dr. T. S. West, personal interview, St. Christopher's Hospice, Sydenham, England, October 3, 1975.

completely pain-free, comfortable, and fully alert until the moment of death. How is this achieved?

Physical pain

Physical pain can be defined as that constant or occasional discomfort ranging from a mild toothache—and dying cancer patients do get toothaches—to the severe and chronic debilitating pain so familiar to those who have treated the advanced-stage cancer patient. In her paper, "The Treatment of Intractable Pain in Terminal Cancer,"[4] Cicely Saunders states that "pain itself is the strongest antagonist to successful analgesia and if it is ever allowed to become severe, the patient will then increase it [pain] with his own tension and fear."[5] Once the patient has been allowed to continually experience the severe physical pain associated with his illness, he becomes anxious and fearful that he will never again be pain-free. This generalized anxiety and loss of confidence in the caregivers' ability to lower the patient's pain threshold in turn increases the patient's susceptibility to pain and he becomes trapped in the all too frequent downward spiral of the intractable pain syndrome.[6]

Since physical pain influences and is influenced by the three other kinds of pain, a careful assessment of the possible symptoms that trouble the patient must first be made. Once an assessment has been made—which is by itself a highly specialized art—the appropriate intervention strategies can be initiated. This usually starts with the immediate removal of *all* the annoying symptoms of the patient's already diagnosed cancer. The goal, it must be remembered, is to keep the patient pain-free, comfortable, and mentally alert until death occurs. The success in achieving this goal is not so much a question of the specific drugs used as it is of the principles underlying their use. Several cardinal principles of controlling physical pain in the terminally ill cancer patient have emerged over the last two decades, primarily through the work of Cicely Saunders and her colleagues with thousands of dying cancer patients, at both St. Joseph's Hospice and St. Christopher's Hospice.[7]

These cardinal principles include the following: (1) the successful management of the cancer patient's pain is both an art and a science; (2) the concept of addiction does not apply in the care of the terminal cancer patient; and (3) there is a need for great flexibility in both the variety of drugs used and in their dosage levels. The skillful management of the terminal cancer patient's physical pain is an art in and of itself. It is an art in the sense that it involves (1) the careful assessment of the patient's symptoms, and this often includes an assessment by other members of the care team, (2) the selection of the appropriate drugs administered at an optimum dosage, and (3) the sensitivity to appreciate that fact that, in the final stages of treatment, the dying cancer patient's needs change rapidly and the medication regimen must keep pace with these changes. The science of treating the patient's physical pain needs includes (1) solid mastery of the drugs used in palliative care and (2) a genuine clinical understanding of their interactions and side effects. It is only through a skillful blending of both the art of knowing how to listen with the third ear to the patient in pain and the science of seeing with the third eye what his or her needs are that the full and proper care of a dying patient can be achieved.[8]

The question of addiction is not an issue in the hospice treatment of the dying cancer patient for two main reasons: (1) the concerns that physicians frequently express regarding accidental addictions are based

---

[4]Cicely Saunders, "The Treatment of Intractable Pain in Terminal Cancer," *Proceedings of the Royal Society of Medicine,* 56(3):1-7, March 1963. Hereafter referred to as Saunders, "Intractable Pain."

[5]Ibid, p. 2.

[6]Dr. Cicely Saunders, personal interview, St. Christopher's Hospice, Sydendam, England, October 3, 1975.

[7]Saunders, "Intractable Pain," pp. 1-7.

[8]Ibid.

primarily on an inappropriate application of the medical school model emphasizing the treatment/cure/get well dimension of medical practice that carries little or no validity when applied to the care of the dying. It is a fact of medical practice that patients sometimes do become drug-dependent, especially if they have had a long and difficult recovery from a curable/treatable illness, and this dependecy sometimes poses a medical management problem. It is also a fact of life that not all patients have curable diseases, and not all of them get well: some do in fact die, no matter how many analgesics are given or are withheld. They die just the same, with or without the nedication. The solution to the concern over addiction seems obvious, yet the issue will undoubtedly continue to be debated in the lecture halls of academic medicine and in the hospitals where the hospice concept has not yet achieved full and complete adoption. (2) Interestingly enough, dying patients are almost never emotionally dependent on their drugs[9] in contrast to findings by researchers using the drug-addiction models depicted in standard medical and pharmacological texts, which have been mainly constructed from data collected on the youthful offender, the diversion of the chronic drug user, and so on. The data base upon which these models have been built, moreover, has totally ignored the whole area of the dying cancer patient's medication needs.

The models used in assessing addiction factors of terminally ill patients are neither valid nor reliable. Dying patients frequently display a surprising amount of dosage reduction behavior once their pain has been brought under control.[10] The central issue is one of care vs. cure and since the dying cancer patient is not going to be cured it seems logical that he or she be cared for compassionately.

There are undoubtedly several drugs that can be employed in the successful treat-ment of physical pain and its related symptoms. While many physicians have their own special set of favorite drugs, there is a decided need for greater flexibility in the variety of drugs (and dosage levels) used in treating physical pain. The pharmacology of cancer, pain control, and related symptomology has mushroomed in the past decade and the variety of analgesics available for treating in the mild, moderate, and severe pain that is so much a part of the cancer patient's clinical course is at times overwhelming. While 30 mg of a particular analgesic may seem high, 60 mg may indeed be the appropriate optimum dosage level when one considers the nature of the illness and the special needs of the individual patient. There is no easy formula.[11]

In treating the advanced-stage cancer patient's physical pain, it is important to remember that analgesics should be given *regularly,* usually every 4 hours. "The aim is to titrate the level of analgesia against the patient's pain, gradually increasing the dose until the patient is pain free."[12] The next dose is given *before* the effects of the previous one have worn off and "before the patient may think it necessary."[13] The notation "P.R.N." on an analgesic medication order, therefore, is inappropriate since this suggests that the patient will ask for his pain medication when he feels he needs it. Since not all terminal cancer patients request pain medication when they experience discomfort for fear of bothering the nurse or of violating a socially acceptable norm, and since the goal of comprehensive pain management involves preventing pain from *occurring,* analgesics are given routinely.[14]

The following adopted drug schedule is presented as *one* example of *some* of the

---

[9]Ibid., pp. 2-3.
[10]Dr. T. S. West, op. cit.

[11]Ibid.
[12]"Drugs Most Commonly Used at St. Christopher's Hospice," unpublished paper, St. Christopher's Hospice, Sydenham, England, January 1975, p. 1. Hereafter referred to as "Drugs, St. Christopher's."
[13]Ibid.
[14]Saunders, "Intractable Pain," p. 2.

approaches used at St. Christopher's[15] in dealing with physical pain and its related symptomology.

Mild physical pain

1. Dextropropoxyphene with paracetamol: 2 tabs every 4 hours or

2. Paracetamol: 2 tabs every 4 hours.

These are also used as adjuncts to stronger analgesics and are often useful in bone pain.

Moderate physical pain

1. Dipipanone 10 mg with cyclizine 30 mg, 1 to 2 tabs every 4 hours. This is a useful analgesic of medium strength and is especially valuable with outpatients or if the patient prefers a tablet to a mixture.

2. Diamorphine and cocaine elixir (B.P.C.), MACS solution in U.S.

B.P.C.

Diamorphine HCl	5 to 10 mg
Cocaine	10 mg
Alcohol (90%)	1.25 ml
Syrup	2.5 ml
Chloroform water to 10 ml	

U.S.

Morphine	10 mg
Cocaine	10 mg
Ethanol	20 mg
Simple syrup qsad	5 ml
Chloroform water to 10 ml	

Unless transferring from another potent narcotic analgesic, the initial dose given is 5 mg. This is given with a phenothiazine, usually as a syrup. Prochlorperazine 5 mg in 5 ml is the one usually added, chlorpromazine 12.5 to 25 mg in 5 ml if sedation is required. These potentiate the effect of diamorphine, and also act as antiemetics and tranquilizers. For outpatients, prochlorperazine or chlorpromazine syrup can replace syrup in the standard mixture when a stable level of analgesia is obtained.

3. Phenazocine 5 mg, 2 to 3 tabs every 4 hours. This is a useful strong analgesic, especially if the patient dislikes the diamorphine and cocaine elixir, or prefers a tablet.

Severe physical pain. Diamorphine and cocaine elixir, 10 to 40 mg, or even 60 mg, every 4 hours is usually effective. If this does not control the pain the patient should be transferred to injections of diamorphine every 4 hours, starting with half the previous oral dose and increasing it until the pain is controlled. The analgesic effect of diamorphine is shorter when given by injection, especially at higher doses. Sometimes therefore it may be necessary to inject the patient every 3 hours.

The phenothiazine should continue to be given, either orally or by injection. Diamorphine alone can be given subcutaneously.

Physical pain and vomiting. The diamorphine and cocaine elixir with phenothiazine may be tolerated and prove effective. However, it may be necessary to give injections of diamorphine and a phenothiazine for a few days; this may need to be prolonged in the case of intractable vomiting, obstruction, or if the patient cannot swallow. Oxycodone pectinate suppositories (30 mg) (1 to 2 every 8 hours) are occasionally used with outpatients to avoid the regular injections of analgesics. (In the United States oxymorphone 5 mg suppositories are used.)

Nausea and vomiting. Probably the phenothiazines are the most useful drugs. Prochlorperazine 5 to 10 mg, promazine 25 mg, or chlorpromazine 25 mg are all useful antiemetics and are listed in ascending order of sedative effect.

They may be given every 4 hours in syrup or as a suspension in the case of promazine. Alternatively, they may be given in tablet form or by I.M. injection. Prochlorperazine suppositories (25 mg) and chlorpromazine suppositories (100 mg) are useful if oral preparations are not tolerated and injections are impracticable—for example, if the patient is at home. These are normally given every 8 hours. If these prove inadequate it is probably better to add a further antiemetic of a different type rather than to increase the dose. Cyclizine 50 mg orally or I.M. (intramuscularly), B.D. (twice daily),

---

[15]"Drugs, St. Christopher's" pp. 1-3.

is often useful, as is metaclopramide 10 mg, especially if given about 1 hour A.C. (before meals).

Obstructive vomiting. It is usually possible to control the pain and vomiting caused by malignant large bowel obstruction in its terminal phase by the use of adequate analgesics and by a combination of antiemetics. In these cases tabs of dioctyl sodium sulfosuccinate 100 mg, 1 to 2 T.D.S. (3 times per day) are sometimes used until it appears that obstruction is complete. Tabs Lomotil 2 Q.D.S. (4 times per day) may have a place in the control of painful colic.

Psychological pain

The dying patient experiencing psychological pain is frequently the frightened or anxious patient, the lonely or depressed patient, or the hurt and angry patient. As he begins his final stage of growth by anticipating his own death, the terminally ill patient often endeavors to set things in balance by attempting to maintain a kind of psychological homeostasis of equifinality[16] with his inner emotional self and *his* perception of the immediate environment. This imbalance or loss of control over his or her life, especially the now new experience of learning how to die, usually calls up a repertoire of coping behaviors aimed chiefly at reducing the stresses of dying and at regaining control over one's life. An early attempt to understand this was presented by Elisabeth Kübler-Ross in her work on a stage theory of dying (denial, isolation, anger, bargaining, depression, and acceptance).[17]

The hospice approach to treating the patient in psychological pain, like its approach to treating the patient in any of the other three kinds of pain, is concerned first of all with the notion that *anxiety, depres-*

sion, and *agitation*—three terms for affective disorders that abound in the psychiatric literature—are normal, fight-flight reactions to coping with dying and death. When viewed as *normal*, given the nature of the illness, as opposed to *abnormal*, as current psychiatric diagnostic procedures would have one believe, depression, anxiety, and agitation take on a very different kind of emotional pain profile. They take on an affective domain pain profile, which, when viewed through the hospice model, suggests that amelioration of the dying patient's psychological pain may best be achieved through a careful analysis of the primary emotional sequelae operating at that particular moment, along with their accompanying secondary symptoms, and then through initiation of the appropriate combination of chemotherapeutic (antianxiety and antidepressive) and psychotherapeutic (clergyperson, therapist, family, friends, etc.) agents.

Thirty minutes of cathartic grieving with a family member, nurse, or skilled therapist can have profound positive effects on a dying patient's depression and concomitant anxiety. Five milligrams of diazepam or fifty of a phenothiazine may do little more than add one additional order the attending pharmacist has to fill and the nurse has to administer. The key to intervening in order to alleviate psychological pain in the dying patient as suggested by the hospice approach is to first acknowledge that in any organic disease or dysfunction there is *always* an emotional pain component operating in concert with or in opposition to the other three types of pain associated with terminal disease. The treatment intervention strategy used in combating psychological or emotional pain must be considered, moreover, in a framework that goes beyond the conventional unidimensional concepts of reactive depression and acute anxiety reaction, and must include a clinical appreciation for the delicate balance between psychological pain, social pain, spiritual pain, and physical pain, and quite possibly existential pain as suggested so

---

[16]The term *equifinality* was introduced in the late 1950s by general systems theorists in an attempt to provide biomedical researchers with a more *dynamic* as opposed to *static* definition of living or "open" systems.
[17]Elisabeth Kübler-Ross, op. cit, pp. 38-137. See also Elisabeth Kübler-Ross (ed.), *Death: The Final Stage of Growth*, Prentice-Hall, Englewood Cliffs, N.J., 1975, p. 161.

eloquently in Martin Buber's concept of the I-thou.[18]

The following chemotherapeutic agents have been proven useful in treating the advanced cancer or psychological pain of dying patients.[19] Their success in removing the symptoms of the stresses associated with the dying process, namely anxiety and depression, lies not so much in their pharmokinetic properties, but in their appropriate combinations and dosages offered within an atmosphere of genuine caring and concern for the patient's well-being.[20]

Depression. (1) Attention to physical and mental distress; (2) antidepressants: amitriptyline 10 to 25 mg T.D.S. if mild sedation is also required, or 25 to 50 mg nocte; imipramine 10 to 25 mg T.D.S. if sedation is not required. Patients with malignant disease should usually be started on a small dose, e.g. 10 mg T.D.S., as larger doses sometimes precipitate confusion in debilitated patients.

Anxiety. (1) Tabs diazepam 2 to 5 mg T.D.S.; (2) tabs promazine 25 mg T.D.S. or chlorpromazine 25 T.D.S.; (3) I.M. or I.V. diazepam 10 mg is of use in acute panic states or prior to some procedure that distresses the patient, e.g. catheterization.

Confusion. In mild confusion chlorpromazine 10 to 25 mg Q.D.S. may be adequate. In severe restlessness and confusion, injection chlorpromazine 25 to 100 mg may be needed or injection methotrimaprazine 25 to 50 mg. These may be given with opiates or in conjunction with diazepam if necessary.

Insomnia. Nonbarbiturate sedatives are preferred, chloral glycerolate (chloral hydrate in the United States), tabs dichloralphenazone (ethchlorvynol in the United States), or tabs nitrazepam (flurazepam in the United States). It is sometimes useful to add chlorpromazine 25 to 50 mg either with the hypnotics or in the early evening.

Social pain

Social pain may be defined in two ways: (1) it may be defined as a patient's mild-to-severe discomfort with man's inhumanity to man—a common theme in the history of all technocratic civilizations; or (2) it may be defined as simply a patient's discomfort with the level and intensity of his or her interpersonal relationships, especially if one is in the process of dying. Extensive research by Colin Murray Parkes[21] and others concerned with the process of anticipatory grief, grief, grief work, and bereavement has clearly documented the importance of the need for the dying patient and his or her family to finish any unfinished interpersonal business including learning how to say good-bye to one another for the last time.

This unfinished interpersonal business becomes of immense importance in the final days of the dying patient's life. Should the dying patient be denied the opportunity to resolve or attempt to resolve such interpersonal business, i.e., to put some kind of closure on his or her social/interpersonal relationships with family and close friends, it can cause tremendous social pain for both the patient and his or her family. This kind of pain frequently appears as a passive-depressive presenting set of symptoms that all too often gets diagnosed as psychological pain and is inappropriately treated with an antidepressive agent, which in turn only further separates the dying patient

[18]Martin Buber, *I and Thou*, 2d ed., Scribner's, New York, 1958, pp. 3-137. See also Avery D. Weisman, "Misgivings and Misconceptions in the Psychiatric Care of Terminal Patients," *Psychiatry*, **33:**72, February 1970. The author visited St. Christopher's Hospice in Sydenham, England, in October 1975 through a special grant from the Smythe-Sollenberger family to observe firsthand the care provided patients in that facility.

[19]"Drugs, St. Christopher's," pp. 4-5.

[20]Dr. T. S. West, personal interview, London, England, October 9, 1975.

[21]Colin Murray Parkes, "The First Year of Bereavement: A Longitudinal Study of the Reaction of London Widows to the Death of Their Husbands," *Psychiatry*, **33:**444-467, November 1970.

from his need to resolve, with the help of those around him, any pressing social/interpersonal concerns with family and friends. This does not mean that it is necessary or even desirable to hold a party around the patient's deathbed—although some cultures do it routinely—but that well-timed, well-planned selective social interaction is a vital and necessary part of appropriate social pain intervention. Since the dying patient and his family (and this could include his adopted family of medical caregivers) in their transactions with one another over a period of time have worked out a highly patterned, balanced system of social exchange, which constitutes a unit of care,[22] full consideration must be given to the social concerns of the dying patient and his family when any assessment is made regarding the nature and level of their verbal and unverbalized social pain.

The hospice approach in dealing with social pain, as determined by the patient's needs, is to facilitate (in the necessary and proper doses) *quality* social interaction. This helps the patient live more fully until he or she dies. Through the process of preventing the takeover of social pain (isolation) the caregiver performs the vitally important function of preventive psychiatry of providing additional opportunities for the grieving process to begin, i.e., anticipatory grief, before the patient dies. This also affords the caregiver with another opportunity to participate in a rich and personally rewarding experience in caring. As far as the man's inhumanity to man theme of social pain is concerned, it is already being dealt with right here and now on a one-to-one basis with any dying patient fortunate enough to have a caregiver who knows about social pain in the broader context and who will hear him or her out.

Spiritual pain

To date there is no clear-cut definition of what constitutes spiritual pain, particularly

as it relates to the dying. Spiritual pain is as different for each patient as is the patient's specific religious, racial, or cultural background. When Alaskan Indians die, for example, they "exhibit a willfulness about their death,"[23] as demonstrated by their active participation in its planning and in the time of its occurrence, that shows a remarkable power of personal choice. They frequently initiate their final dying rituals by calling their whole family and their close friends together, and then, when everyone is assembled, they tell the story of their life and pray for all the members of their family.[24] Spiritual pain for the Alaskan Indian might be the fear, or the reality, of not being able to participate in his or her own dying process because of the effect of sleep-producing drugs or the existential crisis of dying alone, without the comfort of meaningful praying, singing, and interacting with family and friends before death.

In sharp contrast to man's Westernized view of dying and death, Hindus and Buddhists see death and dying as anything but "the endless time of never coming back,"[25] or "the absence of presence."[26] Hindus view death as both a necessity and a blessing—a necessity in the sense that "without the establishment of an operative balance between the workings of the powers of birth and death, the world of living beings would soon choke to death on the excessive creativity of the creator himself."[27] Buddhists, by contrast, see death and dying as "a cutting off of the life-force or a total nonfunctioning of the physical

---

[22]Edward F. Dobihal, "Talk or Terminal Care?" *Connecticut Medicine*, **38**:366, July 1974.

[23]Murray L. Trelease, "Dying Among Alaskan Indians: A Matter of Choice," in Elisabeth Kübler-Ross (ed.), *Death: The Final Stage of Growth*, Prentice-Hall, Englewood Cliffs, N.J., 1975, p. 33.
[24]Ibid., p. 34.
[25]J. Bruce Long, "The Death That Ends in Hinduism and Buddhism," in Elisabeth Kübler-Ross (ed.), *Death: The Final Stage of Growth*, Prentice-Hall, Englewood Cliffs, N.J., 1975, p. 53. Hereafter referred to as Long, "Hinduism and Buddhism."
[26]Ibid. See also, Richard Lamerton, "Care of the Dying 7," *Nursing Times*, **69**:88 January 18, 1973.
[27]Ibid., p. 64.

body and the mind.''[28] This life-force[29] is not destroyed at death, but is temporarily displaced to continue to function in another (unspecified) form. Every birth is a rebirth in linear fashion according to Buddhist doctrine, occurring immediately or 49 days after death.[30] Hindu doctrine holds that ''it is an individual's *Karma* that is the fundamental cause of birth and death . . . and for the time being, until all creatures have liberated themselves from the law of rebirth, a provision must be made both for the coming-to-be and the passing-away of things, for the sake of the well-being of the world''—a blessing.[31]

Although Hindus and Buddhists are not in concurrence on whether there is a real self that survives from one lifetime to the next, both belief systems generally agree that ''the most effective method of *conquering* [italics added] death is to accept death as the chief fact of life and as the main signal that all the things you hoped for will be utterly destroyed in due course and that once you come to be able to neither long for nor fear death, you are beginning to transcend both life and death and coming into unity with the Changeless Absolute.''[32]

Spiritual pain for the practicing Buddhist or Hindu—should he or she ever have any—might be as expressed in the sermon of the thirteenth-century Zen master Dogen:

To find release you must begin to regard life and death as identical to Nirvana neither loathing the former nor coveting the latter. It is fallacious to think that you simply move from birth to death. Birth, from the Buddhist point of view, is a temporary point between the preceding and succeeding; hence, it can be called ''birthlessness.'' The same holds for death and deathlessness. In life there is nothing more than life, in death nothing more than death: we are being born and dying at every moment.[33]

Jewish tradition, on the other hand, specifically views the period of dying *(Goses)* and terminal illness *(Shechiv Mera)* as a time when loved ones should surround, comfort, and encourage the patient.[34] Jewish law provides for death with dignity and meaning by ''allowing the dying person to set his house in order, bless his family, pass on any message to them he feels important, and make his peace with God.''[35]

The deathbed confessional is viewed as an important element in the transition to the world to come. The dying patient is to be instructed to recite the confessional according to the limitations of his physical and mental condition. ''And one says (to the patient), 'Many have confessed and have not died and many who have not confessed have died, as a reward for your confession you will live, and whoever confesses has a portion of the world to come.' '' (Yoreh Deah 378)

This deathbed scene is thus structured to give the terminally ill and dying patient an outlet for expression of natural concerns and anxieties, yet within a reassuring framework which never attempts to be deluding.[36]

Each of these procedures—repentance, confession, the ordering of one's material affairs, the blessing of family, and ethical instruction—takes into account the theological, practical, and emotional needs of the terminal patient. They enable the patient to express fears, find comfort and inner strength, and communicate meaningfully with those close to him.[37]

Contemporary programs to alleviate the distress of terminally ill and dying patients are very much in consonance with teachings of the Jewish tradition which stress the normalcy of these events of the life cycle. The patient's emotional equilibrium is maintained, with the continued support of family and community, who perform the mitzvah of ''Bikkur Cholim''—visiting the sick with a sensitivity nurtured by their religious

---

[28]Ibid., p. 65.

[29]It is interesting to note how frequently the term *life-force* or the notion of life-force appears in the recorded transcripts of psychiatric patients undergoing therapy, even dying ones.

[30]Long, ''Hinduism and Buddhism,'' p. 65.

[31]Ibid., p. 64.

[32]Long, ''Hinduism and Buddhism,'' p. 71.

[33]Ibid., p. 70.

[34]Rabbi Zachary I. Heller, ''The Jewish View of Death: Guidelines for Dying,'' in Elisabeth Kübler-Ross (ed.), *Death: The Final Stage of Growth,* Prentice-Hall, Englewood Cliffs, N.J., 1975, p. 39.

[35]Ibid., p. 38.

[36]Ibid., p. 40.

[37]Ibid., p. 41.

tradition. When death, the natural end of human existence, inevitably does come it is accepted as the degree of human mortality by the Eternal and Righteous Judge.[38]

Spiritual pain then, for the dying Jewish patient, could include any accidental thwarting of his or her reconciliation with God, any blocking of confession, or any interference with the ordering of the patient's material affairs, the blessing of family, and the passing on of ethical imperatives as laid down in the finest of Jewish law and tradition.

Regardless of the form (unspecified anxieties, etc.) or function (passive or active existential crises) of spiritual pain, it must be recognized as such and treated appropriately by the appropriate person (not by drugs)—which may or may not be the hospital chaplain, visiting priest, rabbi, or resident Zen master. The important point is that clergymen or clergywomen by virtue of their particular religious teachings and training are highly skilled listeners, especially in those times of profound spiritual silence that are an inherent part of the dying patient's experience as he moves through the various stages of his illness. They are unquestionably the key caregivers and supporters of patients experiencing spiritual pain. The clergyperson's role in relieving spiritual pain and effecting a kind of spiritual healing is simply to be present, to minister to the spiritual/religious needs of the patient and his family and to meet the related spiritual needs of the medical caregivers on a P.R.N. basis. The clergyperson's job, unlike that of the immediate hospice staff, does not end with the patient's death, but continues through the period of the funeral and the ensuing grief work done by the patient's family long after the 6-month follow-up by the medical social worker.[39]

The clergyperson may choose to work either directly with the patient and his or

her family through the religious medium of confession, communion, prayer, etc., or indirectly through other members of the care team as a counselor/consultant, or both. The approaches and the options are as varied as are the patients. To be able to *see* and *hear* (diagnose) the dying patient in spiritual pain and to minister to that pain by hearing confession, offering communion, praying with the patient, or by participating in his singing rituals (as in the case of the Alaskan Indians) is to reduce that patient's suffering and alleviate his or her pain—a worthy calling for a man or woman of the cloth and a vital function in the case of the dying.

PHILOSOPHICAL AND ORGANIZATIONAL COMPONENTS OF HOSPICE CARE

In addition to the fourfold approach to pain control so central to the hospice concept there are eight other major components or characteristics of hospice care that distinguish it from other programs of terminal care. These eight components comprise the basic philosophical and organizational framework of an authentic hospice program and are described briefly below.

The provision of care by an interdisciplinary team

The successful care of the dying patient and his or her family must utilize an interdisciplinary team approach. Interdisciplinary or multidisciplinary team care must not be a synonym for fragmented care in which the bewildered patient does not know who is in charge or who is dealing with which problems. Authentic hospice care mandates that the multidisciplinary team sit down together at regular conferences, usually weekly, to work out a plan of care for the patient and his or her family and to learn something of each other's specialized (professional) language code. This is of particular importance when the team comprises members with divergent racial and cultural backgrounds. The team includes the dying patient, his immediate

[38]Ibid., p. 43.
[39]Colin Murray Parkes, op. cit.

family, his primary physician, his nurses, the medical social worker, volunteers, and appropriate clergypersons.

Service availability to home care and inpatients on a 24-hour-a-day, 7-day-a-week, on-call basis with emphasis on availability of medical and nursing skills

Although most Americans (98 percent) now die in either a hospital or extended-care facility (i.e., nursing home), the increasing trend among more and more Americans is toward dying at home in their own bed surrounded by loved ones, as was the custom in this country before the turn of the century. In order to provide hospice care for those choosing to die at home, 24-hour-a-day, 7-day-a-week skilled and supportive services—with an emphasis on visiting nurses and homemaker services—must be available to patients and their families. All too often medical emergencies occur at night and on weekends when nursing or medical services are scarce.

Such was the case of a husband who reluctantly placed his wife in a convalescent home for the final 3 months of her life because the stresses of coping with the unavailability of inhome nursing service were overwhelming. Upon admitting his wife to the facility, he recalled with vivid horror the time her gastrostomy tube fell out at 3:00 a.m. one weekend and how he desperately tried replacing it according to telephone instructions from an unknown emergency room physician. Although actual case examples like this one are fortunately in the minority, they do occur. The availability of a 24-hour-a-day, 7-day-a-week nursing service not only eliminates the possibility of such unfortunate events from occurring, but also allays the already burdened family's fear that no one will be there to help when it is needed most.

Home care service in collaboration with inpatient facilities

A true hospice program has both a strong home care program and an inpatient facility or back-up beds of some kind. Since there are already some three dozen hospices throughout the British Isles and Europe, each with its own unique program of home care, there is little need for constructing a rationale for building more hospices. In America, however, there are presently no free-standing inpatient hospice facilities, although there are a growing number of home care programs with limited numbers of back-up beds, or specialized hospice type units within existing hospitals and extended care facilities. While these back-up bed arrangements present a special set of problems (i.e., reimbursement, visiting hours, presence of pets at the patient's bedside, room design, coordination of care team, etc.), these arrangements are deemed by many hospice authorities as only temporary until more appropriate *care* guidelines are incorporated into the legal, medical, and economic policies and regulations governing the bulk of health care facilities in the United States.

Other alternatives, of course, include building hospices and then linking them up with existing community-based home health agencies (HHAs)—the result, a bonafide hospice program. Until such true hospice programs become a reality in America, the trend over the next several years will be toward developing strong home care programs, using volunteers extensively, and establishing a system of back-up beds in one or two local hospitals that agrees to accept *any* medical insurance carried by the patient and agrees to take an *active* role in meeting the special needs of the patient and family placed in its care. It is in this particular component of hospice care that most of the necessary legislative changes will occur, the greatest modifications in our system of health insurance will be seen, and about which no doubt the liveliest of academic discussion will ensue.

The patient and family together regarded as the unit of care

It is a fundamental principle of hospice care that nothing we do as caregivers should serve to separate someone who is dying from his or her family and, even though there will undoubtedly be moments of difficulty and despair, it is of paramount importance that the family come through to the end together. Because most people in America die in hospitals or extended-care facilities, the traditional and familiar home setting with all its comforting presence is absent from the process. The absence of family members—including children and grandchildren—and the familiar home setting more often than not works to the social and psychological demise of the patient long before he or she dies physically. Maintaining meaningful interaction for the advanced cancer or dying patient with his family, through either face-to-face social exchange, telephone conversations, letters, audio-tape cassettes, or other electronic means helps the patient—especially the older patient—stay in touch with life until he dies. It is therefore vital that the family be the unit of care and receive full and proper attention.

A bereavement follow-up service

In a genuine hospice program, care does not end with the death of the patient but is extended to provide a program of emotional support for the surviving family members during their bereavement. Families must be visited on both a regular and an emergency basis right through the time of death of the family member and on into the mourning period. Because the social and psychological loss of a loved one can sometimes be so emotionally devastating to surviving family members—particularly spouses—assistance must be given in an attempt to prevent any further unnecessary suffering.

In the first year after the loved one's death, for example, there is a documented vulnerability of the survivors to illness[40] as reflected in a 40 percent increase in the mortality rate of widows. Other less well studied (consequently less-understood) illnesses include increased alcoholism, reactive depression, cardiac dysfunction, psychotropic drug addiction, and long-term detrimental effects to children caused by the loss of a parent, especially if the death was sudden and unexpected. Research by Colin Murray Parkes[41] and others suggests that simple friendly visits by *trained* caregivers with the survivors gives them an opportunity to *express* (not *ventilate*) their grief and discuss the terminal illness including the death itself, and that this can go a long way toward mitigating the ill effects of bereavement.

The first few bereavement visits are typically made by the primary nurse who was involved in the direct care of the patient before his or her death. This provides the family with a caregiver who was close to the patient when he or she died and provides the family with someone who can discuss with them such often-asked questions as, "Should we have kept her at home?" "Should we have taken him to the hospital?" "Was it worth continuing with that unpleasant treatment for so long?" "Should we have pressed him to continue with chemotherapy?" "Why didn't she go to the doctor as soon as she felt the lump?" Many of these questions can easily be answered in the course of frank and open discussions. Ideally, much of this follow-up bereavement counseling—which in one sense is a very specific form of preventive psychiatry—could be done by adequately trained volunteers. The need in this aspect of hospice care is great, the possibilities many.

Extensive use of volunteers as an integral part of the hospice care team

Fundamental to the continued success of any hospice program is the extensive use of trained volunteers. While the wise use of volunteers has in the past been conspicuously absent in the United States from the care of the dying and their families,

[40]Thomas H. Holmes and Richard H. Rahe, "The Social Readjustment Rating Scale," *Journal of Psychosomatic Research*, **11**:213-218, August 1967.

[41]Colin Murray Parkes, op. cit.

there is at present a resurgence of interest in the use of volunteers for such purposes (as evidenced by the emergence of the professionally trained volunteer) and this has provided a welcome change in our thinking about and in our care of the dying. Trained volunteers provide two primary services to patients and their families: (1) they provide such vital household services as helping with transportation, light housework, shopping, babysitting, laundry, letter writing, etc., and (2) perhaps even more vital, they provide friendship to the dying and to the family by giving of themselves in a basic, person-to-person sort of way that seems to help keep the patient and his or her family from falling through the many psychological and social cracks professionals pride themselves on successfully filling.

There are many models of volunteer programs for the terminally ill and the one that will undoubtedly serve as the key model for training volunteers for most hospice programs in the United States and Canada is the highly successful SHANTI Project. According to its founder, Charles Garfield, the project "was developed on a shoestring budget and in just 2 years of operation has provided emotional support to thousands of patients and families facing a life-threatening illness."[42] Its success as a training model for volunteers interested in working with the fatally ill and their families is grounded in the notion that, through caring counseling and emotional support during a time of severe illness or grief, the presence of another human can be helpful in generating the emotional strength needed to cope with sorrow and stress.

Volunteers are indeed the vital thread that ties the whole hospice program together and extensive use of them is absolutely essential if the full and proper care of the dying and their families is to be achieved and if the label "hospice care" is to be applied in describing the services rendered.

---

[42]Personal interview, Santa Barbara, Ca., October 9, 1976.

Central administration and coordination of services

It is essential that a hospice program have its own autonomous central administration and system of coordination of patient services. All too frequently well-intentioned community health care agencies join forces to provide care for the terminally ill and their families only to learn that much of their success is highly dependent on how smoothly the simple logistics of record keeping, team leadership, distribution of supplies and caregivers, communication, etc. are carried out. Many acute-care hospitals and extended-care facilities are now employing personnel whose specific function is to coordinate inpatient and home care services in order to ensure some measure of continuity of care for the patient once he or she is discharged from active treatment. This is a step in the right direction toward providing a comprehensive program of terminal care, but it must be well conceived (i.e., it must use a general systems theory approach) and carried out by dedicated caregivers with the thought in mind that it is only a first step in moving toward a *completely* centralized administration and system of coordination of services for the dying.

Knowledge and expertise in the control of symptoms (physical, psychological, social, spiritual)

At the outset of this chapter, we identified the four types of pain frequently experienced by terminally ill patients and their families and suggested some rather specific intervention strategies caregivers could employ in their work with the dying and the bereaved. It was also stated that the role of the hospice caregiver in alleviating the patient's pain—which is in some *way always* tied to the family's ability to deal with pain, or to the stresses associated with an impending loss (death) of a family member—was to tease out through careful observation and inquiry the specific pain components operating at that moment and to then apply the appropriate intervention(s).

For many medically oriented caregivers this suggests that all pain has its beginnings in a physical trauma of some sort. While real *physical* pain must be respected as such and adequate analgesics given (e.g., the Brompton mixture, etc.) in addition to competent nursing care (e.g., bowel, bladder, oral, and skin care, etc.) to ensure the patient's complete physical comfort during the final days of his or her life, not all pain has its origin in human tissue. The pain associated with terminality is often psychosocial and spiritual in origin and it can indeed become intense enough to hurt and to cause such specific secondary physical symptoms as blood in the urine or stool, nonspecific tachycardia, migraine, spastic colon, TMJ disorders, and a whole range of other psychosomatic illnesses.

One such example is that of a 32-year-old male of Latin descent who was referred to the author not long ago for therapy when his urologist could find no physical or clinical basis for the presence of blood in the patient's urine (the symptom). Upon only one visit it was learned that the man's ex-wife[43] was dying of cancer and because he had been asked by her to tell their son about her illness he had become uptight and resented having to be the one to tell his oldest boy about his mother's impending death. It is a clinically documented fact that when sphincter muscles become constricted or tight (probably due to stress) they can cause irritation pain and even bleeding.

It took no major mental exercise on the patient's part to begin to understand the what and when (not why) of his passing blood and within a few days his urine content returned to normal and during a followup telephone conversation a week later he reported having easier bowel movements and no more constipation. In this particular case the patient was male, in his 30s, a father, once divorced, although remarried, and, as he himself indicated, uptight no doubt as a direct consequence of being placed in the position of having to impart the information of his ex-wife's illness to their son and of worrying about the effect all this would have on his present marriage and his two children. There are literally thousands of cases like this one and, although it was easily handled, it clearly underscores the principle that psychological pain is a distinct and unique category of pain quite different in origin, coding, usage, and treatment, from the category of physical pain and physical pain control. A demonstrated knowledge and expertise in symptom control is central to the whole concept of hospice care and if these skills are appropriately applied they can have profound effects on the *quality of life* for the dying.

---

[43]Given the data that many Americans are children of divorced parents and, according to current statistics, will themselves stand a good chance of being divorced, it is important that this be kept in mind when any assumptions are being made about the makeup of a particular patient's family.

BIBLIOGRAPHY

Abram, Harry S.: "Psychological Responses to Illness and Hospitalization," *Psychosomatics,* **10:**218-224, July–August 1969.

Amacher, Nancy Jean: "Touch Is a Way of Caring," *American Journal of Nursing,* **73:**852-54, May 1973.

"At Home with Death," *Newsweek,* January 6, 1975, pp. 43-44.

Baer, Eva, Lois Jean Davitz, and Renee Lieb: "Inferences of Physical Pain and Psychological Distress: I. In Relation to Verbal and Nonverbal Patient Communication," *Nursing Research,* **19:**388-392, September-October 1970.

Baqui, Mufti, Rabbi B. Joseph Hackney, and Rabbi M. Levenstein Bow: "Jewish and Muslim Teaching Concerning Death," a St. Joseph's Hospice occasional paper, London, England.

Barnett, Kathryn: "A Theoretical Construct of the Concepts of Touch as They Relate to Nursing," *Nursing Research,* **21:**102-110, March-April 1972.

Barton, David, Joseph H. Fishbein, and Frank Stevens Jr.: "Psychological Death: An Adaptive Response to Life-Threatening Illness," *Psychiatry in Medicine,* **3:**227-236, July 1972.

Brodsky, Carroll M.: "The Pharmacotherapy System," *Psychosomatics,* **11:**24-30, January-February 1970.

Bronzo, Anthony and Gerald Powers: "Relationship of Anxiety with Pain Threshold," *Journal of Psychology,* **66:**181, July 1967.

Buber, Martin: *I and Thou,* 2d ed., Scribner's, New York, 1958.

Cook, Mark, Lalljee Cook, and G. Mansur: "Verbal

Substitutes for Visual Signals in Interaction," *Semiotica,* **6**(3):212-221, 1972.

Cramond, W. A.: "The Psychological Care of Patients with Terminal Illness," *Nursing Times,* **69**:339-343, March 15, 1973.

Craven, Margaret: *I Heard the Owl Call My Name,* Dell, New York, 1973.

Cronk, Hilary M.: "The Business of Dying," *Nursing Times,* **68**:1100, August 31, 1972.

Crowther, Clarence Edward: "Care Versus Cure in the Treatment of the Terminally Ill," unpublished doctoral dissertation, University of California, Santa Barbara, December 1975.

de Groot, M. H. L.: "The Clinical Use of Psychotherapeutic Drugs in the Elderly," *Drugs,* **8**:132-138, 1974.

Dobihal, Edward F.: "Talk or Terminal Care?" *Connecticut Medicine,* **38**:364-367, July 1974.

Driver, Caroline: "What a Dying Man Taught Doctors About Caring," *Medical Economics,* **50**:81-86, January 22, 1973.

"Drugs Most Commonly Used at St. Christopher's Hospice," unpublished paper, St. Christopher's Hospice, Sydenham, England, January 1975.

Ekman, Paul and Wallace V. Friesen: "The Repertoire of Nonverbal Behavior—Categories, Origins, Usage and Coding," paper presented at the University of California Medical Center, Langley Porter Neuropsychiatric Institute, San Francisco, October 1967.

Enelow, Allen T., (ed.): *Depression in Medical Practice,* Merck, Sharp & Dohme, West Point, Pa., 1971.

Feifel, Herman, (ed.): *The Meaning of Death,* McGraw-Hill, New York, 1959.

Feinstein, Alvan R.: "Biologic Dependency, 'Hypothesis Testing,' Unilateral Probabilities, and Other issues in Scientific Direction vs. Statistical Duplexity," *Clinical Pharmacology and Therapeutics,* **17**:499-513, April 1975.

Formby, Father John, Reverend Michael Hickey, and Reverend A. Gordon Jones: "Christian Teaching Concerning Death," A St. Joseph's Hospice occasional paper, London, England.

Gladman, Arthur E.: "The Role of Non-Verbal Communication in the Development and Treatment of Emotional Illness," *Psychosomatics,* **12**:107-110, March-April 1971.

Goldberg, Harold L.: "Sleep Disturbances Accompanying Clinical Depression/Anxiety," Clinical Cassette Series, Pfizer, New York, 1972.

Gordon, Audrey: "The Jewish View of Death: Guidelines for Mourning," in Elisabeth Kübler-Ross (ed.): *Death: The Final Stage of Growth,* Prentice-Hall, Englewood Cliffs, N.J., 1975, pp. 44-51.

Hart, Betty and Ann W. Rohweder: "Support in Nursing," *American Journal of Nursing,* **59**:1398-1401, October, 1959.

Heller, Rabbi Zachary I.: "The Jewish View of Death: Guidelines for Dying," in Elisabeth Kübler-Ross (ed.), *Death: The Final Stage of Growth,* Englewood Cliffs, N.J., 1975, pp. 38-43.

Hinkle, Lawrence E., Jr.: "The Concept of 'Stress' in the Biological and Social Sciences," *The International Journal of Psychiatry in Medicine,* **5**:335-357, Fall 1974.

Hinton, John: *Dying,* Penguin, Baltimore, 1972.

Hoffman, Esther: "Don't Give Up on Me!" *American Journal Of Nursing,* **71**:60-62, January 1971.

Huszar-Bronner, Judith: "The Psychological Aspects of Cancer in Man," *Psychosomatics,* **12**:133-138, March-April 1971.

Johnson, Betty Sue: "The Meaning Of Touch in Nursing," *Nursing Outlook,* **13**:59-60, February 1965.

Joyce, C. R. B.: "The Issue of Communication Within Medicine," *Psychiatry in Medicine,* **4**:357-363, October 1972.

Kavanaugh, Robert E.: *Facing Death,* Penguin, Baltimore, 1972.

Kram, Charles and John M. Caldwell: "The Dying Patient," *Psychosomatics,* 10:293-295, September-October 1969.

Krant, Melvin J. and Ned H. Cassem: "Anxiety/Depression: Terminal Disease," *PROBE* Audio-Tape Series, Wallace Pharmaceuticals, Cranbury, N.J., 1973.

Kron, Thora: "How We Communicate Nonverbally with Patients," *Nursing Research,* **68**:21-23, November 1972.

Kübler-Ross, Elisabeth: *On Death and Dying,* Macmillan, New York, 1969.

—: "What Is It Like to Be Dying?," *American Journal of Nursing,* **71**:54-61, January 1971.

—: *Questions and Answers on Death and Dying,* Macmillan, New York, 1974.

—: *Death: The Final Stage of Growth,* Prentice-Hall, Englewood Cliffs, N.J., 1975.

Lamerton, Richard: "Care of the Dying 2," *Nursing Times,* **68**:1544-1545, December 7, 1972.

—: "Care of the Dying 3," *Nursing Times,* **68**:1578, December 14, 1972.

—: "Care of the Dying 4," *Nursing Times,* **68**:1642-1643, December 28, 1972.

—: "Care of the Dying 5," *Nursing Times,* **79**:16, January 4, 1973.

—: "Care of the Dying 7," *Nursing Times,* **69**:88-89, Janurary 18, 1973.

—: "Drugs for the Dying: The Treatment of Terminal Pain," *St. Bartholomew's Hospital Journal,* **79**(1):353-354, 1975.

Lazarus, Richard S.: "Psychological Stress and coping in Adaptation and Illness," *The International Journal Of Psychiatry in Medicine,* **5**:321-333, Fall 1974.

Liegner, Leonard M.: *St. Christopher's Hospice—Site Visit Report: Care of the Dying Patient, 1974,* Columbia University, Department of Radiology, College of Physicians and Surgeons, New York, 1974.

Long, J. Bruce: "The Death That Ends Death in Hinduism and Buddhism," in Elisabeth Kübler-Ross (ed.), *Death: The Final Stage of Growth,* Prentice-Hall, Englewood Cliffs, N.J., 1975, pp. 52-72.

MacKinnon, Bernard L.: "Death and the Doctor,"

The Journal of the Maine Medical Association, **63:**169-171, August 1972.

McNulty, Barbara: "The Needs of the Dying," lecture given to the Guild of Pastoral Psychology, Sydenham, England, January 1969.

—: "Care of the Dying," *Nursing Times,* **68:**1505-1506, November 30, 1972.

Miller, Sara and Stuart Miller: *First Report of the Program in Humanistic Medicine 1972-1973,* Institute for the Study of Humanistic Medicine, San Francisco, 1973.

Morison, Robert S.: "Dying," *Scientific American,* **229:**55-74, September 1973.

Mount, Balfour M.: "Death and Dying: Attitudes in a Teaching Hospital," *Urology,* **4:**741,747, December 1974.

—: "Death—A Part of Life," *CRUX, A Quarterly Journal of Christian Thought and Opinion,* **11**(3):3-13, 1973-1974.

Mowbray, R. M.: "The Hamilton Rating Scale for Depression: A Factor Analysis," *Psychological Medicine,* **2:**272-280, August 1972.

Nadelson, Dr. Theodore: "Anxiety/Depression: Clues to Their Recognition," *PROBE* Audio-Tape Series, Wallace Pharmaceuticals, Cranbury, N.J., 1972.

Nolen, William A.: "Fewer Pills and More Conversation," *PRISM,* **1:**29-81, October 1973.

Parkes, Colin Murray: "Effects of Bereavement on Physical and Mental Health—A Study of the Medical Records of Widows," *British Medical Journal,* **2:**274-279, August 1964.

—: "The First Year of Bereavement: A Longitudinal Study of the Reaction of London Widows to the Death of Their Husbands," *Psychiatry,* **33:**444-467, November 1970.

—: "Psycho-Social Transitions: A Field for Study," *Socal Science and Medicine,* **5:**101-115, April 1971.

—: "Components of the Reaction to Loss of a Limb, Spouse or Home," *Journal of Psychosomatic Research,* **16:**343-349, August 1972.

Pozos-Bonilla, Randolfo: "The Santa Barbara Hospice: An Anthropological Perspective on the Planning and Development of Special Services for the Terminally Ill," unpublished paper, University of California, Berkeley, Department of Anthropology, May 1975.

Rees, W. Dewi: "The Distress of Dying," *Nursing Times,* **68:**1479-1480, November 23, 1972.

Rogers, Carl R.: "The Characteristics of a Helping Relationship," address delivered at the APGA Convention, St. Louis, Missouri, March 31-April 3, 1958.

Saunders, Cicely: "The Treatment of Intractable Pain in Terminal Cancer," *Proceedings of the Royal Society of Medicine,* **56:**1-75, March 1963.

—: "Watch with Me," *Nursing Times,* **61:**1615-1617, November 26, 1965.

—: "The Need for In-Patient Care for the Patient with Terminal Cancer," *Middlesex Hosptial Journal,* **72:**1-6, February 1973.

—: "The Need for Institutional Care for the Patient with Advanced Cancer," unpublished paper, St. Christopher's Hospice, Sydenham, England.

—: "Terminal Care," in K. D. Bagshane (ed.), *Medical Oncology,* Blackwells, Oxford, 1973.

Scott, Patrician Cumin: *Some Information for Those Caring for Patients,* St. Christopher's Hospice, Sydenham, England, 1974.

Simpson, Michael A.: "What Is Dying Like?" *Nursing Times,* **69:**405-406, March 29, 1973.

Strode, Orienne Elizabeth: Program Bulletin for "Human Dimensions in Medical Education," The Center for Studies of the Person, La Jolla, Ca., Summer 1975.

St. Christopher's Hospice Annual Report, Sydenham, England, 1973-1974.

Tanner, E. R.: "A Time to Die," a St. Joseph's Hospice occasional paper, London, England.

Thompson, Captane P.: "Prevention in Psychiatry," *Nursing Times,* **61:**1620-1621, November 26, 1965.

Torrey, E. Fuller: *The Mind Game: Witchdoctors and Psychiatrists,* Bantam, New York, 1973.

—: *The Death of Psychiatry,* Penguin, Baltimore, 1974.

Trelease, Murray: "Dying Among Alaskan Indians: A Matter of Choice," in Elisabeth Kübler-Ross (ed.), *Death: The Final Stage of Growth,* Prentice-Hall, Englewood Cliffs, N.J., 1975, p. 33.

Twycross, Robert G.: *The Dying Patient,* Christian Medical Fellowship Publications, London, 1975.

Watts, Alan W.: *Psychotherapy East and West,* Ballantine, New York, 1961.

Weisman, Avery D.: "Misgivings and Misconceptions in the Psychiatric Care of Terminal Patients," *Psychiatry,* **33:**68-75, February 1970.

West, T. S.: "Approach to Death," *Nursing Mirror,* **139**(15), October 10, 1974.

Whybrow, Peter C.: "The Use and Abuse of the 'Medical Model' as a Conceptual Frame in Psychiatry," *Psychiatry in Medicine,* **3:**333-342, October 1972.

Zung, William K. and Thomas H. Wonnacott: "Treatment Prediction in Depression Using a Self-Rating Scale," *Psychiatry,* **2:**321-329, October 1970.

40

The Shanti Project: a hopeful scenario for the dying

ELLEN GOODMAN

We have all been born. We will all die. These are simple truths, yet the experience is rarely so simple. For each of us the quality of these inevitable times will vary with the kinds of persons we've been in our lives, who will be around as we are dying, and the immediate cause of our deaths. For most of us these "simple truths" remain in the safety of the distant future; for others they do not. These others are the people who have learned that they have a terminal illness, that they are dying . . . now. For them, their families, and their friends, death has become as immediate as life, as immediate as their feelings of fear, confusion, anger, and alienation.

What can we expect when the prospect of our own deaths has changed from a distant possibility to a present probability? This year 75 percent of us who die in the United States will end our days in hospitals or nursing homes. We can expect unfamiliar surroundings and procedures, intense conflicting feelings, and inadequate emotional support. There are many reasons for this grim picture. Among them is the culture in which we live. Our culture teaches us to deny death and the dying while it has made available to us great technologic and medical advancements that prolong the time of our living and our dying. Many therapeutic treatments offer us precious time in which to come to terms with our deaths, the feelings we are experiencing, and the relationships important to us—time to share our

fear, sorrow, love, and growth. Yet this gift can weigh heavily when offered by a culture that insists on ignoring the psychologic realities of dying. Many of us will be left alone in our fear and will have no one with whom to share our last days.

The Shanti Project is one hope for change toward a different scenario for the dying. Shanti is a Sanskrit word that means inner peace. The Shanti Project is a volunteer counseling service that offers caring, ongoing support to patients and families facing life-threatening illness. The project provides free counseling services to the San Francisco Bay Area community and was founded and directed by Dr. Charles Garfield, a clinical research psychologist at the University of California Medical Center's Cancer Research Institute.

Garfield, an internationally known authority on the psychosocial aspects of life-threatening illness, was concerned with the inadequate support available to the dying, their families, and the health care professionals who work with them. Along with others who shared his concern, Garfield searched for an inexpensive and flexible alternative for dealing with the emotional needs of people facing life-threatening illness.

Stewart Brand, who developed the *Whole Earth Catalogue,* came up with the simple concept that has since formed the basis for Shanti's community service operation. Brand's suggestion was that a group of volunteers who had the interest, ability, and time to work with the dying could be organized and reached at a central telephone number. The volunteers could be matched with a client whose needs they are best equipped to meet and then go out into the community to visit with clients anywhere support was needed.

This idea became a reality in February of 1975, when the first Shanti telephone line was installed. In the beginning there were only 14 volunteers. That number has since grown to nearly 100, with volunteer counselors providing more than 50,000 counseling hours per year, totally without cost to the clients.

Shanti's services are available to anyone who desires to use them. The process is simple. There are no forms to fill out. All one needs to do is call. A 24-hour message tape is available for anyone who calls outside of office hours—9:00 to 5:30 on weekdays—or when other lines are busy. A member of the Shanti staff discusses the caller's situation and needs in detail and then makes the necessary contact with an appropriate Shanti volunteer.

The problems of those who call are varied. But the one commonality among all callers is a need for someone to listen, to give feedback, and to be willing to do what needs to be done. In general the requests for counseling services come from four different kinds of clients.

The first are patients who desire one-to-one counseling, companionship, and emotional support. These people want an advocate who will be a constant contact in the often bizarre and rapidly changing medical world they now face on a daily basis. Often the request is for someone to help break the news of illness to other members of the family.

Recently Shanti received a call from a mother whose 7-year-old son was dying of leukemia. She said she needed help. "We have three other children in the family. They know that Danny is very sick but we haven't told them that he is dying. I want to tell them; I'm afraid they will be angry and hurt if we don't tell them ahead of time. We've been dealing with the knowledge that our son might die for 3 years now. It's been so frightening for us. We want the other kids to know but don't know how to tell them. We need someone to talk to before we talk to them.''

A second group requests volunteers to spend time with an entire family in which one member is suffering from a life-threatening illness or for a volunteer to work with just one member of a patient's family. Often the strain of dealing with a life-threatening illness interferes with communication between patient and family at a time when such communication is desperately wanted and needed. Sometimes the volunteer is there to facilitate communication among the family members. At other times he or she is there to support the rights and feelings of the patient's family or spouse, who, without caring support and validation for their own feelings, may withdraw from the patient out of fear, sorrow, and a sense of helplessness.

A third group of callers are themselves survivors of the death of a family member or close friend. They are suffering from the trauma of separation with its pain, fear, and loneliness. Unfortunately they are suffering in a society that does not want to be reminded of death. Too often they are told to mourn quietly and quickly, never given the opportunity to work through their loss. One caller said, "My 22-year-old daughter was raped and murdered 6 months ago. I'm working on my Ph.D. in sociology but I'm still finding it hard to concentrate. I miss my daughter terribly. Even professionals tell me I should be over it by now, and my friends don't want to talk about it anymore. I think it scares them. It scares me! Sometimes I think I'm going crazy."

This woman has been led to believe that she should have been able to "get over" the trauma of her daughter's sudden, violent death and 22 years of mothering in 6 short months. This kind of call is all too common. Fortunately, however, Shanti volunteers look on grief counseling and ongoing emotional support for survivors as a vital part of their work. They are there for as long as they are needed.

Finally there are those callers who work with the dying outside the usual institutional setting. They call for support, back up consultation, or just someone with whom to talk. These calls come from clergy, private duty nurses, teachers who tutor sick children at home, and others who have intimate contact with the dying, who share their emotional pain, and who come to care very much for them. Often these people have no one immediately available to deal with *their* sadness.

It takes special kinds of people to respond to these calls and become involved in the lives and deaths of the callers, and the Shanti volunteers are indeed special. They have varied backgrounds and personal beliefs, but all of them share a willingness, strength, and sensitivity to confront humanely the realities involved in dying. They are chosen for their compassion, introspection, and healthy sense of self. Most important is their willingness to let each person die in his or her own style and their awareness that there is no "right" way to die.

All volunteers make an 8- to 10-hour weekly commitment to the project and agree to at least 1 year of participation. It is this level of involvement and caring that allows Shanti to provide the personal and continuous care so important to Shanti clients and so frequently unavailable from other sources.

In addition to providing counseling for people who call, the Shanti project serves two additional functions. The first is to offer training programs to health care professionals, the clergy, and the lay public. It is an important part of the Shanti program to share its particular skills with all groups who have need of them and to publicize the emotional and social issues involved in dealing with the terminally ill and their families.

The second function is to act as a model for others who wish to develop similar services in other parts of the country. Garfield is currently assisting nearly 50 groups modeled after the Shanti Project. The Shanti staff is currently preparing a manual describing its methods of selection, training, and supervision of volunteers and its philosophy and organization. Garfield is conducting institutes and seminars to assist others who wish to use the Shanti experience to help establish volunteer counseling in their own communities. Similar groups have already been formed in California and other areas throughout the country.

The Shanti Project is an independent, nonprofit organization. Its financial support has come through donations from public and private foundations, as well as from private individuals and memorial gifts. The Shanti Project is grateful for all such expressions of support for the work it is doing and for the ideas it advocates. The service the Project provides is a continuing one, as is the need it seeks to meet. At some point in our lives, each of us shall experience both illness and death. Through the efforts of groups such as the Shanti Project there is hope that these experiences will occur in an environment rich in support and understanding.

For further information contact Dr. Garfield at 106 Evergreen Lane, Berkeley, California 94705.

41

A problem solving approach to terminal illness for the family and physician

DAVID M. KAPLAN and NETTA GRANDSTAFF

In a growing number of circles of our society there is the realization that we have not paid enough attention to the late phases of living, which include death, dying, old age, and chronic illness, or to the impact that these experiences have on all of us as human beings—young and old alike. This conference is itself a testimony to the fact that physicians and health professionals have neglected until recently these stages of living and that we need to do considerably more to modify our attitudes and increase our knowledge and skills in these areas.

The attention of this conference is focused on the dying patient; on how he and those close to him may be helped to cope more effectively with the final phases of living. But, it is critically important to note that for most of us it is too late to cope successfully with dying and death if our first attempt to do so occurs only days, weeks, or months from the end itself.

The existentialists remind us that coming to terms with death should take place long before we experience terminal illness. Camus,[3] for example, maintains that life is lived more fully with the knowledge that death is an ever-present reality and not

something to face reluctantly only after we become old and feeble.

The task of teaching ourselves and our children these facts of living is obviously a community responsibility and not that of any one group in our society. However, physicians and health professionals do have opportunities to help people accept and adapt to unwelcome changes in life, long before terminal illness occurs.

The diagnosis of a chronic illness, for example, gives us an earlier opportunity to learn to reconcile ourselves to death. This is true, partly because such illnesses convey to us intimations of our mortality but also because these disorders require us to accept disagreeable limitations as well. The experience of adapting to disabilities, to unwelcome restrictions, and to the losses inherent in a serious illness constitutes a rehearsal of what we must face later on in preparing ourselves for death. One woman who lived through and wrote about her experience with breast cancer concluded:

I have made death's acquaintance. And however horrendous and premature the meeting was, I think it will have softened the shock of our eventually living together, whenever that happens. I hope it won't be soon . . . the peek at death has given me some new information about life, all of which has made me better at it than I was before. And, with some more practice, I would get better still. If I don't have a recur-

Presented at the Second National Training Conference for Physicians on "Psychosocial care of the dying patient"—Doctor-Patient Relationships in Terminal Illness—on June 2 to 4, 1977.

343

rence of cancer and die soon, all I've lost is a breast, and that's not so bad.[9]

Needless to say, we human beings have considerable difficulty in accepting limitations of any kind, and as a result many of us fail to live as fully as possible with chronic illness. The woman who delays having a breast lump examined by her physician for months or years after its discovery; the man who survives a heart attack without making any changes in critical habits including his drinking, eating, smoking, working, or exercising; the parent who magically expects heart surgery to correct an infant's mental retardation; and the glaucoma patient who fails to renew prescriptions for essential eye medication are but a few examples from a long list of common failures to accept or adjust realistically to threatening, disabling diseases long before we die from them.

Those investigations that have focused on early human reactions to chronic disease indicate that the failure to cope realistically with the implications of serious disease at the outset is closely linked to the subsequent failure to manage the late phases of the same illness.[5] In other words, early unrealistic responses to serious illness become bad habits that are reinforced and entrenched with the passage of time.

The importance of focusing our clinical attention on human adaptation to illness in the early phases is underscored by the additional finding that the negative consequences of unsuccessful adaptation are not visited on the patient alone but also have a major impact on other members of the family.[4,6]

The implication of family members in the process of accommodation to illness occurs because a serious disease in one member requires complementary adjustments by all family members. The process of individual adaptation takes place in an arena in which every member of the family influences and is influenced by every other member. The family is potentially an enormous resource of support if it acts to reinforce effective coping efforts among its members. Con-

versely, when it fails to encourage realistic adaptation for whatever reasons, the family seriously interferes with individual coping attempts and weakens its traditional responsibility for stress mediation. Serious illness is a family affair, and by that token family involvement in it is an opportunity for every member of the family to learn some important lessons about living and dying.

For these reasons, the early detection of unsuccessful coping reactions to illness is as important to prevention and to rehabilitation as is the early detection of disease itself. We must one day come to regard adaptational failures as medical challenges that are worthy of more serious attention than they have been given so far.

Because human adaptation to disease has been a neglected area of medical investigation, the resources available to physicians and other health personnel to prevent or to correct adaptational failures are limited and largely ineffective. Indeed with the present state of knowledge, we have difficulty even in deciding what is good adaptation and what is not.

Those theoretic approaches to problems of adjustment on which clinicians drawing heavily have a common denominator, that is, the idea that adaptation to illness is determined largely by premorbid variables. The sociologic approach posits one or more factors of social background as the primary influence in adaptation outcome, for example, class, race, or education. In the psychiatric model, illness outcome is presumed to be determined by the presence or absence of individual psychopathology. Both of these conceptions of human adaptation are oversimplifications because they ignore the process of adjustment itself in which situational factors play in important role. The process of adaptation acts as an intervening variable and exerts a strong influence on illness outcome.

Bard and Sutherland comment on the inadequacy of personality theory in explaining patient reactions to mastectomy in breast cancer:

It has been said that the "mature" woman will have less reaction to mastectomy than the "neurotic" woman with an abnormal investment of emotion in her breast. If the mature woman is defined as one who has less reaction and therefore has a "normal" investment in her breasts, then this statement is circular and must obviously be true. Unfortunately, the impact of mastectomy, as of other mutilating surgery, cannot often be predicted prior to the event.

The rather moralistic fashion of dividing personalities into the mature and immature, the normal and the neurotic, seems to have less and less meaning as our understanding of the dynamics of adaptation deepens. These appear more and more to be abstract entities better designed to fit into theories than to describe real people. They add nothing to our understanding of dynamic processes. The emphasis should be placed on understanding the *meaning* of the specific experience to the individual patient in his total life adaptation rather than on an abstract personality type can withstand any experience abstractly regarded as stressful.[1]

There are no simple methods of resolving the problems associated with maladaptive responses to illness, but there is a way of conceptualizing such problems that may result in effective interventions. This relatively new theoretic approach is concerned with the process of adaptation itself rather than with premorbid factors.[7] The process of individual adaptation to change is conceived of as a complex but decipherable attempt at problem solving. It is the problem-solving process that is at the heart of adaptation and of more effective interventions.

In this approach to human adaptation, individual coping responses to illness are conceived of as attempts to resolve specific and immediate coping tasks posed by an illness, whatever the individual's history may be.[5] These coping efforts are coherent responses that can be identified readily and their efficacy judged by how well they resolve the problems and tasks of adaptation and by the extent to which they are associated with good rehabilitative outcome.

The substance of this problem-solving model lies in detailed knowledge of the nature of successful coping behavior. The quintessential question to ask about an individual struggling to cope with a serious illness is not Is he psychologically healthy? but Are his attempts to cope effective? Personality theory has not shed much light on our understanding of the process of human adaptation to change, nor has it produced effective methods of intervention in these situations.

The concept of problem solving may connote to many an intellectual exercise having little, if anything, to do with human emotions. In this presentation cognition is an important part of the problem-solving process, but so are the emotions that are aroused by an illness that threatens cherished activities, causes suffering and disability, and involves painful sacrifices. The individual ability to handle the emotions generated by illness is an essential ingredient of effective problem solving. The temptation to avoid disturbing emotions such as sadness, anger, fear, and anxiety rather than allowing these feelings to run their course is a cause of much, but not all, ineffective coping.

Finally problem solving involves individual decision making. There are, for example, two major sets of decisions that have to be made in the breast cancer problem-solving process. One group of decisions relates to the phase of obtaining physical care for the disease, that is, those decisions that determine how quickly the problem is brought for treatment and the form that treatment will take.

The other set of decisions embraces those interpersonal relationships that are mobilized to (1) obtain physical care and (2) meet the patient's and family's needs for information, emotional support, and reassurance during the process of adapting to this life-threatening illness. One may succeed in obtaining good physical care quickly, which offers the best chance for long-term survival, without also making those coping decisions that are associated with a good psychosocial outcome.

It is important to note that there are op-

timal periods of time for making these decisions. If one fails to reach a decision in the
appropriate time period, one is likely to
suffer the consequences in lower levels of
rehabilitative achievement and long-term
disruption of important family and community relationships. These problem-solving
decisions are the distillates of the adaptational process; they provide the criteria by
which the effectiveness of each person's efforts to cope with illness can be evaluated.

Let us now apply the problem-solving
model of adaptation to a specific illness,
that is, to breast cancer.* The process of
adaptation to breast cancer begins with a
woman's acknowledgement of the existence of a breast lump. Her awareness or
suspicion of a growth constitutes the first
coping task. Not uncommonly, a lump of
moderate or of large dimensions may exist
for some time without being recognized.
Again, the failure to acknowledge a tumor
constitutes a coping decision, that is, one
way to deal with the problem. In this instance further problem solving is obviated
until such time as the lesion is knowledged.

The woman who accomplishes the first
task of recognizing the existence of a breast
lump goes on to face the second coping
task, that is, evaluating the potential risk of
her tumor. There are women who have not
learned that a breast may be cancerous; for
them the lump is not a threat and there is no
need to evaluate its significance. Further
problem solving does not occur for these
women until an awareness of the potential
threat of the lesion is realized.

For the woman who has learned that a
breast lump may be cancerous, an assessment is made of the potential risk she runs
from her lesion. There are basically three
kinds of decisions that can be reached in
such lump evaluations. One decision is to
conclude that the growth is not cancerous,

for example, it may be perceived as the result of an infection or associated with the
menstrual cycle or viewed as a benign lump
in a woman who has had a history of non-
cancerous breast lesions. The second possible decision is to concede the possibility
of malignancy but to judge the risk to be
only potential and not immediate. Usually
this decision is accompanied by a "wait and
see" attitude while a home remedy or
prayer or other action is resorted to in the
hope that the lesion will disappear. Weeks
or months may go by before this attitude is
changed. The third option is to decide that
the lump risk is immediate and requires an
early examination by a physician or some
other healer. (We will assume for the purpose of this presentation that the patient's
contacts are with physicians.)

This process of decision making, which
first occurs following the discovery of the
breast lesion, is repeated (typically) two
more times—once after an initial examination by a physician who is not a surgeon and
again after a second examination by a surgeon.

After each medical examination, the
physician or surgeon makes one of three
recommendations that closely parallel the
decisions a woman has to make independently on lump discovery. The physician
may decide (1) that the lump is not cancerous, (2) that the lump needs to be examined
again after a specified time interval, or (3)
that the tumor should be referred to a surgeon for further examination. In the case of
the surgeon, the third choice is to recommend a biopsy. The patient can respond to
each medical recommendation by concur-
ring, by disagreeing, and/or by seeking another medical opinion.

When the patient decides to go ahead
with a biopsy, there are several decisions to
be made in the event that the tissue proves
malignant: (1) The patient may agree to a
biopsy without any further treatment commitment; (2) the patient may decide against
any treatment after biopsy or to have only
nonsurgical treatment (for example, radiation implant, chemotherapy, or radio-

*The work described is the result of a current investi-
gation supported by the American Cancer Society
(Division of Clinical Social Work, Stanford University
Medical Center), whose goal is the development and
evaluation of psychosocial interventions for the breast
cancer patient and her family.

therapy); (3) if she elects surgical removal of the cancerous tissue, she may agree to one-stage surgery (biopsy and mastectomy performed in one operation) or to two-stage surgery (the first surgery limited to the biopsy followed, usually after a brief interval, by a second surgery for the mastectomy); (4) she may decide to have the type of mastectomy recommended by her surgeon or elect to have an alternative form of mastectomy; and finally (5) she may or may not accept the recommendations for adjuvant treatment following surgery.

The implications for intervention of these decisions are not difficult to infer. Those decisions that ignore or overlook the existence of a breast lump are clearly hazardous. Since each woman is primarily responsible for lump discovery on her own, the appropriate intervention is educational in nature, that is, teaching women that lumps may be cancerous and urging them to conduct regular self-examinations. Our efforts to educate in this area have not met with outstanding success so far.

Those decisions that dismiss lumps as benign without careful examination and biopsy or that put off medical examinations for more than a few weeks are also risky. Again, educating women, family members, and physicians about these risks is an important aspect of breast cancer intervention.

The second, concurrent group of decisions that each woman makes as she decides whether to recognize a breast lump or not and what to do about it concerns those other persons whom she involves in her decision making; specifically, which persons she involves, when she involves them, and how she involves herself with them, that is, for what purposes.

There are many reasons for involving other people in the problem-solving process: (1) to gather the data needed to make decisions, (2) to find support for those decisions that are made, (3) to seek comfort for the many fears associated with breast cancer, particularly the threat of death and disfigurement, and finally (4) to allow others who are close to the patient the time to prepare themselves for the possibility and implications of malignancy as the woman with a lesion must prepare herself. The woman who acknowledges the existence of a potentially cancerous breast lump goes on to make these decisions. Although there may be variation in how they are reached, the decisions made by each individual fall into identifiable patterns and into recognizable subsets that can be identified as adaptive or maladaptive; whether or not decisions are adaptive can be empirically verified by subsequent assessment once the crisis is over.

There are many issues and fears that may preoccupy a woman once she discovers a breast lump. These critical issues and fears are the essence of the coping task whose resolution is the main business of the adaptive process. Pattison lists eight fears of the dying patient: fears of the unknown, of loneliness, of sorrow, of the loss of one's body, of the loss of self-control, of suffering and pain, of the loss of one's identity, and of physical and mental regression.[8] The woman with a breast lesion may be concerned with one or more of these fears and others besides; the loss of her good health to a life-threatening chronic disease, the possibility of not surviving surgery, and the disfigurement following mastectomy. Once surgery is over, there is the additional worry about whether cancer cells will be found in the lymph glands and, if they are a fear of the effects of adjuvant treatment.

Our study observations indicate that those concerns that center on (1) disfigurement following breast amputation and (2) the loss of one's good health to a disease that may eventually cause death should be confronted and substantially resolved before surgery is performed. Successful resolution implies accepting these two concerns as real possibilities that one must be prepared to live with—not to like. If these issues are denied or not resolved prior to surgery for any reasons, the full rehabilitation of the woman may not be achieved or may be delayed for years even when the prognosis of the illness itself is a favorable one.

Why is it so important to achieve a substantial resolution of these two problems before surgery? In the course of any crisis, one's normal activities and responsibilities vis-à-vis others are suspended while the individual is given a brief time to solve the new problems and to come to terms with a new reality, with a new set of circumstances imposed by a serious illness.

Whether a woman can achieve the resumption of most of her responsibilities, consistent with the limitations of having a serious disease, depends on how quickly and how successfully she comes to terms with her new self. Many women do resume highly satisfying lives within weeks of lump discovery despite the fact that they no longer have intact healthy bodies and have to live with the knowledge of possible recurrence of a life-threatening disease for the rest of their lives. Many women do not.

If these coping tasks, that is, acceptance of disfigurement and of the disease's threat to life, are not resolved before surgery, it will be extremely difficult for the woman to take up the job of fashioning a new life, part of which involves picking up old responsibilities and activities. The longer one is preoccupied with tasks that need to be resolved effectively and quickly, the greater is the risk that important activities and relationships may deteriorate or be lost altogether. A woman, for example, who cannot accept the fact of disfigurement before surgery will not be able to resume sexual relations with any measure of pleasurable anticipation or satisfaction for herself or her partner. The woman who fails to successfully resolve these particular coping tasks early is apt to be preoccupied and/or inhibited by these problems until they are resolved. She will be unable to pick up the pieces of her life and put them together into a new, viable and satisfying way of living.

Unfortunately one does not have unlimited time to resolve threatening and disruptive changes. Nature abhors the vacuum created by an illness and permits only a temporary suspension of the normal responsibilities of being a wife, a mother, etc. If the vacuum is not filled within a fairly brief time, family and community relations that existed prior to the illness may never again be reconstituted or, if they are resumed, may continue only in attenuated and unsatisfying forms.

There are a number of accounts written by women who have had breast cancer describing their particular experiences and their efforts to cope with the disease and its implications. Two of these reports will be reviewed to illustrate the problem-solving approach to adaptation described in this paper.

Mrs. B. reports that she had been in the habit of routinely examining her breasts for years before she discovered a lump. She had grown children at the time. She had just been sworn in as Special Assistant to the President's Council on Environmental Quality and was about to represent the United States in Moscow for the meetings of a joint U.S.A.-U.S.S.R. committee on environmental protection. She immediately saw her personal physician, who recommended further examination by a surgeon although he thought the lump was probably benign. Since Mrs. B. had no sense of concern at that time and had a full work schedule, she and the surgeon agreed to do the biopsy after her return in 6 weeks from her European trip. She told no one else about her lump but went on to make the planned trip.

While abroad she experienced pain and burning sensations in her breast and she began to be worried. Surreptitiously, after her return home, she read about breast cancer and asked her brother, a hospital administrator, for information. She did not wish to alarm her family, particularly her mother. She found it difficult to talk to her husband but she felt he should be prepared for the possibility of cancer, which she was beginning to think about seriously. She was told in her initial medical examination that the chances of finding a benign lump were 60 to 40 in her favor. But now she began to face the fact, with her husband, that the tumor might be malignant, no longer comforted by the 6 to 4 odds, presumably, in her favor.

By the time she entered the hospital for the biopsy, she felt apprehensive. She recalled several close friends, three of whom had died because the cancer was not found in time and several others who had had a mastectomy and survived. One friend had signed papers without understanding she had given permission for a mastectomy. She only expected a biopsy. Mrs. B. decided to have two-stage surgery in the event of malignancy. Her physicians outlined the surgical choices, favoring a modified radical mastectomy. Mrs. B. elected to have a simple mastectomy with nodal dissection (which is a modified mastectomy) on the assumption that the cancer had probably not spread to the lymph glands; at this point in considering the type of surgery she could elect, she also faced the possibility that her life might be shortened if the malignancy had metastisized. In that event, she decided she "would live as long as she was supposed to." Her biopsy was positive and when she recovered she began to accept the fact that she had cancer and the imminent loss of her breast. She cried for the first time, alone, and with her two daughters as she recovered from the biopsy surgery in the hospital.

Fortunately, the pathology report following surgery indicated no nodal involvement. After the mastectomy, Mrs. B. decided, with her family's agreement, to write about her experience for the benefit of other women. She concluded her account by attributing her good psychological recovery to her family's support during the "unexpected, traumatic experiences of the last several weeks."[2]

Mrs. B's early decisions to put off surgery so that she might attend the Moscow conference and her failure to inform any family members of her predicament are not examples of effective coping in our experience. On the contrary, these decisions reflect her early failure to prepare herself or others for the possibility of malignancy and breast amputation. Apparently these early decisions reflected less an inability to face unpleasant reality than an understandable desire to accomplish an important and unique work assignment. Mrs. B. demonstrated her ability to cope effectively once her government assignment was out of the way.

Although she wisely sought medical advice before taking her trip abroad, her failure to enlarge the circle of those informed of her lesion at that time may well have served the function of lessening the chances that someone might have sought to dissuade her from her trip.

Once she returned from abroad, her coping efforts improved considerably. She began to prepare herself and others in the family for a possible diagnosis of cancer. She achieved this preparation by electing two-stage surgery, which gave her further time to come to terms with cancer and her disfigurement following surgery. She mourned the loss of her health to a chronic disease with its ever-present threat of death and the loss of her intact body as a result of breast amputation. Had she chosen one-stage surgery instead, Mrs. B. might not have provided the time she and her family needed to prepare for her cancer. Fortunately her family responded with realistic and firm support to which Mrs. B. correctly attributed an important part of her good psychologic recovery from her trauma.

The second personal account of the breast cancer experience is more detailed and gives us the opportunity of reviewing another woman's early coping patterns along with outcome revealed months after surgery.

Ms. R.'s husband discovered her breast lump during sexual intercourse. She was 38 years old at the time, with no children. She went immediately to her physician who, after examining her mammograms decided there was no need to worry. He diagnosed the lump as a benign cyst.

Almost a year after her first examination,

Ms. R., following her physician's earlier recommendation, returned for a second medical examination. Her decision to return was influenced by the publicity given to Mrs. Ford's and Mrs. Rockefeller's mastectomies and the realization that early detection could save one's life. This time, the mammography examination prompted a physician to recommend that the lump be surgically removed. Ms. R. fleetingly thought about the word "cancer" but dismissed this diagnosis as a real possibility. She was convinced by her history of excellent health and a strong sense of invulnerability that the biopsy was merely a "nuisance interruption." She did little, if anything, to anticipate possible bad news from a biopsy.

Ms. R. later wondered at being so "pigheadly unafraid" prior to surgery but she was convinced at that time that "bad things don't happen to me." Prior to seeing the surgeon, she acknowledged that she had not come to terms "with what might happen to me." She could not seriously worry about something that probably would not happen. She reminded herself of the odds, 10 to 1 in favor of the lump being benign.

The surgeon told her following his examination that there was a "good chance of a malignancy"; Ms. R. reacted with shock to this news. She came very close to fainting. She cried briefly but after leaving the surgeon's office she reminded her husband that "it still might not happen." During the weekend of waiting for surgery scheduled for the following Monday, Ms. R. decided that keeping busy ("with trivia") would best get her through the waiting period. She shopped and spent time with friends. She left instructions for her husband to tell her parents only if cancer was discovered. She did get as far, psychologically, as fearing the loss of her breast. Her husband, she realized later, had gone beyond that to consider that she might die as the result of cancer. She did not consider any issue other than her fear of breast loss nor did she accept emotionally the possibility of breast loss prior to surgery.

The evening before surgery, her surgeon discussed possible options should the biopsy prove positive. He recommended a "modified radical" and gave Ms. R. the choice of one- or two-stage surgery. She thought two-stage surgery was "stupid" and gave the surgeon permission to do what he thought best. Her uppermost concerns, at this point, were her fears of not surviving surgery and of disfigurement.

In the days of hospitalization after surgery, Ms. R. enjoyed the attention and concern of many friends. She acted bravely and cheerfully, playing the part of Pollyanna with visitors. She enjoyed, particularly, visits from an old suitor who indicated his continued, serious interest in her. But she rejected a visit from a Reach-to-Recovery volunteer.

She refused to look at the breast wound, realizing that to do so would shatter her precarious "tough" pose. In the hospital, she "didn't feel much of anything." In her own words, she realized intellectually what had happened but not emotionally. Even the good news from pathology indicating that her lymph nodes were clear brought little reaction from her—a numbness of all feelings characterized her during the hospital stay of 8 days.

The first night at home was the occasion for an abortive attempt at love making. She endured sex because her "husband needed it," but the effort ended disastrously when he felt her intact breast. The next day the bottom fell out of her "brave" act. She realized that she was not healthy any more. Her chances for long-term survival had dropped from 96% to 80%. She was very angry that the lump had not been taken out a year earlier. Finally, for the first time since the operation she began to cry. She became acutely aware of the possibility of dying of cancer and sought comfort from her husband; she continued to cry profusely. Finally, Ms. R. realized that the fear of dying must be borne—that there was no alternative to bearing this fear. She felt rage, self-pity, and frailty, feelings she had not experienced earlier.

Sex with her husband was something she continued to dread because she no longer found herself attractive. She felt deformed, and that killed any sex urge she might have had. She continued to be unable to look at her wound. She made a tentative visit to obtain a breast prosthesis and was so upset at the prospect of wearing one that a month passed before she could again consider the kind of prosthesis she might prefer.

She returned to work 8 days after leaving the hospital but this did not work out; she felt strange and exhausted. Two weeks after surgery, she forced herself to look at her wound and found the experience devastating. She no longer slept naked as had been her custom.

While her relationship with her husband was deteriorating, she continued to become seriously involved with her old boyfriend. She was unable to let her husband see her wound for a few weeks. When she did show it to him, his attempts to reassure her did not comfort her.

One month after surgery, she left her husband to live with her old suitor. She left stealthily, without any warning or discussion with her husband. She was aware that her marriage had not been perfect. On the other hand, she recognized that it had held real satisfaction for both partners. It was her fear of her husband's infidelity based on earlier incidents that caused the separation. About 5 months later, despite continued protestations of his continuing love, her husband agreed, reluctantly, to a divorce. It was a painful experience for Ms. R. Soon after the divorce, her relation with her new partner began to go sour over his desire for children, which put her at some risk of cancer recurrence. The planned marriage was delayed. Their relationship deteriorated further and finally ended 8 months after it began.

Nine months after surgery, Ms. R. was living with her mother after the unexpected death of her father and because she was lonely. She resumed contact with her ex-husband on a tentative basis, both consider-ing remarriage but neither one being willing to move precipitously to reunite.[9]

Ms. R. was unable to prepare herself for the possibility that she might have cancer before her surgery. She did not consider the prognostic implications of having cancer until she left the hospital some 8 days after surgery. She got as far as contemplating breast amputation with considerable repugnance but no acceptance. In the hospital she repressed successfully almost all unpleasant feelings, only to have these feelings, fears, and frightening thoughts overwhelm her once she came home.

Sexual relations proved totally impossible because she felt herself to be physically unattractive. Again, we have observed that feeling better about oneself and one's body comes only after mourning one's losses, which Ms. R. did achieve some months after surgery. However, she did not achieve acceptance of her disfigured body before terminating a meaningful marriage and catapulting herself into a new relationship with another man, which also fell apart after 8 months.

Ms. R.'s decision to terminate her marriage while she was in the throes of coping with cancer and the results of her surgery violates an important coping principle, namely, that one is better advised not to make major changes in one's life until one resolves an existing crisis. The motto to follow in such situations is "don't just do something;—stand there."

If our observations of the importance of solving the breast cancer problems of disfigurement and life-threatening disease prior to surgery hold up in our continued investigation, and we expect that they will, perhaps, the most critical intervention will consist of identifying those women who are unable to achieve this problem resolution on their own in the critical presurgery period and of developing techniques to resolve these coping tasks as expeditiously as possible.

This goal is not unlike the situation that confronts a physician called on to treat a child with an acute infection, for example, septic sore throat. He must diagnose the disease and introduce antibiotics during the acute stage to prevent permanent damage to vital organs. If suitable treatment is not instituted rapidly, the risk of complications and sequelae will increase considerably. Some significant treatment time can be gained for those women who have not made progress in their resolution of early coping tasks by electing two-stage surgery. However, the extension of time gained in this manner represents an opportunity but not a guarantee that the time will used effectively for problem solving.

REFERENCES

1. Bard, M., and Sutherland, A.: Psychological impact of cancer: IV. Adaptation to radical mastectomy, Cancer, July-August 1955.
2. Black, S. T.: Don't sit home and be afraid, Mc Call's, February 1973.
3. Camus, A.: The myth of Sisphus and other essays, New York, 1955, Alfred A. Knopf, Inc.
4. Grandstaff, N.: The impact of breast cancer on the family, Front. Radiat. Ther. Onc. **11:**146-156,
5. Kaplán, D.: Problem conception and planned intervention. In Health and disability concepts in social work education, proceedings of a workshop conference sponsored by the School of Social Work, University of Minnesota, April 1964. Reprinted in Glaser, P., and Glaser, L.: Families in crisis, New York, 1969, Harper & Row, Publishers, Inc.
6. Kaplan, D., Smith, A., Grobstein, R., and Fischman, S.: Family mediation of stress posed by severe illness, Social Work, July 1973.
7. Lindemann, E.: Symptomatology of management of acute grief, presented at Centenary Meeting of The American Psychiatric Association, Philadelphia, May 15-18, 1944. Reprinted in Am. J. Psychiatry **101**(2): September, 1944.
8. Pattison, E. M.: The living-dying process. In Conference proceedings for First National Conference for Physicians on Psychosocial Care of the Dying Patient. April 29-May 1, 1976, University of California School of Medicine, San Francisco.
9. Rollin, B.: First, you cry, Philadelphia, 1976, J. B. Lippincott Co.

42

Life-threatening illness in families

RICHARD BURNHAM JONES

All my reading and thinking about death and dying did little to ease my fears and awkwardness as I faced the reality of my first meeting with a terminally ill patient. To put it simply, I did not know what to expect. I was afraid to see this "person who was going to die." What could I do that would make any difference? What could I say that would alleviate his emotional turmoil?

It was a beautiful day as I stood on the steps of the hospital mentally going over what might happen in this introductory encounter. I felt that I would have to be very careful in what I said. All of the rules about meeting someone for the first time seemed irrelevant. Even such an innocuous subject as the weather would be taboo since I was the healthy one able to enjoy the day, whereas this man whom I did not know would most likely never be able to do so again.

Many of my fears proved unfounded, and the meeting went fairly well. With time and experience I have gradually become more comfortable talking with people facing the prospect of death. It is not surprising, though, that many family members struggling with the imminent death of a loved one share my initial concerns. Even nurses, doctors, clergymen, and others who come in contact with the dying on a regular basis are frequently uncertain about how to react or help.

Why do so many of us have such a negative reaction to the mere mention of death?

For most of us death is a topic that brings to mind negative images: pain, suffering, fear. Death and dying are therefore subjects to avoid or speak of in hushed tones. Even with the increased interest in death and dying manifest in the United States in the past few years, most people continue to ignore and deny death. Formed by a culture that worships youth and applauds achievement, we spend considerable amounts of money and energy repeating, "Progress is our most imporant product." Death is not an event that is consistent with this attitude. Life is productive and forward moving; dying and death are not. In short, death is an inadmissible part of life in our culture.

Moreover, much of our fear of death results from a cultural image of what death is like: violent and frightening. These aspects of death do exist, and our society clearly has a morbid fascination with them. There is nothing newsworthy in a person's peaceful acceptance of his or her life and death. What sells is sensationalism, the extraordinary, not the commonplace or norm. The actual experience of dying may be much less frightening than we imagine it to be. Our fear of death has perhaps become more awesome than the prospect of death itself.

Given our cultural rejection of death, it is easy to understand why patients, their families, and their nurses and doctors often wish to avoid such an unacceptable subject. What is especially ironic and sad is that, because of apprehensions about dying, they tend to bring about the very thing they fear—an alienating, frightening experience in which family ties fall apart, doctors and nurses treat only the medical necessities, and patients feel hopeless and isolated.

Each family has its own fears and feeling of frustration. The Sandburgs (fictitious name) illustrate what can happen in a family when the wife and mother is diagnosed as having metastasized cancer and a life expectancy of approximately 6 months. Married for many years, the Sandburgs have three children, ages 17, 15, and 11. Mrs. Sandburg has been in and out of the hospital for the last month undergoing test after test as well as a regime of chemotherapy and radiation treatments. She is now hospitalized.

The family arrives at the hospital and files into the mother's room; after exchanging the initial salutations, no one speaks. This family, like many other American families, has rarely experienced dying or death before. They may have heard of a relative's death or attended a funeral, but they have had little experience with dying. They simply do not know how to handle the situation and do not know what to say to each other.

Finally Mr. Sandburg breaks the silence by saying to his wife, "You look much better today. You're feeling fine, aren't you? Why pretty soon we'll be able to take you out of here." Mrs. Sandburg in fact looks very weak and pale and has lost a considerable amount of weight. She knows, even though she has not been told directly, that her illness is very serious and that she may be dying. She also knows that, except for a possible short visit home, she will probably not leave the hospital.

The family visits for a while, talking about nothing in particular, and then Mr. Sandburg pats his wife on the shoulder and kisses her, and they say goodbye. Carolyn, the 11-year-old, is the only one to show much emotion; she has been crying softly away from the others.

What is happening in this family? They used to be so close and now they act like strangers with each other. I asked Mrs. Sandburg why she looked so depressed after her family left and she said, "It's as if I don't know who they are anymore." After we had talked for some time and gotten to know each other, she explained that she is trying to protect her family from her awareness that she may be dying. "If they react this way now, how would they react if I were to let them know how I really felt?" Her family in turn has already been told of her diagnosis, but they are trying to protect her by not discussing it.

The Sandburgs are having a difficult time dealing with the realities of a terminal illness, and understandably so! In a very real way the Sandburgs are victims of the shared attitudes of our culture.

The same avoidance of death extends to those who work in health care facilities such as hospitals and nursing homes. Various studies indicate that nurses and doctors spend less time with terminally ill patients, take longer to answer their call buttons, and speak to them with averted looks.[9]

Part of the problem is the health care system itself for it is exactly that—*health* care, not *dis*-ease care. In institutions committed to healing, dying is viewed as a failure. Although our medical system has improved methods for early detection and treatment of many diseases, it has neglected and at times ignored the emotional aspects of patient care. It is not unusual to find hospital charts with reams of information about a person's physical functioning with no mention at all of how he or she may be reacting emotionally. Those who are dying can become dehumanized in a technologic society until they cry out, as a client of mine did, "I am not a cancer; I am a person!"

In the rush to find new ways to prolong life and cure illness, the willingness to preserve the quality of individual human lives seems to lag. The last months or years of a person's life are a time to be alive; they can also be especially meaningful for both the terminally ill patient and his or her family. The closeness and sharing of family ties can be intensified and the power of emotions—sadness, joy, love, anger, tenderness—heightened.

How can a caregiver assist terminally ill

patients and their families in facing the prospect of death? There are five fundamental guidelines for working effectively with patients and families facing serious illness.

1. Deal with your own feelings of mortality.
2. Be willing to get involved in a personal way.
3. View the family as the unit of care and as an integral part of the counseling.
4. Provide a supportive and open environment.
5. Be aware of the emotional energy required to work with the terminally ill and their families and seek a personal support system.

FACING ONE'S MORTALITY

It is no accident that dealing with one's own feelings about death is the first guideline, for it is a prerequisite to all the others. It is perhaps the most important and least tangible of the qualities needed by the caregiver.

If a counselor has unresolved feelings and attitudes about death, these attitudes will be communicated in some way to the patient and the patient's family. Openness of communication is essential, and problems will occur if any aspect of your personality prevents you from relating honestly and openly. Indeed it is in exactly those areas in which the counselor is afraid or unwilling to accept his or her own emotions that communications inevitably break down.

Fear of being in contact with those who have a terminal illness is a main source of difficulty. My fear of seeing my first client is a symtomatic effect of our cultural attitudes about death. A counselor or health professional must strive to accept a reality of death fashioned from actual experiences rather than allowing preconceived fears and anxieties to interfere with their contacts with the terminally ill.

To "work through one's mortality" is of course easier said than done. It is a rare person who allows himself even a glimpse of what his own death may be like. But it is not necessary for a counselor to have had a near-death experience or to have somehow transcended his or her own death. What is necessary is to examine and be aware of feelings or fears that could create a barrier in relating to patients. This "working through" may take the form of experiencing the death of a loved one. There is, in addition, increasing opportunity for those who work with patients facing life-threatening illness to participate in seminars or conferences on death and dying or to get supervision from experienced people in the field.

Counselors should come to understand and accept their own feelings about death. This does not mean, though, that they will or should become dispassionate. Quite the contrary, it is likely that caregivers involved with terminally ill patients will feel a range of emotions and share many of these feelings with their clients.

THE IMPORTANCE OF "GETTING INVOLVED"

It would be hard to overestimate the importance of relating to patients and their families in a personal way. As a therapist, nurse, doctor, or member of the clergy, it is often easy to relate to others from the safety of a role. This stance may seem convenient. It requires no involvement, no risk; one is simply doing a job. However, it prevents a person-to-person contact between the counselor and the patient or other family members. It often perpetuates the patient's feeling of isolation and helplessness. People who are dying often have an uncanny ability to see through insincerity! Being well-meaning, taking care of needed tasks, or even making frequent visits may not be enough. The patient and family may need someone with whom they can share their intense feelings.

There is no simple technique that can be used to help patients and families with the crisis that dying produces. In fact too many techniques or "how to" methods are dangerous because they tend to create a distance between the caregiver and the family. The need of those facing death and their families is for someone who understands and cares and is willing simply to be with them during this stressful time.

Helping persons must be authentic and encourage family members to be authentic, too. Sometimes this is difficult or embarrassing. For example, when the Sandburg children came to visit their mother, they were feeling very strange and frightened to see her so ill, but they were afraid to say so. If someone had dared to say, "Gee, Mom, hospitals make me feel uncomfortable," she could have said, "Yeah, your fidgeting is making *me* feel uncomfortable too!" This may have alleviated some of the tension and opened a pathway for them to talk more openly about their mutual fears.

In almost all cases, it is important for the patient to be told of his or her condition. The deception that takes place when patients are not told is usually only thinly veiled: They are aware of the medical procedures, the often-constricted conversations with nurses and doctors, and the sad and pained reactions of visiting family members and friends. Patients fear the worst, even if they are unwilling to admit it to themselves and need a source of comfort and solace. Family and staff, afraid of saying the wrong thing, tend to avoid the terminally ill patient. Although staff and family mean well, their conspiracy of silence is usually the worst possible solution.

Telling patients the truth about their illness is essential, but I emphasize that it must be done with sensitivity. Health workers should explain the situation to their patients but with the awareness that they will absorb only as much as they really want to know. This allows the patient to retain some sense of hope about the future. If patients know about their medical condition, they can participate in their own treatment and develop a sense of trust toward the hospital staff. Moreover they can better understand the reactions and difficulties their family members face.

Dealing honestly with a patient and his family means being able to admit one's own feelings and openly discuss the truth of the situation. It also means being able to accept the other person as someone with unique qualities as well as with less desirable personality traits very much like oneself. True understanding of another person comes from being with that person in a real way—from the reciprocal sharing and caring about true feelings.

THE FAMILY AS THE UNIT OF CARE

In the United States, most people die in an institution; 75% die, not at home in a familiar environment, but in a hospital or a nursing home.[5] These institutions are designed to meet the medical needs of patients, but they rarely provide a comfortable, relaxed, caring environment in which a person's *total* needs are taken into consideration. Too often family members are viewed as meddlers, in the way, rather than as allies essential to the process of caring for the patient. In addition many hospitals have rules that exclude children from visiting their parents. These restrictions can be a source of great sadness and trauma to both parent and child; they can also leave lasting scars on a child who was unable to see his or her parent before the parent's death.

Recognizing these problems is the first step toward improving the situation. Ideally, helping the patient to be comfortable would include allowing him or her to remain at home as long as possible. However, because most terminally ill patients require hospitalization at times, health workers should consider family members as an important part of the support system and encourage them to spend as much time as possible with the patients. The family knows the patient best and can therefore be a great source of comfort. The mood of family members affects the patient more than anything else; their continued care and concern are high on the list of factors that determine the patient's emotional adjustment to a limited life expectancy.[10]

Unfortunately, though, even when given the opportunity, many families find it difficult to provide the support and caring that seem to be their natural function. The acute emotional and physiologic changes experienced by the patient are often exacerbated by the reactions of family and friends. Those who were once close to the dying person may communicate in a guarded and cautious manner, visit the person less frequently, and stay shorter periods of time.

Even though the family can provide support for the patient, the family may also be undergoing a painful upheaval. The caregiver must recognize the enormous stress that a terminal illness produces in a family and help them deal with the crisis so that they in turn can provide support to their loved one.

If we view the family as an entity unto itself, we see that it is a living, functioning system. The family members for a period of many years have established routines of being together, each person with his or her own particular role in the system. When one member of a family is terminally ill, the other members face not only the death of that person but also the psychologic death of the family. The life of the family—its familiar patterns of interrelationships—comes under attack.

Stresses affect each family differently, depending on the nature of both the stress and the family system. In the Sandburg family, for example, under the stress of the mother's illness the family unit was disintegrating. The children, husband, and wife/mother consciously and unconsciously sought to deny the pain and difficulties they all faced.

It is interesting to project how this same family might have reacted to another stressful event. Let us imagine that, instead of confronting a death in the family, they faced the aftermath of a fire that had destroyed their home while they were on vacation. Hearing the terrible news, the Sandburgs would cut their vacation short and drive home as quickly as possible. Despite the shock and depression of seeing the charred rubble of their home and all their possessions, they would all pitch in to help with the tasks of finding a temporary place to live, looking for a new home, etc. Later, even though the loss still caused them much pain, they would have grown much closer to

each other as a result of working, crying, and remembering together. In contrast to their response to Mrs. Sandburg's serious illness, this family might well react to the news of a fire with a willingness to talk openly and share their fears and hopes.

How unfortunate that most families, like the Sandburgs, are unable to respond in this way when death comes to the fore. Most families try to maintain their familiar interpersonal balance. When the stress becomes so great that it upsets that balance, the family may attempt to regain its comfortable pattern by simply pretending that nothing has happened.

The Wilsons are a family attempting to deal with Mrs. Wilson's serious illness. Fred and Laura Wilson have been married for 18 years and have one son, David, age 12. Two years ago Laura had developed a malignant tumor in her breast and underwent a mastectomy. She was doing fine until 9 months ago when, during a routine examination, her doctor found a mass in her liver; it was malignant. The cancer had spread through her bloodstream.

The family's reaction to this news was almost imperceptible—at least on the surface. But it is very difficult for a family to experience such stress and successfully deny or suppress the emotional pain. Something has to give. In this case, the steam valve was David. He had been told about his mother's illness, but, except for the initial transmission of the news, the family rarely talked openly about the subject. As a result, David harbored many unanswered questions.

David began to behave unusually—"acted out" the tension the family was feeling but not acknowledging. He refused to go to school and missed so much that he had to be held back a year. His grades plummeted, he argued violently with his mother, and in general he created a ruckus. Fred and Laura sought help for what they perceived as their son's problems, and I began working with them in intensive family therapy.

Of course the problem was not that the son was an incurable delinquent. The problem was that the whole family system had been shaken, but the son was the only one expressing the tension. Laura's latest diagnosis had created an enormous strain on the family and upset its balance. Past unresolved and unexpressed anger and frustration had begun to surface. The parents began to argue.

Feeling that this strain might drive his parents apart, David created a diversion. By becoming a problem child, he focused the attention on himself. His parents would have to argue with him rather than with each other, and that would ensure that the family would stay together. His staying home from school also tended to cement a mutual dependency between him and his mother.

The parents in turn refused to discuss their feelings toward each other, revealing how angry and upset they were only through their behavior. For example, instead of telling Laura that the constant bickering between her and David was driving him crazy, Fred Wilson worked late at the office most nights. This upset Laura because, at this time of her life more than at any other, she needed to be reassured that she was loved and appreciated.

What can a caregiver do to ease a situation such as this? The goal is to improve communication among family members and to help them deal more openly with their emotions. It is not necessary to focus immediately on the patient's illness and what it means for them. Ultimately their fears and pain about this will probably surface, but often this cannot and should not be confronted head on. The counselor can be most effective by dealing with whatever emotions arise, not by having an agenda of what he thinks the family should be feeling.

With the Wilsons, the immediate problem was the relationship between the parents. David had lodged himself between them in hopes of preventing their arguing. Once he could see that they could argue openly and discuss their differences and frustrations in a constructive way without separating, much of the tension in the family—and David's acting-out symptoms—disappeared.

With the improved communications in the family, their interpersonal problems subsided. David is back in school getting all As and Bs and may be promoted back to his original grade. The extreme interdependency of David and his mother has been replaced by a genuine liking and respect for each other. Both Laura and Fred are increasingly able to give and receive affection between each other as well as with David. David and his father are getting to know each other better than they ever have before.

Now with a great deal of trust built up from the more open and supportive family environment, the Wilsons are beginning to share some of their feelings about Laura's illness. Whether it has to do with her increased emotional health or not is uncertain, but Laura's tumor has diminished in size to a point at which the physician can no longer feel it, and tests indicate that the cancer has not spread to other organs. As of this writing, Laura is continuing to receive chemotherapy and is beginning to accept herself more as a person.

Sooner or later, death comes to all of us; we have no choice in that. The choice—for the individual and his or her family—is whether to pretend that the reality of death does not exist or to acknowledge and express the grief. As painful as it may sometimes be, if a family strives to stay emotionally close as death approaches, their closeness and support can be a great comfort for the dying patient. This caring is likely to become one of the few remaining aspects of life that holds meaning for the dying person.

PROVIDING A SUPPORTIVE ENVIRONMENT

The ability to feel comfortable and show concern in what for many is an uncomfortable situation is one of the most important qualities of a caregiver working with seriously ill patients and their families. A willingness to talk in an open manner about death does much to bring relief and hope to a seemingly hopeless situation. Even acknowledging that "Yes, this is awful, painful, unfair," can provide support for the family and patient.

Occasionally it is helpful simply to be with a patient and family. Touching or being willing to sit quietly a while with someone who is very weak can make all the difference in the world. Too often we feel that to be helpful we must do something. This is, however, not always true in caring for patients and families facing death.

For example, a 78-year-old man who was dying of a brain tumor wanted his family to sit in his hospital room and watch TV with him. The family was very uncomfortable with this because they felt they should be visiting: talking with him and trying to cheer him up. The patient, however, wanted his family to relate to him as a person and not as a "dying patient."

To discuss only the patient's condition or impending death separates the patient from the rest of life and effectively relegates him or her to a position of the already dead. To do so is to commit an act of emotional violence.

The caregiver can also provide assurance that, even though the stress is great and the emotions powerful, much can be done. Sometimes there are legal and financial worries as well as emotional strains, and the caregiver's ability to help and sympathize can put the family at ease.

Family members can experience more pain and loneliness than the patient. One day I went walking with the husband of a woman who was seriously ill, and I mentioned that his wife seemed to be getting much attention and support—visiting family members, etc.—while he was getting little notice. I wondered if he got much support from anyone. He was a proud, stoic man, yet this question brought the only tear I had seen him shed.

The family needs support not only during the person's illness, but also after the patient's death. Grieving, which is a psychologic necessity, can be very difficult, especially if a person is unprepared for it or does not realize that it can be a long, lonely, confusing process.

In our society, grieving, like terminal illness, is a subject people avoid. This unfamiliar nature of the grieving process makes it hard for those who are mourning to prepare for their reactions. Often friends and neighbors expect a bereaved person to get over the death of a life-long spouse in a few months. The idea that one can "get over" someone with whom one has lived all those years in just a few short months is absurd. With those around telling one to cheer up, it is reassuring if someone can say that it is natural to still feel depressed and lonely. Grieving is often accompanied by symptoms such as shortness of breath, frequent crying, tiredness, lack of concentration, insomnia, lack of appetite, and a preoccupation with the image of the dead person. Just knowing that these are normal reactions can provide much solace.

A grieving person may experience a confusion of emotions and as a result feel overwhelmed at times. Anger is quite common. Embarrassment and elation after a person has died are emotions most people neither expect nor wish to admit, yet they too are not uncommon. If the death has been a particularly difficult one, a feeling of euphoria may come soon after the person has died.

It is important for caregivers to be accessible to a family going through the confusing and painful experiences of the grieving process. Frequently spouses or children or other relatives have no one else to turn to because their friends are all trying to cheer them up. Grieving persons should be encouraged to form new relationships and go out, but only when they are ready. A period of readjustment to life without their loved one must first run its course.

In addition to being accessible to the family members in the first months after a person has died when the grief of the family may be the most acute, the helping person should call on the family again 6 to 9 months after the person has died. This is frequently the most difficult period for the family, although why this is so is unclear. They may be experiencing conflicting emotions at this stage—beginning to feel better about life but feeling guilty for feeling this way. The caregiver can give the survivors permission to feel all right about themselves and their future lives. Another source of difficulty during this period may be that the surviving family members are finally beginning to comprehend what "I will never again see this person" really means. Up to this point they may not have fully felt the impact of the death because of the shock or the need to meet the crisis.

IMPACT ON THE CAREGIVER

Working with those who have a life-threatening illness and their families is difficult and can take its toll emotionally. Facing the reality of a terminal illness, being with someone who is deteriorating rapidly toward death, or seeing someone in intractable pain can be very stressful. Most health professionals rarely discuss the unpleasant aspects of caring for patients in their final days.

Nurses, the front line of the hospital staff, see dying and death almost every day and may become emotionally drained as a result. Professionals dedicated to helping others by reducing their suffering often begin to treat those with whom they work in a detached, unfeeling, and dehumanized way. Part of the problem lies in the job itself. Nurses usually have the most contact with dying patients and their families and shoulder much of the responsibility for patient care, but they have little authority to make the changes or decisions they believe necessary. Many institutions have an extremely high ratio of patients to staff, which creates further problems. Powerlessness, overwork, and mandatory unpopular shifts all contribute to an emotional and physical overload.

The first step toward change is to recognize that there is a problem. If a nurse gets involved emotionally with his or her patients and shows this emotion (for example, cries on the ward), administration and other staff members will likely consider him or

her unable to "take it" or "unprofessional." Many other staff members may have similar feelings, but their fear of negative reactions from colleagues prevents them from talking about it. Thus most health workers who come into frequent contact with the dying tend to hold in their feelings. The lack of communication makes them think they are the only ones who feel the way they do and causes them to conclude there must be something wrong with them.

One of the ways a caregiver can get help is to seek the support of the institution for which he or she works. Support groups can be organized in which nursing staff and other health workers responsible for patient care get together to discuss problems and receive feedback from others. Such groups can generate effective peer support. Just having a place to talk openly about problems and proposed solutions without fear of reprisal can do much to relieve the tension. In realizing that one is not alone and that others experience the same feelings one can help prevent the same problems from occurring again and again. Support groups may also run workshops or arrange for guest speakers on topics that are of particular concern.

If possible, health care professionals should pressure their institution to reduce the work load of staff members working under great stress. The more patients a person has, the less time he or she has to take care of anything more than the basic necessities. The resulting neglect of the patients' other needs causes frustration among both patients and staff. The impossibility of easing this frustration deprives staff members of a sense of satisfaction and reward from a job well done.

In addition there may be community support groups available that can take some of the work load off the staff. Community groups can also provide support for the families of patients and the patients themselves.

Caregivers might also devise ways for getting out of the stressful situation for short periods of time; coffee breaks or scheduling less trying work for a part of each shift can provide some relief. Social outlets that enable staff members to get to know each other apart from the work situation are also useful. Regular vacations to "recharge one's batteries" are helpful. Physical exercise or other life-affirming activities are also important.

A basic problem in working with those suffering from a life-threatening illness is that ultimately the patients will die, and this makes it painful to get involved. Many health workers question the wisdom of becoming close to a person who is only going to die anyway: "Why put yourself through the ringer time and time again and get involved if you're only going to get hurt?"

The problem with this attitude is that, if one does not allow oneself to get to know another person, one simply will not matter for them. One will not "care" for them, other than perhaps making sure the I.V. is properly hooked up and the bedpan emptied. The patient and his family will reciprocate by not offering that person the appreciation, the gratitude, and the occasional smile that could make the work worthwhile.

Health-care professionals need rewards and satisfactions from their jobs. If we do care and get involved, we have the satisfaction gained from doing our job well and the appreciation of both patient and family. In addition, we have the opportunity to do what few people can: give the patient and his or her family support when death is approaching.

Most important of all, I have found in my work with terminally ill persons and their families that I have a lot to learn from someone who is facing death. Sharing as a person reviews his life and attempts to uncover its meaning is a very powerful and intimate experience. Perhaps this is the greatest gift those who are dying have to give: teaching us how to be truly alive and how to live each day to its fullest.

CONCLUSION

In our society death is repudiated, moved out of sight, and infrequently discussed. This results in a lack of awareness of what death is like. The patient and his family suffer from this ignorance when they suddenly must confront life-threatening illness. They desperately need comfort and help in coping with their feelings of dismay and disbelief. There is a great deal that we—as nurses, doctors, therapists, clergy, or other caregivers—can do to provide this help.

First, the caregiver must understand and accept his or her own feelings about mortality. This allows the helper to deal with his fears or other emotions that may interfere with open, honest communication. Second, the caregiver must be willing to "get involved" with those they are helping. Becoming involved means not only encouraging patients to open up their feelings, but also being able to share one's own feelings. Honesty and caring are the qualities that enable people to trust one another and to talk about even the most difficult, painful things.

Third, the caregiver should encourage the family to be there for the patient, not only to visit in a formal way but to maintain their close family bond and to continue the life of the family. Too often the family is forgotten and feels out of place in the face of hospital procedures. Yet the succor the family provides cannot be replaced by hospital staff.

The family, in this stressful situation, also needs support and understanding. Thus the fourth guideline is to provide a supportive environment. We must take our lead in the care of the terminally ill from the family and patient. If they are unable to talk about their fears, the caregiver must respect that boundary but also be available to share other aspects of their lives. The need to assist the family also continues after the family member has died. Providing understanding during the grieving process is an important part of total care.

The final guideline is for the caregiver to get his or her own personal support. Being with patients and families facing death can be an emotionally difficult task. If the caregiver becomes depressed, drained, or insensitive, his or her ability to give comfort and understanding to the patients and their families will be impaired. It is important for helping persons to get what they need to "recharge their batteries," whether it be appreciation from patients, time off, or a shoulder to cry on occasionally.

When a person is facing death, it is time to encourage the family to face this awesome reality together and to remember and share what joys, sorrows, and other experiences the family has had together. It is a time for saying goodbye and for sharing how much we care for that person. It is also a time, however, for the family to continue to live for that is what is most difficult—to live with the awareness that death is nearing.

Separation and loss in all forms teach us how to be in the world as well as how to prepare for death. Personal losses that we all face force us to confront our grief and emptiness. To live fully is to experience life in all its aspects—the joys and wonders as well as sorrow and pain. Birth, death, love, and separation are all of one cloth; they are all part of life. To accept this is to achieve wholeness and maturity.

REFERENCES

1. Ackerman, N.: Treating the troubled family, New York, 1966, Basic Books, Inc., Publishers.
2. Bandler, R., and Grinder, J.: The structure of magic, Palo Alto, 1975, Science and Behavior Books, Inc.
3. Becker, E.: The denial of death, New York, 1973, The Free Press.
4. Frankl, V. E.: Man's search for meaning, New York, 1963, Pocket Books.
5. Garfield, C. A.: Elements of psychosocial oncology: doctor-patient relations in terminal illness. In Garfield, C., ed.: Psychosocial care of the dying patient, New York, 1978, McGraw-Hill, Inc.
6. Haley, J.: Strategies of psychotherapy, New York, 1963, Grune & Stratton, Inc.
7. Haley, J.: Uncommon therapy, New York, 1973, W. W. Norton & Co., Inc.
8. Hillman, J.: Suicide and the soul, New York, 1973, Harper Colophon Books.
9. Kastenbaum, R., and Aisenberg, R.: The psychology of death, New York, 1972, Springer-Verlag New York, Inc.
10. Kubler-Ross, E.: Death: the final stage of growth, Englewood Cliffs, N.J., 1975, Prentice-Hall, Inc.
11. Laing, R. D.: The politics of the family and other essays, New York, 1972, Vintage Books.
12. Luthman, S., and Kirschenbaum, M.: The dynamic family, Palo Alto, 1974, Science and Behavior Books, Inc.
13. Rosenthal, T.: How could I not be among you? New York, 1975, Avon Books.
14. Satir, V. M.: Conjoint family therapy, ed. 2, Palo Alto, 1968, Science and Behavior Books, Inc.

43

Research on ascorbic acid and the dying patient

LINUS PAULING

An optimal intake of vitamin C, considerably larger than the dietary allowance recommended by the Food and Nutrition Board of the United States National Academy of Sciences-National Research Council, may significantly enhance and prolong the life of patients dying from cancer. It may also be the key to making robust longevity the rule rather than the exception for human life.

In support of this thesis I should like to report mainly on observations made by Ewan Cameron in the course of his efforts to obtain some control of cancer and to decrease the suffering of patients with advanced and terminal cancer. His most effective work along these lines has involved the use of vitamin C in the form of ascorbic acid, sodium ascorbate, and calcium ascorbate.

Ewan Cameron has been Consultant Surgeon or Senior Consultant Surgeon in Vale of Leven Hospital, Loch Lomondside, Scotland, since 1952. Of the 375 beds in Vale of Leven Hospital, 100 are in the surgical unit. All 100 beds are in the administrative charge of Cameron, and 50 of them are in his complete clinical charge—the other 50 being in the clinical charge of the second Consultant Surgeon of the hospital.

Paper presented at the Second National Training Conference for Physicians on Psychosocial Care of the Dying Patient: Doctor-Patient Relationships in Terminal Illness, June 2 to 4, 1977.

The two Consultant Surgeons are assisted by a changing group of four Surgical Registrars, who are qualified surgeons on assignment for terms of six or twelve months from one or another of the Glasgow teaching hospitals. The surgical Registrars are assisted by residents and interns. Although some cancer patients are initially treated in the medical or gynecologic unit, there is a tendency for cases of advanced cancer of all kinds (except leukemia and some rare childhood cancers, which are dealt with in a pediatric hospital in Glasgow) to end up in the surgical unit. In fact Cameron oversees the treatment of probably 90 percent of all cases of cancer in the Loch Lomondside area.

For a number of years Cameron sought some way of improving the lot of cancer patients. In 1966 Pergamon Press published his first book on the subject, *Hyaluronidase and Cancer,* in which he advances the thesis that a significant amount of control over cancer might be achieved by finding a way of strengthening the natural protective mechanisms of the human body. He points out that many malignant tumors synthesize the enzyme, hyaluronidase, which when it diffuses into the surrounding tissues catalyzes the degradation of the hyaluronic acid in the intercellular cement of these tissues, thus weakening them and permitting them to be infiltrated by the growth of the malignant tumor.

A natural inhibitor of this enzyme is

363

physiologic hyaluronidase inhibitor. Cameron advanced the idea that it might be possible to stimulate the production of hyaluronidase inhibitor, which would then inhibit the action of the enzyme and possibly permit the growth of the malignant tumor to be stopped. He strove for a number of years to find some substance or mixture of substances, mainly hormones, that would achieve this result, but without success.

Several years after the publication of *Hyaluronidase and Cancer,* Cameron and Douglas Rotman developed the idea that ascorbic acid might participate in the synthesis of hyaluronidase inhibitor.* Moreover the intercellular cement contains, in addition to hyaluronic acid, fibrils of collagen, and an increased intake of ascorbic acid should increase the number of collagen fibrils and thus strengthen the intercellular cement. I suggested that such a reinforcement of the intercellular cement might be one way of achieving the partial control of cancer advocated by Cameron.

In November, 1971, on the basis of these arguments, Cameron cautiously began some trials with patients with advanced cancer. A number of reports on these trials has been published. In the main study reported so far,† 100 patients with advanced cancer who received vitamin C (sodium ascorbate), usually 10 grams per day, were compared with 1000 control patients who were matched for sex, age, and type of cancer and were treated in the same way, except for the ascorbate, in the same hospital. As of June, 1977, the ascorbate-treated patients had lived on the average 5.1 times as long as the matched controls. Sixteen of the 100 ascorbate-treated patients were still alive at that time, whereas all of the 1000 matched controls had died.

One of the first observations made by Cameron and his associates was that patients who received ascorbate suffered much less pain after beginning the ascorbate treatment than other patients. Pain is one of the principal causes of suffering in dying persons, and its alleviation could be of great value. In 1973 Cameron and his associate G. M. Baird reported* that in the first 100 ascorbate-treated patients, five were in considerable pain from multiple expanding skeletal metastases, and before commencing ascorbate treatment these five had been receiving regular large doses of opiate analgesics (morphine or diamorphine) for periods of weeks or months. The pain of one patient with multiple spinal and thoracic cage metastases was inadequately controlled on a dose regime of 30 milligrams morphine sulphate administered intravenously every three to four hours. Within five to seven days after commencing the ascorbate treatment, four of these five patients claimed to be completely free of pain, and the fifth, with a sacral metastasis, required only mild analgesics for comfort. The control of pain by ascorbate has been observed many times since then.

It is interesting that not one of the five patients who had received regular morphine or diamorphine injections for appreciable periods of time prior to the institution of ascorbate therapy experienced any withdrawal symptoms or made any request that his opiate regime be continued.

Cachexia and anorexia also contribute greatly to the suffering of dying patients. In 1974 Cameron and Campbell, in reporting in detail on the first 50 ascorbate-treated patients,† stated that the great majority of ascorbate-treated patients experienced some degree of subjective benefit usually

*The Lancet:, 542, 1972
†Cameron, E., and Pauling, L.: Supplemental ascorbate in the supportive treatment of cancer: prolongation of survival times in terminal human cancer, *Proceedings of the National Academy of Sciences, U.S.A.* **73:**3685-3689, 1976.

*Cameron, E., and Baird, G. M.: Ascorbic acid and dependence on opiates in patients with advanced disseminated cancer, *International Research Communications Systems*
†Cameron, E., and Campbell, A.; The orthomolecular treatment of cancer. II. Clinical trial of high-dose ascorbic acid supplements in advanced human cancer, *Chemico-biological Interactions* **9:**285-315, 1974.

first noticeable approximately the fifth to tenth day after beginning the treatment. This subjective improvement was noted in even the most unfavorable situations. The appetite of the patients returned, they became livelier, and many of them were able to return to their homes and resume their ordinary occupations. I believe that vitamin C in large doses might control cachexia and anorexia in patients who are dying of other diseases as well.

Cameron and Campbell reported that the usual response of patients with advanced cancer, who received 10 grams per day of ascorbate, was the subjective evidence of benefit, usually apparent by approximately the fifth to tenth day of treatment, and that in many patients this response was very striking. The patients then entered a stage of increased well-being and general clinical improvement.

Objective evidence confirmed that some retardation of tumor growth had been achieved. The objective evidence of benefit included the relief of particularly distressing pressure symptoms, such as pain from skeletal metastases, a slowing down of the rate of reaccumulation of malignant effusions, a trend toward improvement in malignant jaundice, and relief from respiratory distress. Sometimes this phase of clinical improvement was of brief duration, but sometimes it lasted for weeks or months; in a few patients it has been so prolonged and accompanied by such convincing evidence of objective benefit as to indicate that the ascorbate treatment can induce permanent regression.

However, the majority of patients, in whom the treatment was introduced in the terminal phase of the illness, was not so fortunate. "After a variable period of sustained clinical improvement the malignant activity reasserts itself, and the patient dies from his original disease. The mode of death was, however, unusual in many of these patients. After a period of comparative well-being and apparent tumor quiescence, the patient may very suddenly enter a rapid terminal phase with a precipitous downhill

course and death within a matter of days from fulminating cancer. We are unable to offer any explanation for this "rebound effect" of abrupt translation from apparently restrained to totally uncontrolled "explosive" dissemination. We have observed this particular sequence of events in a significant number of patients in this series, and have come to recognize the general pattern of something distinct from the usual steady downhill course of terminal cancer."*

Cameron has emphasized to me that in his opinion the patients with terminal cancer who received 10 grams of ascorbate per day experience much less suffering and lead much more satisfying lives than those who do not receive ascorbate. The period of rapid decline culminating in death is far shorter than the usual period of decline in terminal cancer patients and is accompanied by much less suffering. I think that it is likely that a similarly large dosage of vitamin C could likewise improve the well-being and decrease the suffering of people who are dying of other diseases.

There is much evidence to support the thesis that large doses of vitamin C may greatly benefit the dying person. The evidence, in fact, indicates that large doses are needed to ensure the well-being of all people, no matter what the state of their health may be. Several biochemists have discussed the arguments about the optimal intake of ascorbic acid, including especially Irwin Stone in *The Healing Factor: Vitamin C Against Disease*.† I summarized these arguments in my books, *Vitamin C and the Common Cold*‡ and *Vitamin C, the Common Cold, and the Flu*.§ One of the arguments most convincing to me is that almost all species of animals continue to manufacture ascorbate even though they get many

---

*Cameron and Campbell, p. 314.
†Stone, I.: The healing factor: vitamin C against disease, New York, 1972, Grosset & Dunlap, Inc.
‡Pauling, L.: Vitamin C and the common cold, San Francisco, 1970, W. H. Freeman Co. Publishers.
§Pauling, L.: Vitamin C, the common cold, and the flu, San Francisco, 1976, W. H. Freeman Co. Publishers.

times the amount recommended for human beings in their diet of plant foods. The amount manufactured by different animals is proportional to body weight and averages approximately 10 grams per day for 70 kilograms body weight. The dietary allowance for adult humans recommended by the Food and Nutrition Board of the National Academy of Sciences-National Research Council, U.S.A. is 45 milligrams per day. Animals accordingly manufacture approximately 200 times as much ascorbate as is recommended for humans by the Food and Nutrition Board. I do not believe that animals would make this large amount of ascorbate if it were not valuable to them.

The Food and Nutrition Board has set the Recommended Dietary Allowance in terms of the intake that is needed to prevent scurvy. I agree that 45 milligrams per day for an adult human is probably enough to prevent scurvy in almost everyone, but I think that it is likely that most people need an intake 100 to 200 times that large to maintain the best possible health with the greatest resistance to disease. There is a considerable body of epidemiologic evidence showing a negative correlation between intake of vitamin C and incidence of cancer and other disease. The quantitative evaluation of this evidence indicates to me that the length of the period of well-being and the length of life might well be increased by as

much as 20 years through ingesting the optimum of vitamin C as compared with ingestion of the Recommended Dietary Allowance of 45 milligrams per day. A person who ingests the optimal intake and has an increased length of the period of well-being and of life will ultimately die; that is, he or she will in the course of time become a dying patient.

Cameron's observation of patients with terminal cancer has caused him to conclude that death for the ascorbate-treated patients involves less suffering than for other cancer patients. Moreover it has been observed that people who die at an advanced age often experience a death with very little suffering.

An old friend of mine, a chemist interested in vitamins, died last month. He was in fine shape at age 90 with good energy and a lively interest in his business and in the progress of science. He worked in his office one day, went home, went to bed, and failed to awaken the next morning. I venture to suggest that this sort of peaceful death might be the rule, rather than the exception, for those people who achieve the best of health by ingesting the optimal amounts of vitamin C and other nutrients and who live to a ripe old age because of their good nutrition. Perhaps better nutrition is a solution to the problem of the suffering of the dying patient.

44

Depersonalization in the face of life-threatening danger: a description

RUSSELL NOYES, Jr., and ROY KLETTI

Persons suddenly threatened with death have often reported a variety of mental phenomena as part of a progressive deviation from normal consciousness. These have been described by people rescued at the last moment from drownings, falls, and similar accidents. Some anecdotal reports of subjective experiences during mortal danger exist in autobiographical as well as clinical sources (Noyes, 1972). However, the first study of them was undertaken in 1892 by Albert Heim, who accumulated the accounts of over 30 survivors of falls in the Alps. He claimed that in nearly every instance a similar mental state developed, which he characterized dramatically as follows:

There was no anxiety, no trace of despair, no pain; but rather calm seriousness, profound acceptance, and a dominant mental quickness and sense of surety. Mental activity became enormous, rising to a hundred-fold velocity or intensity. The relationships of events and their probable outcomes were overviewed with objective clarity. No confusion entered at all. Time became greatly expanded. . . . In many cases there followed a sudden review of the individual's entire past; and finally the person falling

often heard beautiful music and fell in a superbly blue heaven containing roseate cloudlets. [Heim (Noyes and Kletti, 1972, pp. 46-47)]

What follows is a descriptive analysis of 114 accounts of near-death experiences obtained from 104 persons.

The accounts of the experiences were collected in several ways: 16 persons were personally interviewed when it was learned that they had survived extreme danger; another 38 responded to mountaineering journal advertisements for accounts of subjective experiences during dangerous falls; 39 offered unsolicited reports of their experiences in response to news items regarding this inquiry; and finally, 11 accounts were obtained through a variety of personal contacts. Each person was encouraged to submit a detailed account of his experience and complete a brief questionnaire.

The questionnaire was completed by 85 persons. It contained 40 questions calling for "yes" or "no" answers. The first four dealt with factors presumed to influence the experience. The first asked each person whether or not he believed he had been about to die during his accident. Three more questions dealt with the meaning attached to the experience. The remainder inquired about a variety of subjective phenomena commonly reported during depersonalization and mystical states of consciousness.

The life-threatening circumstances responsible for the experiences reported were

Reprinted from Psychiatry **39**:19, 1976. Copyright © 1976 by The William Alanson White Psychiatric Foundation, Inc. Reprinted by special permission of The William Alanson White Psychiatric Foundation, Inc. This investigation was supported in part by NIMH Grant No. MH12631.

367

as follows: falls, 47; drownings, 16; automobile accidents, 14; serious illnesses, 10; battlefield explosions, 6; cardiac arrests, 5; allergic reactions, 4; and miscellaneous accidents, 12. Accounts were obtained from 70 men and 34 women having a mean age of 33 years. The average (median) age of respondents at the time of their experience was 24 years. The data presented in this article were gathered informally and those who offered their experiences may have been prompted to do so by curiosity about them. In spite of this bias, the accounts are of great interest and, in view of their numbers, warrant serious consideration.

FINDINGS

The frequency with which various subjective phenomena were reported during moments of extreme danger is shown in the table. Persons who had believed that they were about to die (column 1) experienced them more frequently than those who had not thought themselves close to death (column 2). A number of distinct elements were particularly characteristic of the ex-

perience, and following a presentation of examples, will be described in detail. These include altered perception of time, lack of emotion, feeling of unreality, altered attention, sense of detachment, loss of control, revival of memories, and ineffability.

Example 1

A 24-year-old stock car driver experienced two potentially fatal racing accidents in a single year. The first happened on a straightaway as he was traveling over a hundred miles an hour. In the course of the accident his car was thrown 30 feet in the air and turned over several times before landing on its wheels. He said:

> As soon as I saw him I knew I was going to hit him. I remember thinking that death or injury was coming but after that I didn't feel much at all. It seemed like the whole thing took forever. Everything was in slow motion and it seemed to me like I was a player on a stage and could see myself tumbling over and over in the car. It was as though I sat in the stands and saw it all happening. I realized I was definitely in danger but I was not frightened. While I was up in the air

Subjective phenomena during extreme danger

Subjective phenomena	Percentage of subjects*		
	Death believed imminent N = 59	Death not believed imminent N = 26	Total N = 85
Altered passage of time	80	65	75
Unusually vivid thoughts	71	62	68
Increased speed of thoughts	69	68	68
Sense of detachment	67	56	64
Feeling of unreality	67	54	63
Automatic movements	64	52	60
Lack of emotion	54	46	50
Detachment from body	54	38	49
Sharper vision or hearing	49	38	46
Revival of memories	47	12	36
Great understanding	43	24	37
Colors or visions	41	24	36
Sense of harmony or unity	39	24	35
Control by external force	37	25	32
Objects small or far away	36	33	35
Vivid mental images	36	12	29
Voices, music, or sounds	25	14	23

*Based on those completing questionnaire.

I felt like I was floating. . . . I saw flashes of color and distinctly remember blues, greens, and yellows. Everything was so strange. . . .

As soon as I left the ground, I seemed to leave reality and move into another world. At that point I noticed how much sharper my vision was. I could see things more clearly and distinctly than at any time in my life. I remember being upside down and, looking backwards, I saw the man who won the race pass under me. That guy was looking up and I can still see the amazed look on his face. The whole experience was like a dream but at no time did I lose my sense of where I was. . . . It was like floating on air. . . . Finally, the car pancaked itself on the track and I was jolted back to reality.

This account illustrates the slowing of time, lack of emotion, sense of unreality, feeling of detachment, and heightening of certain perceptions, coupled with a dulling of others. The author's use of metaphors to describe his experience is noteworthy; his description has an ''as if'' quality throughout.

Example 2

A 21-year-old college senior described her reaction when, as a result of swerving to miss an oncoming automobile, she lost control of her car. Seeing a bridge abutment looming ahead, she knew she was about to die. And at that point:

. . . despite the horror of the situation, I entered a calm dreamlike state accompanied by a feeling of being at peace with everything. Then I saw an endless stream of past experiences—there must have been hundreds—go through my mind. All sound seemed to blur into an indescribable monotone and all of this became superimposed upon the scene actually taking place. I cannot remember specific thoughts or experiences that passed through my mind, but there were many and they were all pleasant. During all of this, time stood still. It seemed to take forever for everything to happen. Space too was unreal. It was all very much like sitting in a movie theater and watching it happen on the screen. I didn't feel like a participant much of the time. . . .

This young woman gives a typical description of the altered perception of time and space, lack of emotion, and sense of detach-

ment. The redirection of her attention toward memories of past experiences that blotted out environmental perceptions is also noteworthy.

Example 3

A 24-year-old mountain climber described the mental events which accompanied two falls, either one of which might have resulted in his death. Having lost his footing during a descent, he attempted a self-arrest but lost his ice axe in the process. Finding himself helplessly exposed to a 2,000-foot drop, he reported:

I seemed to lose hope of saving myself but somehow reacted with an instinct for survival, grabbing whatever I could with my hands. Perhaps my subconscious mind initiated this reaction because consciously I was aware of negative thoughts. Losing my ice axe seemed to put control of the situation in the hands of God. . . . I felt intense fear; my thoughts speeded up; time slowed down; and my attention was redirected toward survival and deeply imbedded memories. . . . My mind seemed to alternate between perceiving and thinking. While perceptions were being registered, my thinking seemed to stop; and, while thinking, my data-gathering processes were at work, but perceptions were not registered in my memory. I saw and heard the events of my fall in vivid detail. . . . Some of my thoughts were of future events. I pictured my companion and myself falling 2,000 feet to our deaths. I thought of my mother and what she would think if I were dead. Other thoughts included spiritual perceptions. I felt closer to God. I developed an understanding of death as something beautiful, a realization that stands out yet today as profoundly important. At times my thoughts were so intense that my senses seemed numb. Memories of earlier dangerous experiences were revived but were not vivid.

This account illustrates the heightening, narrowing, and redirecting of attention that were characteristic of the experiences reported. A revival of memories and phenomena having religious significance are briefly mentioned.

Example 4

Religious significance also appeared in the account of a 14-year-old boy who accidentally shot himself in the chest. The religious content was enriched by visions that he recognized as unreal at the time. He said that as soon as he shot himself:

I became aware of a burning pain in my stomach and a deafening ringing in my ears, but the thing I noticed especially was the odor of gun smoke, which was painfully strong. Everywhere I looked I saw a deep blue color. I found myself lying on the floor and I believed I was going to die. My father rushed in then and urged me to get up, but he didn't seem to be speaking to me at all. Then the room filled with people that weren't actually there, including my girlfriend, a cousin, and my grandmother. They all appeared as they normally would, but none seemed to notice me. When I got up and walked out (I fell once before reaching the car), it seemed to me that strength came from a force outside myself. It affected my mind as well as my body, and I think it enabled me to hold onto life.

When I reached the car, my attention became riveted on memories of my early life. They began when I was about three and continued up to the present. I saw myself in a high chair at age three. I was with my father under a bridge when we caught a prize paddlefish. I saw myself with friends. The memories were pleasant but made me sad, realizing that this was the life I was leaving. They were very clear, almost as though I were actually living them. Many were events I had not recalled before. They must have been moving extremely rapidly although they did not seem to at the time. My thoughts were speeded up and time seemed stretched out. I felt numb and detached from what was going on around me. . . . In the emergency room I found myself outside of my body, as though I were standing off to one side. I saw myself as plainly as if I had been there; I appeared to be in pain.

This dramatic account provides an illustration of each of the elements listed above. The youth's descriptions of early memories (panoramic memory) and of detachment from his body are particularly vivid.

Example 5

A mystical extension of the phenomena so far described may be found in the following account. A 22-year-old woman, in a serious suicide attempt, took an overdose of barbiturates. The alteration in conscious-

ness produced by the drug no doubt influenced the development of the mystical experience, in addition to her awareness of impending death. Not long after taking the overdose she began to feel drowsy and then:

. . . as I went deeper, reality vanished and visions, soft lights, and an extreme feeling of calm acceptance passed over me like waves. The waves seemed to massage a part of me, but not my physical body. I saw lovely things and took leave of the phases of my life. I said goodby to myself as I watched the various stages. I felt close enough to grab onto some sort of wheel which I would become one with, yet add to. I would be filled with the wisdom of things I'd wondered about but would be myself no longer. I would diffuse, burst apart. I felt close to knowing all and accepting a long rest and lasting peace. My experiences were close to being in no time at all, almost as though time were at a standstill. Things were very far away, almost in another world. I couldn't touch them. My strength was centered but scattered. I was stronger because of being more whole, because I was no longer me as I had once known myself. I had a feeling of becoming part of a greater whole, a feeling impossible for me to describe exactly. It was a loss of identity, and not a feeling I could relate to the realm of human experience.

In this account many of the components—such as alteration in time and space, detachment, and recall of early experiences—are recognizable but in extreme, symbolic, or ineffable form.

CHARACTERISTIC ELEMENTS

The most frequently reported subjective phenomenon experienced during extreme danger was an apparent slowing of time (75%; see table). This was outer or environmental time, as opposed to inner time, which was perceived as being correspondingly increased in speed. Not only did elapsed time seem drawn out, but events seemed to happen in slow motion. Yet in contrast to the outward slowing, individuals described their thoughts as speeded up (68%) and expressed amazement at the number of thoughts or mental images that passed through their minds in a matter of seconds. These two aspects of the experience of time were generally described together and were clearly related to one another.

Lack of emotion was a striking feature of the experience for 50% of those completing the questionnaires. Many experienced fear momentarily upon the recognition of extreme danger. However, they soon found themselves calm. Nearly half reported no fear at all despite the gravity of the situation. A third acknowledged feeling as though a wall existed between themselves and their feelings. Emotions were not entirely blocked out, however, for 52% reported fear; 37%, sadness; and 30%, anger. Rarely painful, these emotions were dampened and, when recognized at all, were of minimal intensity. Under the circumstances described, most respondents found themselves calm and peaceful. In fact many described their emotional state as pleasurable and 23% even experienced joy. A 67-year-old physician, recalling his narrow escape from drowning 50 years earlier, said, ". . . once I realized I could not rescue myself, an indescribable feeling of calmness and serenity came over me that I have often wished desperately to experience again." And a 30-year-old mountaineer who lost his footing in a creek that was plunging down the side of a mountain claimed that, having resigned himself to his fate, "I had no more feeling of anxiety. In fact, at that moment I became elated." As in both of these instances, pleasurable emotions generally appeared when the person gave in to his presumed fate. Anger, on the other hand, was more commonly reported by persons who persisted in rescue efforts throughout the period of danger.

More than half (63%) of those completing questionnaires indicated that they had felt strange or unreal during their experience: 31% felt as though the world about them were unreal; a smaller number reported feeling as though the accident were not actually happening to them. Despite this sense of separation from reality, an appreciation of it was maintained throughout. This fact was clear from the metaphorical language used in describing experiences and repeated use of the phrases "as if" and "as though." A landing craft commander who was nearly killed when an enemy ammunition stockpile blew up beside him felt "as if I were sitting on a cloud looking down upon the whole scene, past, present, and future. Tremendous explosions were occurring all around me but faded and became a minor part of the whole experience." Thus, while removed from reality, he nevertheless maintained his contact with it.

Attention appeared to be heightened and narrowly focused. During a fall which he expected to be fatal, a 19-year-old mountain climber reported:

Not only were my thought processes speeded up, but I was aware of a definite and intense deviation from normal consciousness. The intense fear and subconscious hope of survival instinctively forced a concentration of my thoughts on rescue efforts and a redirection of my whole mind onto whatever might be necessary to prevent the potential plunge. For example, if I had been cold, I would not have felt it. If I had been hurting myself, I would have felt no pain. . . . My vision was very active and alert.

Thus, within the immediate focus of attention, whether on perceptions or mental images, objects became increasingly vivid, whereas outside this focus perceptions and sensations were dulled or obscured entirely. So long as an individual persisted in efforts to rescue himself, this vastly increased alertness was directed, as necessary, toward accomplishing this end. A jet pilot during the Vietnam conflict claimed that his altered state of mind saved him from almost certain death when his plane was improperly launched. He said:

. . . when the nose-wheel strut collapsed I vividly recalled, in a matter of about three seconds, over a dozen actions necessary to successful recovery of flight attitude. The procedures I needed were readily available. I had almost total recall and felt in complete control. I seemed to be doing everything that I could and doing it properly.

Many persons felt, as in the case of this jet pilot, that they performed feats, both mental and physical, of which they would ordinarily have been incapable. However, once such efforts were given up, attention seemed to turn inward, leading to further reflection upon unalterable circumstances and life's approaching end.

A sense of detachment was reported by a majority of persons surviving these moments of extreme danger (64%). One mountain climber noted that although his fall of 30 feet had not taken long, he found "ample time in a peculiarly calm and impersonal way" to think that he would probably die. "It is difficult," he commented, "to describe the odd third-person viewpoint I seemed to have during the fall." Many spoke of feeling like observers rather than participants in the events taking place. Half (49%) claimed to have experienced a feeling of being detached from their bodies. Occasionally this detached, "observing" self was described as traveling outside of space and time.

A majority of subjects (60%) reported a sense of loss of control, consisting of feeling as though movements or thoughts were mechanical or automatic. A more exaggerated sense of loss of control took the form of feeling in the presence or under the control of an outside force (32%). A young woman claimed that when she had been on the verge of death following a serious automobile accident that occurred as she was on her way to her honeymoon, she "felt the presence of someone or something with the power of life and death within me. . . . I talked to the being and said that my life had been so gratifying that if it were my time to go, it was acceptable to me."

A dramatic accompaniment of many near-death experiences was a revival of memories (36%). This occurred largely among persons expecting to die (see table) and commonly took a form called panoramic memory. Scenes of early life passed through the person's mind rapidly "as though on a conveyer belt" or "like a film sprung loose from the camera," suggesting

a loss in the continuity of images, one from the next. The scenes depicted were vivid and were often accompanied by emotions appropriate to their content. All were memories of presumed actual events, some of which had not previously been recalled. Most were pleasurable, although painful remembrances were also reported. One young woman who had suddenly been confronted with the probability that complications of a serious automobile accident would be fatal said:

. . . my life passed before me in a way that took me right back to my childhood. I remembered the smell of pudding my mother used to make, the smell of the old house, and feelings I had then. These were things long forgotten. The memories were beautiful and I was happy to have experienced them.

Very early memories were reported as often as later ones, and they frequently appeared in sequence.

The ineffable quality of these reactions to moments of extreme danger was repeatedly commented upon: 38% found their experiences hard to describe. Many found language inadequate to communicate experiences that were so foreign. Their difficulty was often compounded by a reluctance to speak of events that might reflect on their sanity or, because of their mystical nature, might invite criticism. However, great personal significance was often attached to these experiences, an aspect discussed elsewhere (Noyes and Kletti, in press).

Mystical consciousness, as it is commonly defined (James, 1929; Stace, 1960), appeared to be an extension or further elaboration of the deviation of consciousness thus far described. It seemed not so much a distinct element of the altered mental state under examination but rather its most extreme progression. Characteristic components of this mystical extension included transcendence of time and space, feelings of unity, loss of will, sense of truth, and intense emotion. For someone who had progressed to this point, not only was the perception of time altered but also the person often perceived of himself as ouside of or beyond time, so that his experience took on a timeless quality. Similarly, space often appeared limitless. Not only did his movements seem automatic, but he frequently felt as though his "will were in abeyance, and indeed sometimes as if he were grasped and held by a superior power" (James, 1929, pp. 380-381). And, finally, separated from his body and freed from the limits of his being, he often became united with the universe.

The following brief account is illustrative of this transcendence of time, space, and individual identity. A 55-year-old man recalled his experience as a soldier during World War II when his jeep was blown up by a German mine. He reported:

Almost immediately after the explosion, I was certain that death had occurred. I experienced no physical sensations, no sense perceptions. Rather I seemed to have entered a state in which only my thoughts or mind existed. I felt total serenity and peace. I had no remembrance of anything, only a realization that life had ended and that my mind was continuing to exist. I had no realization of time passing, only of one moment which never altered. Neither did I have any concept of space, since my existence seemed only mental. I cannot stress strongly enough the feeling of total peace of mind and of total blissful acceptance of my new status, which I knew would be never-ending.

The sense of truth characteristic of this mystical extension of consciousness suggests that an increasing separation from familiar reality develops as the observing self is progressively engulfed by the experience.

A sense of harmony or unity was reported by a third of the subjects who completed questionnaires (35%). Similarly, a third reported a feeling of great understanding (37%). It is noteworthy that the mystical extension of this experience occurred almost exclusively in persons in whom some alteration in cerebral functioning might be presumed to have occurred, judging from the circumstances of their experiences. Such an alteration might be assumed, for example, in the case of drownings or serious illnesses but not in the case of falls or automobile accidents uncomplicated by head injuries.

DISCUSSION

The subjective phenomena herein described in reaction to mortal danger are, for the most part, the same ones identified by Slater and Roth (1969, pp. 119-124) in their excellent review of depersonalization. The syndrome, especially as it occurs in patients, has been described by a number of authors (Ackner, 1954; Mayer-Gross, 1935). A classic early description was provided by Schilder in 1928:

To the depersonalized individual the world appears strange, peculiar, foreign, dreamlike. Objects appear at times strangely diminished in size, at times flat. Sounds appear to come from a distance. The tactile characteristics of objects likewise seem strangely altered. But the patients complain not only of the changes in their perceptivity but their imagery appears to be altered. The patients characterize their imagery as pale, colorless, and some complain that they have altogether lost the power of imagination. The emotions likewise undergo marked alterations. The patients complain that they are capable of experiencing neither pain nor pleasure, love and hate have perished within them. They experience a fundamental change in their personality, and the climax is reached with their complaints that they have become strangers to themselves. It is as though they were dead, lifeless, mere automatons. [p. 32]

The syndrome accompanies a variety of mental disorders and altered states of consciousness. It frequently occurs in normal people as well, but since the majority of observations have been made on patients, differences in the phenomena observed in the presumably normal population reported on here are worth examining. It is safe to assume that the syndrome developed as a normal reaction to suddenly-presented, life-threatening danger. It seems clearly to have represented an adaptive, even life-saving, response in many instances. At what point the response may have become disorganized and what phenomena may represent such a breakdown is difficult to determine.

The chief difference observed in persons exposed to extreme danger was an alteration in attention. Depersonalized patients have not reported a heightening of perception but have, instead, rather consistently complained of a generalized dulling or numbing of perception and mental imagery. Likewise, a speeding of mental processes has not been typical of patient reports. While environmental events have seemed to progress slowly for them, they have not described a corresponding acceleration of mental processes. During extreme danger the focus of attention appears to become sharply narrowed. Within a restricted focus, mental images are intensified, even to the extreme of appearing as perceptions. And some sensations and perceptions normally on the periphery of the sphere of immediate attention are excluded from awareness entirely.

A very similar alteration in attention occurs in marijuana intoxication, a comparison specifically referred to by several persons in their accounts. James (1890) likened this change in attention to the effect of observing events taking place through a microscope. Passing at their normal rate, events seen through the high-powered lens would be seen vividly but would appear to flow more rapidly, would take on a two-dimensional quality, and would, at the same time, appear to lose their context within a larger field.

A revival of memories is yet another feature not found among patients suffering from depersonalization. However, as will be explained elsewhere, this particular component appears to be more closely related to life-threatening circumstances than to depersonalization per se (Noyes and Kletti, in press). On the other hand, the vivid, two-dimensional, high-speed qualities of the memories are probably determined by that syndrome. Certainly their occurrence is no myth, though their frequency remains undetermined.

In contrast to Ackner's (1954) character-ization of patients as distressed by the emotional blunting they experience, persons confronted with sudden threats to their lives were gratified at finding themselves calm in the face of the most frightening circumstances imaginable. In fact, many remarked that dying in such a manner would scarcely be distressing. Beyond that, the reaction pattern, by attenuating fear, prevented the paralyzing or disorganizing panic that might so easily have developed in such moments. And, attesting to the effectiveness of this mechanism, many commented that they had been without frightening dreams or anxiety after their accidents and also that they had not found memory of the accident disturbing.

Mystical phenomena, according to James (1929), are transient. They have been reported as a part of brief depersonalization experiences of young people but, not surprisingly, have been absent from the chronically depersonalized states of patients. Naturally occurring mystical states of consciousness commonly develop during periods of intense emotional arousal and alterations in consciousness of various types. Both conditions were frequently present under the circumstances described.

CONCLUSION

From our examination of near-death experiences we may conclude that what Heim (1892) wrote over eighty years ago was substantially correct. He described a syndrome commonly reported by emotionally disturbed patients to which the term depersonalization was later applied. The differences between the subjective experiences of individuals in the midst of life-threatening danger and depersonalization developing among patients may add to our understanding of this curious disorder. Heim intended his presentation as a consolation to the families of victims of mountain-climbing accidents. Similarly, one may today take comfort from the fact that, suddenly confronted by death, he might find within himself the resources for coping with that frightful prospect. In such an urgent moment, strength might be found to effect a rescue, but failing in that, to face life's end with serenity, even acceptance.

REFERENCES

Ackner, B. "Depersonalization. I. Aetiology and Phenomenology," *J. Mental Sci.* (1954) 100:838-853.

Heim, A. "Remarks on Fatal Falls," *Yearbook of the Swiss Alpine Club* (1892) 27:327-337; trans. R. Noyes and R. Kletti in *Omega* (1972) 3:45-52.

James, W. *Principles of Psychology,* Vol. 1; Macmillan, 1890.

James, W. *The Varieties of Religious Experience;* Longmans, Green, 1929.

Mayer-Gross, W. "On Depersonalization," *Brit. J. Med. Psychol.* (1935) 15:103-126.

Noyes, R., Jr. "The Experience of Dying," Psychiatry (1972) 35:174-184.

Noyes, R., and Kletti, R. "Depersonalization in the Face of Life-Threatening Danger; An Interpretation," *Omega,* in press.

Schilder, P. *Introduction to a Psychoanalytic Psychiatry;* Nervous and Mental Disease Publ., 1928.

Slater, E., and Roth, M. *Clinical Psychiatry* (3rd Ed.); Williams & Wilkins, 1969.

Stace, W. T. *Mysticism and Philosophy;* Lippincott, 1960.

Suggested readings

General

Cantor, R.: And a time to live, New York, 1978, Harper & Row, Publishers, Inc.

Hillman, J.: Suicide and the soul, New York, 1964, Harper & Row, Publishers, Inc.

Keleman, S.: Living your dying, New York, 1974, Random House, Inc.

Kushner, R.: Breast cancer—a personal history and investigative report, New York, 1975, Harcourt Brace Jovanovich, Inc.

Leshan, L.: You can fight for your life, New York, 1977, M. Evans & Co., Inc.

Lynch, J. E.: The broken heart, New York, 1977, Basic Books, Inc., Publishers.

Nouwen, H. J.: The wounded healer, New York, 1973, Doubleday & Co., Inc.

Rollin, B.: First, you cry, New York, 1976, The New American Library, Inc.

Rosenbaum, E. H.: Living with cancer, New York, 1975, Praeger Publishers, Inc.

Sontag, S.: Illness as a metaphor, New York, 1978, Farrar, Straus & Giroux, Inc.

Aging

Butler, R. N.: Why survive: being old in America, New York, 1975, Harper & Row, Publishers, Inc.

Comfort, A.: A good age, New York, 1976, Crown Publishers, Inc.

Curtin, S.: Nobody ever died of old age, Boston, 1972, Little, Brown & Co.

Kalish, R. A.: The later years, Monterey, Calif., 1977, Brooks/Cole Publishing Co.

Saul, S.: Aging: an album of people growing old, New York, 1974, John Wiley & Sons, Inc.

Sarton, M.: As we are now, New York, 1973, W. W. Norton & Co., Inc.

Concerning children and parents

Anthony, S.: The child's discovery of death, New York, 1940, Harcourt Brace & Jovanovich, Inc.

Furman, E.: A child's parent dies, New Haven, Conn., 1974, Yale University Press.

Grollman, E. A.: Explaining death to children, Boston, 1967, Beacon Press.

Grollman, E. A.: Talking about death, Boston, 1971, Beacon Press.

Gunther, J.: Death be not proud, New York, 1949, Harper & Row, Publishers, Inc.

Irish, J. A.: A boy thirteen, Philadelphia, The Westminster Press.

Leshan, E.: Learning to say good-bye, New York, 1976, Macmillan, Inc.

Lichtman, W.: Blew and the death of the Mag, Berkeley, Calif., 1975, Freestone Publishing.

Sarnoff-Schiff, H.: The bereaved parent, New York, 1977, Crown Publishers, Inc.

Stein, S. B.: About dying, New York, 1974, Walker & Co.

Death and dying

Brim, O., et al.: The dying patient, New York, 1970, Russell Sage Foundation.

De Beauvoir, S.: A very easy death, New York, 1973, Warner Books, Inc.

Feifel, H.: New meanings of death, New York, 1977, McGraw-Hill Book Co.

Garfield, C. A., ed.: Psychosocial care of the dying patient, New York, 1978, McGraw-Hill Book Co.

Glaser, B., and Strauss, A.: Awareness of death, Chicago, 1965, Aldine Publishing Co.

Glaser, B., and Strauss, A.: A time for dying, Chicago, 1968, Aldine Publishing Co.

Grof, J. H., and Grof, S.: The human encounter with death, 1978, E. P. Dutton & Co., Inc.

Heifetz, M.: The right to die, New York, 1976, G. P. Putnam's Sons.

Kastenbaum, R., and Aisenberg, R.: The psychology of death, New York, 1972, Springer Publishing Co., Inc.

Kübler-Ross, E.: Death: the final stage of growth, New York, 1975, Macmillan, Inc.

Kübler-Ross, E.: On death and dying, New York, 1969, Macmillan, Inc.

Moody, R.: Life after life, New York, 1975, Bantam Books, Inc.

Osis, K., and Harroldsson, E.: At the hour of death, New York, Avon Books.

Pattison, E. M.: The experience of dying, Englewood Cliffs, N. J., 1977, Prentice-Hall, Inc.

Rosenthal, T.: How could I not be among you? New York, 1973, George Braziller, Inc.

Shneidman, E. S., ed.: Death: current perspectives, Palo Alto, Calif., 1976, Mayfield Publishing Co.

Stoddard, S.: The hospice movement, New York, 1978, Stein & Day Publishers.

Sudnow, D.: Passing on, Englewood Cliffs, N. J., 1967, Prentice-Hall, Inc.

Weisman, A.: On dying and denying, 1970, Behavioral Publications.

Fiction

Agee, J.: A death in the family, New York, 1970, AMSCO School Publications, Inc.

Anderson, R.: After, New York, 1974, Fawcett World Library.

Golding, W.: Pincher Mortin, New York, 1968, Harcourt Brace Jovanovich, Inc.

Tolstoy, L.: The death of Ivan Illych, New York, The New American Library, Inc.

Wolitzer, H.: Ending, New York, 1974, William Morrow & Co., Inc.

Grief and bereavement

Caine, L.: Widow, New York, 1974, William Morrow & Co., Inc.

Jackson, E.: You and your grief, New York, 1961 Hawthorne.

Lewis, C. S.: A grief observed, New York, 1961, The Seabury Press, Inc.

Morris, S.: Grief and how to live with it, New York, 1972, Grosset & Dunlap, Inc.

Parkes, C. M.: Bereavement, New York, 1972, International Universities Press.

Seskin, J.: Young widow, New York, 1975, Ace Books.

Index

Home care services in hospice care of terminally ill, 334-335

Home and work, separation between, in coping with burn-out, 118-119

Honesty about terminal illness, 304, 356

Hormones, role of, in resistance stage of stress, 13

Hospice, definition of, 325

Hospice care in terminal illness, 325-339
    pain control in, 325-333
    philosophical and organizational components of, 333-337

Hospital
    admissions to, emotional stress in long-term illness in child due to, 254-255
    areas of, special psychiatric effects of, on patients, 156-160
    environment of
        impact of, on patient, 154-161
        overview of, 155-156
    patient in, 194-197

Hospitalization
    dehumanizing aspects of, 294-295
    for myocardial infarction, psychological management of, 203-209

Hulschnecker, A., on emotional states of patients facing life-threatening illness, 139

Humor in coping with burn-out, 117-118

Hypertension
    definition of, 56-58
    as disease of modern society, 56-74
    essential
        genetic theories of, 60-62
        life cycle development of, 66
        obesity and, 63
        physiology of, 58-59
        salt consumption and, 59-60
        social stress causes of, 63-66

Hypnosis, contribution of, to healing, 81-82

Hysterectomy for cerebral palsy patient, 226-229

I

Ideology, medical, social stress and, 33-44

Iker, H., on relation of life events to cancer, 23-24

Illness
    anatomy of, patient's perception of, 165-174
    dehumanizing aspects of, 294-295
    life-threatening; see also Terminal illness
        personal encounters with, 163-198
    medical, relation of psychological stress to onset of, 17-26
    reasons for, emotional stress in long-term illness in child due to, 254
    relation of social and psychologic factors to, 9-74
    serious, sex and, 236-242
    terminal; see Terminal illness

Imipramine for depression in terminally ill, 330

Individualistic-purposive-involved adaptation to modern society, 67-68

Industrial nemesis, 28

Infarction, myocardial; see Myocardial infarction

Insomnia in terminally ill, management of, hospice approach to, 330

Intensive care unit (ICU)
    doctors and administrators in, 124-125
    environment of, 121-122
    group functioning in, 126-127

Intensive care unit (ICU)—cont'd
    nursing in, psychological stresses of, 121-130
    problems of, solutions to, 127-129
    psychiatric effect of, on patients, 157
    psychological experience in, 125-126
    work load in, demands of, 122-123

Internal resources of dealing with life-threatening illnesses, 142-143

Interpersonal relationships, positive, in prevention of stress-induced disease, 52-53

Interpersonal skills, training in, in coping with burn-out, 114-116

Irrational behavior, evolution of, in renal patient, 223-224

Isolation units, psychiatric effect of, on patients, 156-157

J

Jackson, D. D., on double bind situation, 301

Jaffe, L., on sexuality and terminal illness, 239

Jones, E., on psychodynamics of cancer in Freud, 99-100

Judgment in care of terminally ill, 320-321, 323-324

K

Kastenbaum, R., on emotions of caregivers of patients facing life-threatening illness, 140-141

Katz, A. H., on abnormal reaction to stress, 37

Kavanagh, T., on antecedents to heart disease, 18

Kavetsky, R. E., on relation of life events to cancer, 23

Kidneys
    disease of, chronic, stress in child with, 256
    in essential hypertension, 59

Klopfer, B., on psychosomatic aspects of survival, 5-6

Koroljow, S., on relation of cancer to depression, 105

Kübler-Ross, E., on emotional states of patients facing life-threatening illness, 139

L

Labor, alienation of
    coronary disease and, 37-39
    reduction of, and health, 41-42

Language, body, in communication with terminally ill, 299-300

Leader of patient/family group for stroke rehabilitation, problems and reactions of, 217

Learning during rehabilitation in disabled elderly, 247-248

LeShan, L.
    on emotions of caregivers of patients facing life-threatening illness, 140
    on precursors of cancer, 21
    on psychological aspects of spontaneous regression of cancer, 102
    on relation of life events to cancer, 22-23

Leukemia, child with, death of, 314-317

Levi, L.
    on physiologic effects of piecework, 38
    on relation between time-pressured work and hypertension, 65

Liddell, H., on effects of social support on stress-induced disease, 52

Life
    daily, of child with heart disease, 267-268
    in extremity, 3-7

P

Pain
  as answer to psychic needs, 276
  in burn patient, response of family to, 232-233
  chronic, person in, world of, 274-276
  as communication, 276
  control of
    ascorbic acid in, 364
    hospice approach to, 325-333
  emotional stress in long-term illness in child due to, 254
  killing of, cultural significance of, 29
  in patients on cancer ward, reactions to, 194-196
  physical, control of, in hospice, 326-329
  psychological, control of, in hospice, 329-330
  relief of, for dying patient, 309
  severe, of long duration, world of patient with, 273-279
  social, control of, in hospice, 330-331
  spiritual, control of, in hospice, 331-333
  understanding, 271-289
Paracetamol for pain control in terminally ill, 328
Parens patriae, doctrine of, 280, 282, 285
Parents of chronically ill children, emotional stress and coping behavior of, 259-260
Parsons, T., on Flexnerian medicine in action, 35
Passivity of patient in CCU, coping with stress created by, 191-192
Patient(s)
  cancer
    physician as, perspective of, 175-185
    therapist as, perspective of, 186-190
  on cancer ward
    effect of experiment in self-care on, 134-135
    perceptions of, 194-197
  care of, burn-out syndrome and, 111-120
  in CCU, physician as, observations of, 191-192
  contact with, amount and variety of, in coping with burn-out, 118
  dying; *see* Terminally ill
  elderly, rehabilitation of, psychologic factors in, understanding, 243-249
  facing life-threatening illness, emotional states of, 139
  and family as unit in hospice care of terminally ill, 334-335
  impact of hospital environment on, 154-161
  rights of, 280-289; *see also* Bioethics
    in terminal illness, 296
  in severe pain of long duration, world of, 273-279
Patient-family groups in rehabilitation of stroke patient, 213-218
Pattison, M., on process of dying, 308
Pearlman, J., on emotions of caregivers of patient facing life-threatening illness, 140
Pendergrass, E. P., on effects of stress on cancer patient, 5
Perception, anxiety effects on, 141-142
Perlman, L. V., on relation of life events to heart disease, 20-21
Personal encounters with life-threatening illness, 163-168
Personal feelings, analysis of, in coping with burn-out, 116-117
Personality
  normal, reactions of renal patient with, 224-225

Personality—cont'd
  of renal patient prior to illness, effect of, on emotional reactions, 219
Phenazocine for pain control in terminally ill, 328
Phenobarbital for dying patient, 309
Phenothiazines for pain control in terminally ill, 328
Physical activity, restriction of, in child with heart disease, 267
Physical conditioning for post-myocardial infarction patient, 209, 210-211
Physical deterioration and sick role in elderly, 245-247
Physical health of staff in coping with burn-out, 119
Physical pain, control of, in hospice, 326-329
Physical symptoms, emotional stress in long-term illness in child due to, 254
Physician(s)
  burn-out syndrome in, 111-120
  as cancer patient, perspective of, 175-185
  emotional stress among, effect of, on patient care, 111-113
  feelings of, about cancer, recognition of, by nurses, 133-134
  in ICU, problems with, 124
  as patient in CCU, observations of, 191-192
  of patient facing life-threatening illness, emotional states of, 139-141
    managing of, 142-145
  of terminally ill, problem solving approach for, 343-352
Pieper, W. J., on relation of life events to cancer, 24
Pituitary, role of, in resistance stage of stress, 13
Preventive medicine, social change as, 40-42
Prochlorperazine for pain control in terminally ill, 328
Promazine
  for anxiety in terminally ill, 330
  for nausea and vomiting in terminally ill, 328
Psychic insults, minimizing, tricks for, 16
Psychobiological aspects of spontaneous regressions of cancer, 99-107
Psychodynamic concept of cancer, 99-100
Psychologic component of illness and injury, 78-79
Psychologic factors
  in rehabilitation, understanding, 243-249
  relation of, to illness, 9-74
Psychologic hazards of coronary-care unit, 146-153
Psychologic impact of long-term illness in child, 254-257
Psychologic management
  of cancer, 103
  of myocardial infarction patient, 201-212
Psychologic pain, control of, in hospice, 329-330
Psychologic reaction to cancer in rehabilitation, 100-101
Psychologic stress(es)
  of intensive care unit nursing, 121-130
  models of, 17
  relation of
    to onset of cancer, 21-24
    to onset of heart disease, 18-21
    to onset of medical illness, 17-26
Psychologic support and survival, 199-249
Psychological dwarfism, 79
Psychology of terminal illness, 293-297
Psychosocial adaptation to long-term physical illness in childhood, 253-263
Psychosocial elements of survival, 3-7